The Biomechanics of the
Foot and Ankle

Contemporary Perspectives in Rehabilitation

Steven L. Wolf, Ph.D., FAPTA
Editor-in-Chief

PUBLISHED VOLUMES

Cardiac Rehabilitation: Basic Theory and Application
Frances Brannon, Ph.D., Mary Geyer, M.S., Margaret Foley, R.N.

Thermal Agents in Rehabilitation
Susan L. Michlovitz, M.S., P.T.

The Biomechanics of the Foot and Ankle
Robert Donatelli, M.A., P.T.

VOLUMES IN PRODUCTION

Pharmacology in Rehabilitation (May 1990)
Charles D. Ciccone, Ph.D., P.T.

Wound Healing: Alternatives in Management (June 1990)
Luther C. Kloth, M.S., P.T., Joseph M. McCullough, Ph.D., P.T. and Jeffrey A. Feedar, B.S., P.T.

Thermal Agents in Rehabilitation, 2nd Edition (July 1990)
Susan L. Michlovitz

Electrotherapy in Rehabilitation (November 1990)
Meryl R. Gersh, M.S., P.T.

The Biomechanics of the Foot and Ankle

Robert Donatelli MA, P.T.
Instructor of Rehabilitative Medicine,
Graduate Programs in Physical Therapy
Emory University Atlanta, GA

Private Practice
Physical Therapy Associates of Metro Atlanta
Atlanta, Georgia

Steven L. Wolf, Ph.D., F.A.P.T.A.
Editor-in-Chief
Professor
Department of Rehabilitation Medicine
Emory University School of Medicine
Atlanta, Georgia

 F.A. DAVIS COMPANY • **Philadelphia**

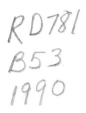

Printed in the United States of America

Last digit indicates print number: 10 9 8 7 6 5 4 3 2

NOTE: As new scientific information becomes available through basic and clinical research, recommended treatments and drug therapies undergo changes. The author(s) and publisher have done everything possible to make this book accurate, up-to-date, and in accord with accepted standards at the time of publication. However, the reader is advised always to check product information (package inserts) for changes and new information regarding dose and contraindications before administering any drug. Caution is especially urged when using new or infrequently ordered drugs.

The Biomechanics of the foot and ankle / [edited by] Robert A. Donatelli.
    p. cm. — (Contemporary perspectives in rehabilitation ; v. 3)
    Includes bibliographical references.
    ISBN 0-8036-2696-7
    1. Foot—Abnormalities. 2. Ankle—Abnormalities. 3. Foot—Abnormalities—Patients—Rehabilitation. 4. Ankle—Abnormalities—Patients—Rehabilitation. 5. Biomechanics. I. Donatelli, Robert. II. Series.
    [DNLM: 1. Ankle joint—physiology. 2. Biomechanics. 3. Foot—physiology. 4. Foot Diseases—therapy. W1 C0769NS v. 3 / WE 880 B615]
RD781.B53 1990
617.5'85—dc20
DNLM/DLC
for Library of Congress
                                                         89-25675
                                                                CIP

Dedication

I would like to dedicate this book to my best friend, Scot Irwin. His love and support have enabled and motivated me to pursue my interest in the area of foot and ankle biomechanics. His friendship has encouraged me to persevere through the good times and hard times in our practice.

Preface

Through our unique evolutionary development, humans have become upright ambulators, each with an individually characteristic gait that is determined, to a large extent, by how weight is transferred to and carried by the lower kinetic chain. The first parts of the lower extremity to contact the ground during the stance phase of gait are the foot and ankle. During this phase, weight-bearing forces are attenuated by the intricate interplay of ligaments, joints, and muscles in both structures. The stability, congruity, and efficiency of these three components describe the foot and ankle's normal biomechanics.

Given the degree to which the normal biomechanics of the foot and ankle influences gait, it should not be surprising that foot and ankle pathomechanics contribute to aberrations in lower extremity progression. What is surprising is how poorly prepared many rehabilitation students and clinicians are to adequately assess foot and ankle pathomechanics, especially since our treatment decisions are influenced by how we view variations in gait. This shortcoming is due, in part, to a lack of suitable instructional materials. While Doctors Root, Weed, and Sgarlato deserve thanks for collectively developing the study of foot and ankle mechanics into a contemporary science for podiatry students, no text has been designed for the unique mission of the physical therapist. *Biomechanics of the Foot and Ankle* was written to bridge the gap between podiatric science and physical therapy management. It combines an analysis of foot and ankle biomechanics with treatment rationales for physiotherapeutic interventions, and problem-solving case formats that emphasize clinical decision making.

In section I, "Biomechanics of the Foot and Ankle," Donatelli establishes the knowledge base needed to develop treatment protocols for mechanical dysfunctions of the foot and ankle. The author's references to the articulations and osteologic landmarks in the normal and pathologic foot are reinforced by ample anatomical illustrations. In the concluding chapter of this section, Corradi-Scalise and Ling offer a concise reappraisal of gait presented within the context of foot and ankle action rather than as a detailed analysis of the entire pelvis and lower extremity.

The chapters of Section II, "Biomechanical Evaluation," reflect the expanded responsibilities of physical therapists in evaluating foot and ankle problems. Following an excellent overview of clinical assessment by Luke Bordelon, Vito and Kalish present x-ray evaluation techniques, and Wooden integrates orthotic construction within the framework of clinical evaluation. Wooden's presentation, moreover, is complemented by Alexander and Campbell's end-of-chapter appendix summarizing contemporary approaches to analyzing foot and ankle movement through the use of dynamic kinematic measurement tools. Finally, the contributions by Greenfield and Schwartz consider the problems faced by clinicians who must evaluate foot and ankle problems in the presence of pathology induced by overuse syndrome and diabetes.

Section III, "Treatment Approaches to Restore Normal Movement," considers orthotics (Donatelli and Wooden), physical therapy (Garbalosa), and surgical interventions (Searle) as therapeutic options in managing foot and ankle dysfunction. The material in each of these comprehensive yet concise chapters is presented in a problem-solving, case analysis format that should challenge as well as inform the reader.

Any rehabilitation professional entrusted with the care and treatment of mechanical abnormalities of the foot and ankle caused by genetic, traumatic, or other pathologies will benefit from this textbook. We hope that its contents, like those of its predecessors in *Contemporary Perspectives in Rehabilitation*, will hold true to the series' philosophy — comprehensive, clinically relevant presentations that are well documented, contemporary, and personally challenging to the student and clinician alike.

Steven L. Wolf, Ph.D., FAPTA
Series Editor

Acknowledgments

Love and thanks to my wife Joni and my daughter Rachel for their patience and understanding. To my brother, Jerry Donatelli and my sister, Linda Donatelli-Schulteiss for their love and support; and Steve Krause for his friendship. Special Thanks to: Agneta for her fine artwork; Irving Miller for his willingness to share his knowledge; Stan Kalish, David Conway, Rick St. Pierre and Joseph Wilkes for their continued support and motivation; Steve Wolf for his support through the development of the book; Dean Currier, Ph.D., P.T., Carolyn Kisner, M.S., P.T. and Cynthia Norkin, Ed.d., P.T., who patiently reviewed the manuscript and who provided much useful advice; and to Jean-François Vilain and his colleagues at F.A. Davis, Herbert Powell, Jr. & Susan McCoy, who shepherded the manuscript from inception to publication.

Contributors

Ian J. Alexander, MD
Department of Orthopedic Surgery
The Cleveland Clinic Foundation, Cleveland, OH

Luke Bordelon, MD
Clinical Professor, Dept. of Orthopedics
Louisiana State University School of Medicine
Director, Foot Clinic
University Medical Center, Fayette, LA

K.R. Campbell, Ph.D.
Department of Musculoskeletal Research
The Cleveland Clinic Foundation, Cleveland, OH

Deborah Corradi-Scalise, MA, PT
Former Assistant Director, Department of Physical Therapy
United Cerebral Palsy Association of Nassau County, Inc., NY
Currently Staff Physical Therapist Stepping Stone Day School

Robert Donatelli, MA, PT
Instructor, Graduate Programs in Physical Therapy
Emory University
Atlanta, GA
Director, Orthopedic and Sports Clinic
Jonesboro, GA
Instructor, Dogwood Institute, Atlanta GA

John Garbalosa, MS, PT
Physical Therapy Associates of Metro Atlanta
Atlanta, GA

Bruce Greenfield, MS, PT
Instructor, Graduate Programs in Physical Therapy
Emory University, Atlanta, GA

Physical Therapy Associates of Metro Atlanta
Atlanta, GA

Stanley Kalish, DPM
Associate Professor, Department of Surgery
New York College of Podiatric Medicine
Attending Podiatrist, HCA/Doctor's Hospital
Tucker, GA
Staff Podiatrist,
Henry General Hospital
Atlanta, GA

Wen Ling, Ph.D., PT
Assistant Professor
Department of Physical Therapy,
New York University
New York, NY

Nathan Schwartz, DPM
Assistant Clinical Professor
Emory University
Atlanta, GA
Private Practice
Windy Hill Hospital
Marietta, GA

Karen Seale, MD
Assistant Professor and Head of Foot and Ankle Surgery Section
Department of Orthopedic Surgery
University of Arkansas
Little Rock, AK

George Vito, DPM
Resident, HCA/Doctors Hospital
Tucker, GA

Michael J. Wooden, MS, PT
Instructor, Graduate Programs in Physical Therapy
Emory University
Atlanta, GA
Orthopedic Physical Therapist
Physical Therapy Associates of Metro Atlanta
Co-Founder, Clinical Education Associates of Atlanta
Atlanta, GA

Table of Contents

Normal and Abnormal Biomechanics

CHAPTER 1

Normal Anatomy and Biomechanics

Robert A. Donatelli, MA, RPT

The study of normal mechanics in the musculoskeletal system is the analysis of forces and their effects on anatomic structures such as bones, muscles, tendons, and ligaments.[1] The study of forces acting on the musculoskeletal structures can be divided between the examination of bodies at rest (static) and bodies in motion (dynamic).[1] Kinetics is the study of the relationship between the forces and the resulting movement of the musculoskeletal structures.[1] This chapter focuses on descriptions of movements and forces acting on the functional joints of the normal human foot and ankle. Since the pre- and post-natal development of the human foot are important in the establishment of an organ of locomotion, the development of the functional joints of the foot and ankle is briefly discussed. Consideration of the ligaments, tendons, and muscles and their influences on movement are also included. A glossary of key terms appears at the end of this chapter.

What is a normal foot? Four of Cailliet's[2] criteria for normalcy are absence of pain, normal muscle balance, central heel, and straight and mobile toes. Adequate distribution of weightbearing forces on the foot while standing and during the stance phase of gait is also an important criterion of normalcy.

The foot is the terminal joint in the lower kinetic chain that opposes external resistance. Proper arthrokinematics within the foot and ankle influence the ability of the lower limb to attenuate the forces of weightbearing. The lower extremity should distribute and dissipate compressive, tensile, shearing, and rotatory forces during the stance phase of gait. Inadequate distribution of these forces can lead to abnormal movement, which in turn produces excessive stress and results in the breakdown of connective tissue and muscle. The normal mechanics of the foot and ankle are the combined effects of muscle, tendon, ligament, and bone function. The coordinated and unified effect of these tissues within the foot, ankle, and lower extremity results in the most efficient force attenuation.

The foot, for the purposes of this chapter, can be divided into three sections: the rearfoot, midfoot, and forefoot. The rearfoot converts the torque of the lower limb. The transverse rotations of the lower extremity are converted into sagittal, horizontal, and frontal plane movements. The rearfoot also influences the function and movement of the midfoot and forefoot. The midfoot transmits movement from the rearfoot to the forefoot, and promotes stability. The movements and function of the midfoot are dependent upon the mechanics of the rearfoot. The forefoot adapts to the ground as the terrain changes, adjusting to the uneven surface. The forefoot accommodation is dependent upon the normal mechanics of the rearfoot.

The bones of the foot are shown in Figures 1-1 and 1-2.

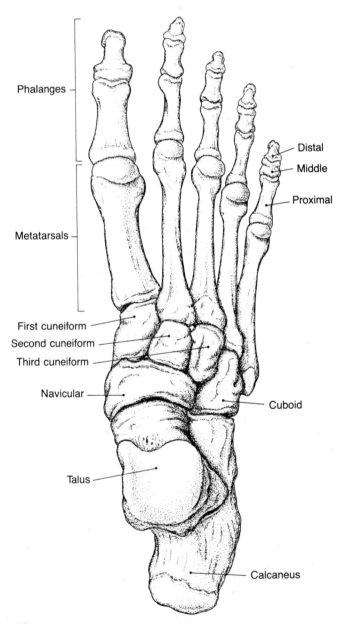

FIGURE 1-1. Dorsal view of the bones of the foot. (FA Davis Co., Philadelphia, with permission.)

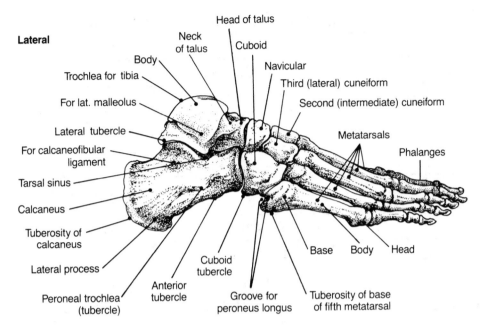

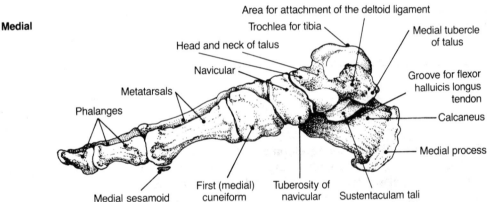

FIGURE 1–2. Lateral (*top*) and medial (*bottom*) views of the bones of the foot. (FA Davis Co., Philadelphia, with permission.)

DEVELOPMENT OF THE HUMAN FOOT FOR LOCOMOTION

Early Development

REARFOOT

The rearfoot is made up of the talus and the calcaneus. The importance of the calcaneus and the talus is apparent from their early development within the fetus and from the evolutionary changes that have enhanced their function. The calcaneus is the first of the tarsal bones to begin ossification (Table 1-1). The ossification center appears between the fifth and sixth fetal month. The talus is the second tarsal bone to ossify, at about the eighth fetal month.[3] The talus and calcaneus have exhibited evolutionary

TABLE 1-1 Ossification Schedule of the Bones of the Foot and Ankle

Bone	Ossification Period	
Tibia (distal epiphysis)	6-10 mo gestation	to 18 yr
Fibula (distal epiphysis)	11-18 mo	to 17 yr
Talus	8 mo gestation	to 17-18 yr
Calcaneus	5-6 mo gestation	to 16 yr (females) 20 yr (males)
Navicular	Boys, 3 yr Girls, 2 yr	to 17-18 yr to 17-18 yr
Cuboid	birth-21 days	to 17-18 yr
Cuneiforms	Lateral, 4-20 mo Medial, 2 yr Intermed., 3 yr	to 17-18 yr to 17-18 yr to 17-18 yr
Metatarsals	1-12 wk gestation 2 or 3-9 wk gestation 4 or 5-10 wk gestation	to 16-18 yr to 16-18 yr to 16-18 yr
Phalanges	Proximal, 1-2.2 yr Distal, 2.5-4.7 yr Intermed., 15 wk gestation	to 13-16 yr to 11.5-14.7 yr to 18 yr

changes associated with the development of the foot into the body's primary weight-bearing, balancing, and propulsive organ.[4] The calcaneus has become quite large (for additional propulsive leverage) and has developed a sturdy tuberosity for increased weightbearing.[4] The talus articulates with the calcaneus on facets parallel to the ground for additional balance and adaptation. The articulations of the talus in humans differ from those of other primates, where the articular facets are steeply sloped.[4]

The calcaneus of the fetus at three months represents an average of 25.3% of the total foot length; in adults it is 35%.[5] The posterior segment of the calcaneus grows faster than the anterior segment, contributing to the mechanical efficiency of the triceps surae. The talar body increases more rapidly in height than in length, contributing to the development of the talocrural joint.

The foot develops in a supinated position. Correction of fetal supination is accomplished by changes in the rearfoot. As lateral rotation of the talar head and neck occurs, the forefoot varus is reduced. The lack of this rotation is the major cause of forefoot varus.[6,7] Another characteristic of fetal supination is a varus calcaneus (inverted position). Three months after birth, the varus angle of the calcaneus is 36.8°, compared with a varus angle of 3.6° in adults.[5] Finally, an adducted position of the forefoot is corrected by changes in the position of the talus and calcaneus. The talar neck-calcaneal angle decreases from 42° at birth to 23° in the adult. The talar trochlear and calcaneal angle reduces from 9° at birth to 1° in the adult (Fig. 1-3).

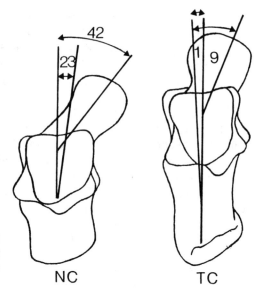

FIGURE 1–3. Talar trochlear and calcaneal angle. Calcaneal angle (NC) is 42° in infant and 23° in adult. Trochlear-calcaneal angle (TC) is 9° in infants and 1° in adults.

MIDFOOT

The midfoot is made up of the navicular and cuboid bones. The midtarsal joint is the major articulation of the midfoot formed by the approximation of these two bones, which articulate with the calcaneus and the talus, respectively. Ossification of the cuboid bone takes place from birth to 21 days of age.[3] The navicular is one of the last of the tarsal bones to ossify, which it does between the second and fifth years.

FOREFOOT

The forefoot includes the cuneiforms, metatarsals, and phalanges. In the fetus, the first metatarsal grows faster than the second. After birth, the first and second metatarsals grow at the same rate. The first metatarsal is shorter and thicker than the second. The intermetarsal angle between the first and second metatarsal bones decreases from 32° at age two months, to 8.9° at age nine months, and 6.2° in the adult.[5] The primary ossification centers of the metatarsals appear between the eighth and tenth weeks of life.

The hallux is the most prominent of the phalanges. Ossification of the medial and lateral sesamoids of the great toe takes place between the ages of 12 and 14 years. By the age of two years, the ossification centers of the medial cuneiform and the proximal phalanges have appeared. Between the ages of two and three years, the ossification centers of the middle cuneiform and middle phalanges appear.

Development During Childhood

The infant foot appears excessively pronated because the medial arch is occupied by a fat pad.[8] The infant foot is very supple. The total range of motion of the subtalar joint is 50°. The ankle joint or talocrural joint exhibits a combined dorsiflexion and plantarflexion range of 20–50°.[9]

From the age of 5 to 10 years in females and 5 to 12 years in males the foot grows .9cm per year. At the age of 10 and 12 years, respectively, the foot is at 90% of the adult size. At the age of 14 and 16 years, respectively, the foot is at the adult size.[8]

By six to eight years of age the bones of the foot assume adult shape.[8] The adult pattern of gait develops between three and five years of age, slightly ahead of the bones of the foot.[3]

In summary, early in the developmental stages the rearfoot largely influences the midfoot and forefoot's form and function. Lack of lateral rotation of the talar head, inadequate reduction in the talar-calcaneal angles, and insufficient changes in the varus angle of the calcaneus can produce deformities of the forefoot and rearfoot. Abnormal pronation and supination in the adult, may be attributed to the imperfect development of the foot within the fetus. The evolutionary changes in the development of the foot are secondary to alterations in function. The foot has become the primary organ of weight-bearing, balance, and propulsion.

FUNCTIONAL ANATOMY
AND MECHANICS OF THE ADULT FOOT

The functional joints of the foot and ankle are the ankle (talocrural), the subtalar, the midtarsal (transverse tarsal), the tarsometatarsal (TMT), and the metatarsophalangeal (MTE) joints.

The rearfoot, midfoot, and forefoot function as a unit during the stance phase of gait. Alterations in any one of these structures will influence the function of the entire foot and ankle during the stance phase. The interdependency and interrelationships of the rearfoot, midfoot, and forefoot are established by muscle and connective tissue structures. Movement of one joint will influence movement of other joints in the foot and ankle. Furthermore, the soft tissue structures establish an interdependency of the foot and ankle to the entire lower limb. Therefore, alterations in the mechanics of the foot and ankle can influence the function of the lower limb.

This section discusses the principles of movement, the specific movements of the joints of the foot and ankle, and their combined function during the stance phase of gait. Special consideration of periarticular stability and muscle function are reviewed.

Principles of Motion

Motion can be divided into two components, translation and rotation.[11] Translation, movement of an object in a straight line, occurs when the line of force passes through the center of the object. Rotation is movement of an object in an arc around a fixed axis. It occurs when the line of force does not pass through the center of the object. The greater the distance between the line of force and the center of the object or center of mass, the greater the rate of rotation.[11] Rotational movement is always perpendicular to the axis of rotation. For example, when a door swings open, the movement of rotation occurs around and perpendicular to the fixed axis of the hinge. Movement is also described according to the body plane in which it occurs (the plane of motion). The primary planes of motion in the foot and ankle are the frontal, sagittal, and transverse planes. The frontal plane movements are inversion and eversion. The sagittal plane movements are dorsiflexion and plantar flexion. The transverse plane movements are adduction and abduction.

The joints of the foot and ankle function as hinges.[10,13] Motion must occur perpendicular to the axis. If not, partial dislocation or impingement may occur.[14] A true hinge joint provides 1° of freedom, or motion, in one plane.[14,15] The interphangeal (IP) joints of the toes provide 1° of freedom, or movement, in one body plane. The MTP joints have two independent axes of motion. Each axis provides 1° of freedom, therefore giving the joints 2° of freedom. The midtarsal, subtalar, and talocrural joints and the first and fifth rays all provide movement in the three cardinal body planes. As described by Root, Orien, and Weed,[14] the fifth ray is the fifth metatarsal and the first ray is the first metatarsal and the first cuneiform.

TRIPLANAR MOVEMENT OF THE FOOT AND ANKLE

The ankle, subtalar, and midtarsal joints, and the first and fifth rays have axes of motion that are oblique to the body planes. The axes of motion are at an angle to three body planes.[14] The movement remains perpendicular to the axis, while the plane of movement occurs at an angle to all three body planes. If movement occurs in all three body planes simultaneously, it is referred to as triplanar motion.[14] The triplanar movements of the foot and ankle are supination and pronation.[14] The three body plane motions in pronation are abduction (transverse plane), dorsiflexion (sagittal plane), and eversion (frontal plane).[14,15] Conversely, supination is a combined movement of adduction, plantar flexion, and inversion (Fig. 1-4).[14,15] The amount of movement occurring in each body plane depends on the position of the axis. For example, if the axis lies close to the frontal plane, more motion occurs in dorsiflexion and plantar flexion. If the axis of motion is closer to the sagittal plane, more motion occurs in adduction and abduction than in dorsiflexion and plantar flexion. Motion at the subtalar joint represents the purest triplanar movement. The oblique axis of the subtalar joint is equidistant from the planes of movement;[10,14] therefore, the amounts of sagittal, transverse, and frontal planar motion are equal during movement at the subtalar joint.

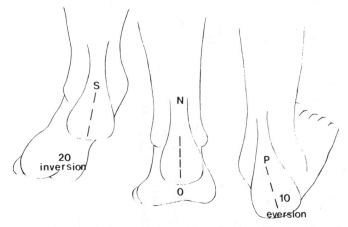

FIGURE 1-4. Open kinetic chain pronation and supination. P, pronation; S, supination; N, neutral.

Rearfoot Stability and Mechanics

ANKLE (TALOCRURAL) JOINT MECHANICS

The tibiotalar, fibulotalar, and tibiofibular joints are three articulations that make up the ankle, or talocrural, joint (Fig. 1-5). The superior surface of the talus bone is wedge shaped and is referred to as the trochlea.[10,11] It may be as much as 6 mm wider anteriorly than it is posteriorly.[10] Dorsiflexion is the close-packed position of the talocrural joint. In the close-packed position there is maximum congruency of the trochlea of the talus with the distal fibula and tibia. The "mortise" is another term used to describe the ankle joint. The mortise is formed by the distal end of the tibia, its medial malleolus, and the lateral malleolus of the fibula.[19]

Hicks[13] and Barnett and Napier[16] identify two axes of ankle joint motion. The dorsiflexion axis is oriented in a downward and lateral direction, and the plantar flexion axis is downward and medial. In the frontal plane, the axis of the ankle joint is observed as slightly distal to the medial and lateral malleoli, in a downward and lateral direction. The oblique anteroposterior inclination of the ankle axis as measured in the transverse plane is called "tibial torsion" or "maleolar torsion."[10] In the normal adult foot the external tibial torsion is 23° (Fig. 1-6).[10]

The triplanar movements of supination and pronation occur at the joints of the ankle because of the obliquity of the axes to the body planes. The trochlea, the dome of

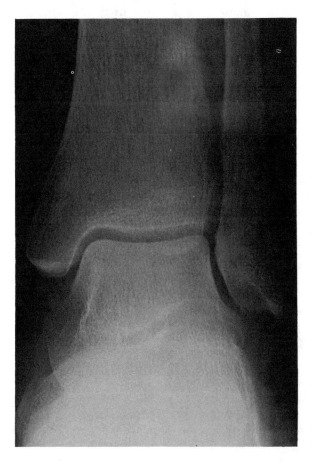

FIGURE 1–5. Ankle joint x-ray (horizontal view) of tibiofibula, tibiotalar, fibulotalar.

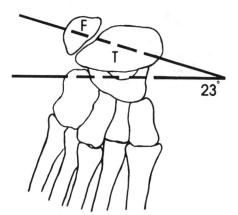

FIGURE 1–6. Malleolar torsion measured by the position of the distal ends of the malleoli, using a goniometer. F, fibula; T, tibia.

the talus, is cone shaped with a medial apex.[5] The cone shape of the trochlea describes two arcs of motion. The small anteromedial arc corresponds to dorsiflexion, and the larger posteriolateral arc corresponds to plantar flexion.[5] The arc of movement during dorsiflexion allows the talus to move into abduction or external rotation, and the plantar flexion arc describes medial rotation or adduction.[5]

From full plantar flexion to dorsiflexion, 1.5 mm of lateral excursion of the fibula and 2.5° of lateral rotation was measured.[5] Throughout the dorsiflexion and plantar flexion range of motion, the malleoli of the fibula and tibia hug the talus for all positions of the joint.[10] Close and Inman[17] measured 1 mm of tibial and fibular malleoli separation during dorsiflexion of the ankle. The dorsiflexion movement was studied during normal walking during weightbearing. The normal range of motion of the ankle joint is 20° of dorsiflexion and 50° of plantar flexion.[18] The most clinically tested movements of the ankle joint are dorsiflexion and plantar flexion;[5] however, the ankle joint is classified as a triplanar joint.[14]

The *closed kinetic chain* ankle movement is influenced by the obliquity of the axis from the tips of the fibular and tibial malleoli. From initial contact to weight acceptance, medial rotation of the lower limb is accompanied by ankle joint plantar flexion and a toe-in position of the foot.[10] During midstance, anterior excursion of the tibia on the talus is initiated as the foot is fixed against the ground.[10] The anterior movement of the tibia on the talus in the closed kinetic chain may be referred to as *closed kinetic chain dorsiflexion*. At heel-off, plantar flexion results in lateral rotation of the leg.

The maximum amount of rotation of the tibia around the oblique axis of the ankle joint is 11°. The average amount of tibial rotation is 19°.[10] The subtalar joint must assist the ankle in accommodating the transverse rotations of the lower limb. The greater the obliquity of the ankle joint axis, the more triplanar movement is available.

ANKLE (TALOCRURAL) JOINT STABILITY

Stormont and coworkers[19] determined that stability of the weightbearing ankle depends on several factors, including the congruity of articular surfaces, the orientation of ligaments, and the position of the ankle at the time of stress. McCullough and Burge[20] added muscle action to the dynamic stability of the weightbearing ankle.

During loading of the ankle, or weightbearing, 100% of inversion and eversion ankle joint stability was accounted for by the joint articular surface; however, in the unloaded or non-weightbearing position, none of the stability was contributed by the articular surface. The three lateral collateral ligaments accounted for 87% of resistance to inversion in the unloaded position. The most important stabilizer was the calcaneo-fibular ligament (Fig. 1-7). The anterior talofibular ligament was the second most significant stabilizer, resisting inversion of the ankle in the non-weightbearing position.[19] The deltoid ligament afforded 83% of the ankle joint stability during eversion in the unloaded condition.[19]

Internal and external rotation of the foot on the leg were generally more stable during weightbearing.[19] The primary stabilizers for internal rotation included the anterior talofibular ligament and the deltoid ligament. External rotation was stabilized by the calcaneofibular ligament. The posterior talofibular ligament was the primary stabilizer

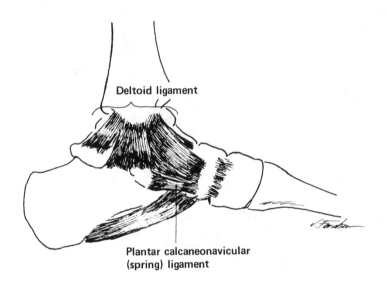

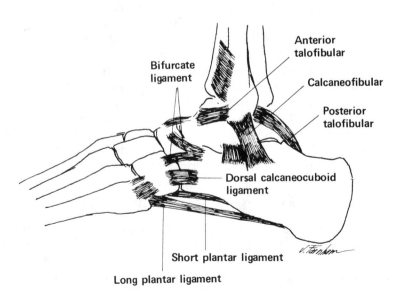

FIGURE 1-7. Medial (*top*) and lateral (*bottom*) ligaments of the posterior ankle/foot complex. (From Norkin and Levangie: Joint Structure and Function. FA Davis, Philadelphia, 1983, p. 339, with permission.)

during plantar flexion.[19] Abnormal talar rotation is prevented by the distal tibiofibular ligaments and the anterior two thirds of the deltoid ligament.[20]

Harper[21] has shown that the excursions of the talus are limited by the medial and lateral structures of the ankle. Tilting of the talus secondary to a valgus stress, anterior excursions, and lateral tilting were the three movements examined in the study. The lateral supporting structures of the joints of the ankle were the major restraint against anterior talar excursion.

Clinically, a positive anterior drawer sign (anterior position of the talus relative to the tibia) and talar tilt can be demonstrated roentgenographically (Fig. 1-8), indicating torn lateral collateral ligaments. The deltoid ligament is the primary restraint to a valgus stress. It is an important factor in preventing rearfoot valgus deformities. Overstretching of this structure can produce flatfoot. The lateral malleolus of the fibula is the primary restraining structure to lateral talar shifts.[21] The lateral malleolus is a key structure requiring reduction and stabilization in the management of ankle fractures.

The final consideration regarding the ankle joint is its weightbearing capability. Frankel[22] reported 11 to 13 cm^2 of weightbearing surface in each ankle. (Each ankle carries 49.3% of the body weight, if the feet represent 1.4% of the total body weight.[11,22]) The weightbearing is shared by the tibiotalar and fibulotalar joints.[11] Lambert demonstrated that one sixth of the 49.3% of body weight is carried by the

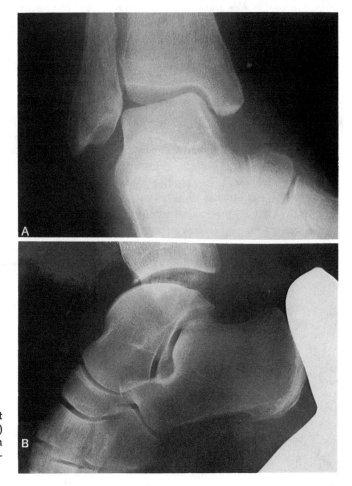

FIGURE 1-8. (A) Talar tilt (1.8B) of 23 degrees and (B) positive anterior drawer sign indicating torn collateral ligaments.

fibula.[23] Because of the large surface area, the load transmission across the ankle joint is less than that across either the hip joint or the knee joint.[11,22] The talocrural joint is a very efficient weightbearing structure.

SUBTALAR JOINT MECHANICS

The talus and calcaneus are the bones that make up the subtalar joint. The subtalar joint is one of the most important joints of the lower extremity and is responsible for the conversion of the rotatory forces of the lower extremity. The mechanics of the subtalar joint dictate the movements of the midtarsal joint and forefoot.

Movement between the talus and calcaneus occurs around an oblique axis. The axis of the subtalar joint extends anteromedially from the neck of the talus to the posterolateral portion of the calcaneus.[10] The average inclination of the axis is 42° from the horizontal and 23° from the midline (Fig. 1-9).

The movement is perpendicular to the axis. Because the axis of the subtalar joint is oblique to three body planes, the motion is triplanar—dorsiflexion, abduction, and eversion for pronation and plantar flexion; adduction, and inversion for supination.

Subtalar joint supination and pronation are measured clinically by the amount of calcaneal inversion and eversion. Root and coworkers[14] describe an inversion to eversion ratio of 2:3 to 1:3, 20° of inversion and 10° of eversion. The midposition of the subtalar joint is subtalar joint neutral. To allow the necessary amount of supination and pronation during the stance phase, the subtalar joint should function as closely as possible to the neutral position (Fig. 1-10). For example, if the calcaneus is everted 10° at heel strike, excessive pronation of the subtalar joint after heel strike will follow. If the subtalar joint is maximally pronated directly after heel strike, torque conversion and shock absorption are significantly reduced.

Bones and soft tissue structures limit the amount of calcaneal eversion and inversion. Inversion is limited by the cervical ligament, calcaneofibular ligament, the peroneus longus and brevis, and the sustentaculum tali striking the talar tubercle.[5] Eversion of the calcaneus is limited by the cervical ligament, lateral process of the talus striking the sinus tarsi surface of the calcaneus, tibiocalcaneal portion of the deltoid ligament, medial talocalcaneal ligament, posterior tibialis tendon and muscle, and the flexor digitorus longus tendon muscle.

In the closed kinetic chain, an important function of the subtalar joint is to act as a torque converter of the lower leg. The transverse plane rotations of the lower kinetic chain are attenuated at the subtalar joint. In addition, the transverse plane movements of the lower limb are dependent upon the oblique subtalar joint axis.[10] For example,

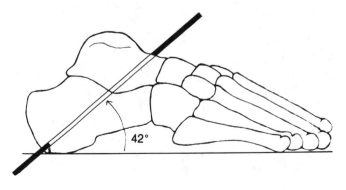

FIGURE 1–9. Subtalar joint axis of motion 42° from the horizontal.

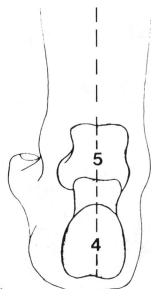

FIGURE 1–10. Neutral position of subtalar joint.

movement of the leg on a fixed foot produces medial and lateral displacement of the lower leg that is accompanied by transverse rotation at the subtalar joint.[10] Figure 1-11 shows how transverse rotation of the lower leg is converted at the subtalar joint. Pronation of the subtalar joint produces internal rotation of the tibia, evidenced by the increased space between the tibia and fibula (Fig. 1-11B). Supination of the subtalar joint produces external rotation of the tibia (see Fig. 1-11D). The space between the fibula and tibia is reduced; the tibia is superimposed over the fibula.

During normal ambulation, the transverse rotations of the lower limb are transmitted to the foot. Sarrafian[5] describes the anterior tibiotalar ligament as contributing to transmission of internal rotation of the tibia to the talus and the posterior talotibial ligament as contributing the transmission of external rotation of the tibia to the talus.

Tibial rotation is clearly demonstrated during the stance phase of walking.[10] The tibia has been found to rotate an average of 19°. The foot does not rotate by moving from a toe-in to a toe-out position during ambulation. Therefore, a mechanism must exist to permit the rotations of the lower limb to occur without movement of the foot. At the beginning of the stance phase, as the tibia rotates internally, the talus plantar flexes and adducts. The talus converts the transverse plane rotations of the tibia into sagittal and transverse plane movements of the talus. The calcaneus simultaneously rolls into eversion to complete the torque conversion. This movement of the talus and calcaneus is closed kinetic chain pronation (Fig. 1-12). During the end of the stance phase, the tibia rotates externally, pushing the talus into dorsiflexion and abduction. Simultaneously the calcaneus inverts to complete the torque conversion. This is closed kinetic chain supination (Fig. 1-13).

The combined closed kinetic chain movement of the rearfoot is important for torque conversion and shock absorption. The obliquity of the ankle joint and subtalar joint axes allows the foot to accommodate for the transverse plane rotations of the lower limb. Talar movement is coordinated at the ankle and subtalar joint. The conical shape of the trochlea and the oblique axis of the ankle joint allow plantar flexion and adduction of the talus immediately after heel strike. As the foot makes contact with the ground, movement occurs around the subtalar joint axis. Subtalar joint closed kinetic chain

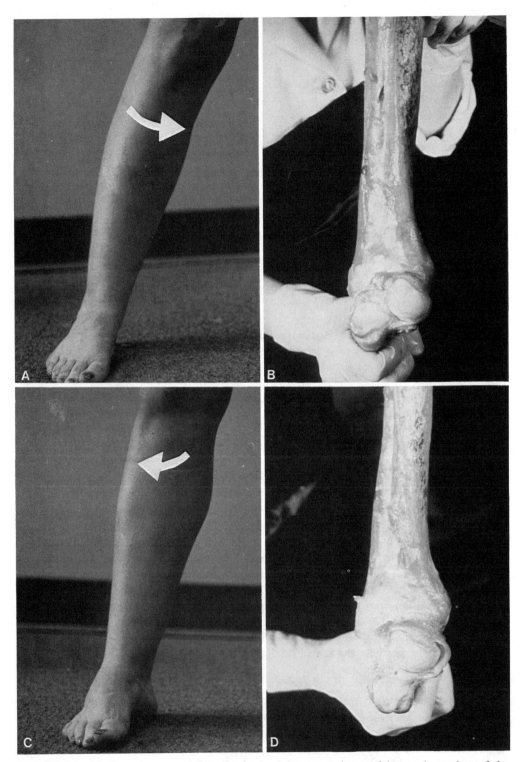

FIGURE 1–11. Transverse rotation of subtalar joint pronation and internal rotation of the tibia. Medial displacement of the tibia (*A*, normal leg; *B*, dissection). Transverse rotation of the subtalar joint supination and external rotation of the tibia. Lateral displacement of the tibia (*C*, normal leg; *D*, dissection).

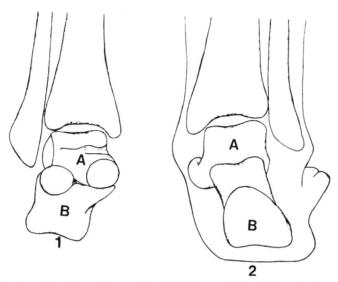

FIGURE 1–12. Anterior (1) and posterior (2) views of closed kinetic chain pronation. A, Talus; B, Calcaneus.

pronation results in plantar flexion and adduction of the talus. In addition, the calcaneus everts to complete the triplanar movement. Therefore, immediately after heel strike the knee flexes, the tibia internally rotates, the ankle plantar flexes, and the subtalar joint pronates as the sequence of events is controlled by the eccentric action of muscle and the tensile strength of ligaments.

As the foot reaches midstance, a reversal occurs at the subtalar joint. In early midstance, the subtalar joint stops pronating and begins to reverse its movement. The tibia moves anterior to the talus. The neutral position of the subtalar joint is reached at midstance. The tibia continues to move anterior to the talus until late midstance. Supination begins during late midstance as the tibia continues to move anterior to the talus. The talus is abducted and dorsiflexed as the tibia externally rotates.

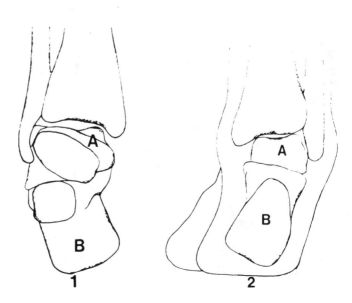

FIGURE 1–13. Anterior (1) and posterior (2) views of closed kinetic chain supination. A, talus; B, calcaneus.

SUBTALAR JOINT STABILITY

The subtalar joint is made up of two articular areas. The posterior articulation consists of the convex calcaneus and the concave talus. The anterior articulations include medial, central, and lateral facets between the talus and calcaneus.[5,24] In a study of 100 calcanei, three different anterior calcaneal facets of the subtalar joint were identified: an ovoid form, a bean-shaped structure with a narrow medial aspect, and two separate articular surfaces.[24] The calcaneus forms an important part of the antero-medial subtalar joint. The sustentaculum tali is the anteromedial aspect of the calcaneus that supports the head and neck of the talus.[10]

Beath and Harris[26] have reported variations in the anteromedial projection of the calcaneus. They classified the support of the anteromedial calcaneus as weak, moderate, or strong. The degree of support is dependent upon how far distally the anteromedial aspect of the calcaneus extends. Excessive plantar flexion and adduction of the talus, components of abnormal pronation of the subtalar joint, are increased by the lack of anteromedial support of the calcaneus. The talus literally falls off the calcaneus in a medial and anterior direction, as a result of weightbearing forces and poor osseous support. Furthermore, the sustentaculum tali forms a fulcrum around which the tibialis posterior, flexor hallucis longus, and flexor digitorum longus tendons pass. The contraction of their muscles gives the hindfoot dynamic stability.[24]

The ligaments of the subtalar joint are important to joint stability. A review of the literature indicates confusion in the description and nomenclature of the subtalar joint ligaments. They can be divided into superficial and deep structures. The superficial ligaments include the lateral and posterior talocalcaneal ligaments. The deep ligamentous structures form a wall that divides the subtalar joint. The deep ligaments include the interosseous, cervical, and axial ligaments.[24] Gray[27] separates the cervical ligament from the interosseous ligament. Viladot, Lorenzo, and coworkers[24] describe the cervical ligament as a portion of the interosseous structure that prevents inversion and eversion.

The ligament in the tarsal canal is the most important ligament formation. The tarsal canal separates the middle and posterior facets of the articulation between the talus and the calcaneus. The ligament of the canal is sometimes referred to as the cruciate ligament of the tarsus, or the axial ligament.[24] Formed mainly by collegen fibers, the axial ligament is very thick and strong. It divides the anterior and posterior subtalar joint and is mainly responsible for limiting eversion.[25] Figure 1-14 (left) shows a dissec-

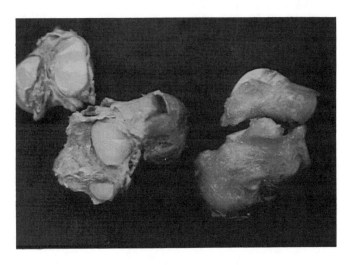

FIGURE 1–14. *Left*, Axilla or interosseous ligament dividing the anterior and posterior facets of the subtalar joint. *Right*, Talus and calcaneus in the normal anatomical relationship, talus superior to calcaneus.

tion of the axial ligament, which divides the subtalar joint, the inferior surface of the talus, and the superior surface of the calcaneus. Figure 1-14 (right) shows the normal relationship of the talus and calcaneus. Overstretching of the axial ligament can result in an acquired heel valgus deformity. Conversely, severe limitations in passive calcaneal eversion may be secondary to lack of extensibility of the axial ligament.

Midfoot Stability and Mechanics

The midtarsal, transverse tarsal, and Chopart's joint are synonymous with the articulations of the calcaneocuboid and the talonavicular joints. The talonavicular articulation resembles the articulation of the acetabulum and the head of the femur. Sarrafian[5] describes the articulation of the head of the talus, the navicular, and the anteromedial calcaneal portion as the "acetabulum pedis." The concave portion of the acetabulum pedis is formed by osseous and ligamentous structures. The floor of the acetabulum pedis is formed by the navicular bone. The convex surface of the head of the talus bone is analogous to the head of the femur.

The calcaneocuboid joint is a saddle, or sellar, joint. As in all saddle joints, the convex and concave joint surfaces are at right angles to each other.[27] The convex joint surface of the calcaneocuboid joint is transverse (or within the horizontal plane) and the concave joint surface is vertical (or perpendicular to the horizontal plane).[5] If the convex and concave joint surfaces are a perfect match, only rotation is allowed to occur.[5] The rotational movement between the calcaneus and cuboid is described as pivotal.[28]

Rotational movements of the midtarsal joint allow the forefoot to twist on the rearfoot. The navicular and cuboid move as a unit with the anterior part of the foot. There is minor relative movement between the navicular and the cuboid.[5,28,29] Therefore, the forefoot, or anterior unit, is capable of moving on the calcaneus and talus by movement of the midtarsal joint.

Manter[28] and Elftman[29] describe two axes of motion at the midtarsal joint (Fig. 1-15). The first axis is longitudinal (extending lengthwise through the foot) and slopes upward and mediad.[14,28,29] Inversion and eversion are the movements occurring around the longitudinal axis.[14,28,29] Clinically, inversion and eversion of the midtarsal joint can be observed in the normal rise and drop of the medial arch of the foot in the weight-bearing position.[28,29]

Manter[28] describes a "screw-like" action of the cuboid and navicular bones rather than a rotation around the longitudinal axis. The "screw-like" action of the cuboid and navicular occurs during closed kinetic chain inversion and eversion. Eversion turns the navicular in a medial direction and displaces it distally.[28] The forward movement of the navicular releases the head of the talus, allowing it to move anteriorly. Forward displacement of the talus is opposed by plantar muscles and ligaments.[28] The forward displacement of the talus and navicular is brought about by pronation of the subtalar joint.[28] The rotational movements of the talus and of the navicular are in opposite directions. For example, observing the right foot from behind, pronation turns the navicular counterclockwise with respect to the calcaneus, and the talus undergoes clockwise rotation.[28]

A rotation also occurs at the calcaneocuboid articulation. During the push-off phase of gait, the pivotal movement of the calcaneus and cuboid allows the cuboid to become fixed. A stable cuboid acts as a fulcrum for the peroneus longus muscle. The peroneus longus pulls around the cuboid, plantar flexing the first ray in the push-off phase of gait.

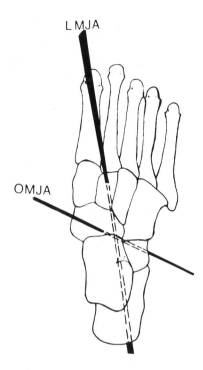

FIGURE 1–15. Midtarsal joint axes: longitudinal midtarsal joint axis (LMJA); oblique midtarsal joint axis (OMJA).

The pivotal movement of the cuboid and calcaneus is accomplished by supination of the subtalar joint.

The second axis of the midtarsal joint is oblique or transverse. Several authors describe the transverse axis of the midtarsal joint as being inclined 52° from the horizontal and 57° from the frontal plane.[14,28-32] Movement at the transverse axis is a combination of dorsiflexion and abduction, and plantar flexion and adduction. Increased motion along the transverse axis occurs with abnormal pronation. In severe cases of flatfoot, the forefoot is dorsiflexed and abducted on the rearfoot.[28] The dorsiflexion component may be compensatory to ankle joint equinus. The increased abduction results from anteromedial displacement of the navicular and talus with rearfoot pronation. Therefore, every degree of subtalar joint pronation produces an increase in midtarsal joint instability.[33]

Rearfoot and Midfoot Closed Kinetic Chain Function

The ankle, subtalar, and midtarsal joints are dependent upon each other during the stance phase of gait. Immediately after heel strike, the ankle plantar flexes, causing internal rotation and adduction of the tibia and talus. The subtalar joint pronates, producing forward displacement of the talus and the navicular. The calcaneus everts, allowing maximum range of motion of the midtarsal joint. The articular surfaces of the navicular and cuboid are more parallel to each other, producing a supple forefoot. During midstance, the tibia advances over the talus in closed kinetic chain dorsiflexion. External rotation of the tibia and abduction of the talus accompanies closed kinetic chain dorsiflexion. During push-off, the subtalar joint supinates, producing a pivotal movement of the cuboid and calcaneus, stabilizing the cuboid. A fixed cuboid acts as a fulcrum for the peroneus longus muscle, facilitating plantar flexion of the first ray or first metatarsal in push-off.

TRIPLANAR MOVEMENTS

The normal mechanics of the rearfoot and midfoot are dependent upon the obliquity of the axes of motion. Because there are wide variances in the direction of the axis of the ankle, subtalar, and midtarsal joints, greater range of motion in one cardinal plane, and restricted movement in another, may be possible from patient to patient.[30,32]

Predominance of motion in one cardinal plane is referred to as *planar dominance.* Variance in the direction of the axis for the ankle, subtalar, and midtarsal joints alters the triplanar motion and determines the planar dominance. For example, if the subtalar joint axis of motion is inclined 68° from the horizontal instead of 42°, movement of the subtalar joint will be increased in the transverse plane and limited in the frontal plane. An individual with these variances will have difficulty compensating for frontal plane deformities intrinsic to the foot, such as forefoot varus.

Conversely, the more parallel the subtalar axis is to the sagittal plane, the greater the amount of inversion and eversion. Patients demonstrating greater ranges of inversion and eversion should be able to successfully compensate for frontal plane deformities and respond better to functional orthoses. Patients who demonstrate reduced ranges of inversion and eversion are less capable of compensating for frontal plane deformities.

The obliquity of the ankle joint determines how much torque conversion is necessary at the subtalar joint. If the axis of the ankle joint is horizontal, it will not function as a triplanar joint. Thus, the movement of the tibia cannot be resolved about the axis of the ankle joint and must take place at the subtalar axis.[34]

Inman[10] reports a heel lift can be therapeutic, and clinically useful for determining the obliquity of the ankle joint axis. In patients with an oblique ankle joint axis, the use of a heel lift increases both plantar flexion and the toe-in position of the foot directly after heel strike. The toe-in position facilitates supination of the foot, reducing the stress of excessive pronation.

The primary planar dominance of the ankle, subtalar, and midtarsal joints will determine the primary planar compensation.[32] The clinical significance of planar dominance becomes evident when selecting a surgical procedure or in determining the foot orthoses perscription. For example, orthotic control of excessive transverse plane motion is difficult. The functional foot orthoses are designed to control frontal plane movement of the forefoot and rearfoot. Controlling a foot with excessive frontal plane movement is easier than controlling one with excessive transverse plane movement. Off-the-shelf arch supports may be somewhat helpful to reducing the symptoms in those patients demonstrating excessive frontal plane movement.[32]

As we become more sophisticated in our understanding of foot function, assessment of the foot's biomechanics will take on added significance. Bordelon[35] describes normal ranges for the cardinal body plane movements of the foot and ankle. Passive motion of the foot in the transverse plane demonstrates 30° of adduction and 15° of abduction. Passive forefoot motion in the frontal plane demonstrates 25° of varus and valgus, or inversion and eversion, respectively. Passive motion of the heel in the frontal plane is 10° of eversion and 20° of inversion. Finally, ankle joint sagittal plane movement is 50° of plantar flexion and 20° of dorsiflexion. The evaluation of planar dominance can begin with these cardinal plane ranges (Table 1-2).

TABLE 1–2 Passive Range of Motion of the Foot and Ankle

Transverse Plane Movement
  30° of forefoot adduction
  15° of forefoot abduction

Frontal Plane Movement
  25° of forefoot inversion (varus)
  25° of forefoot eversion (valgus)

  10° of rearfoot eversion
  20° of rearfoot inversion

Sagittal Plane Movement
  50° of plantar flexion
  20° of dorsiflexion

Forefoot Stability and Mechanics

The normal movement and stability of the forefoot are dependent upon stable metatarsals and good mobility of the metatarsophalangeal (MTP) and interphalangeal (IP) joints. The metatarsal heads tolerate the vertical forces of weightbearing, while the toes stabilize the forefoot dynamically. The forefoot extends from the tarsometatarsal (TMT) joints, or Lisfranc's joint, distally. The tarsometatarsal joints allow flexion and extension of the metatarsal bones and a certain degree of supination and pronation of the marginal rays. Sarrafian[5] describes the supination and pronation of the first and fifth rays as longitudinal axial rotations. The combination of the sagittal motions and the axial rotations of the first and fifth rays results in a supination and pronation twist of the forefoot, as defined by Hicks.[13] A supination twist is a result of first ray extension (dorsiflexed) and fifth ray flexion (plantar flexed) (Fig. 1-16). A pronation twist is a

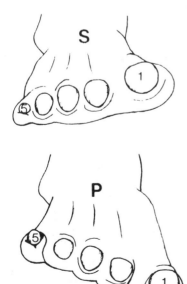

FIGURE 1–16. Forefoot supination twist (S); forefoot pronation twist (P).

result of first ray flexion (plantar flexed) and fifth ray extension (dorsiflexed) (see Fig. 1-16).[5,13]

In a standing position, a high medial arch is produced by external rotation of the tibia, supination of the subtalar and midtarsal joints, and pronation twist of the forefoot. Conversely, a low medial arch is produced by internal rotation of the tibia, pronation of the subtalar and midtarsal joints and a supination twist of the forefoot.[5,13] The forefoot pronation and supination twist is dependent upon the coordinated movement of the midtarsal and subtalar joints. The actual twisting movement of the forefoot results from the reciprocal movement of the first and fifth metatarsals.

METATARSALS

Hicks[13,36] describes the metatarsals as beams supporting the longitudinal arches. The beams are tied together by a "tie rod" or plantar aponeurosis. Upon weightbearing, the metatarsals and calcaneus are forced apart and tension develops within the tie rod.

Perry[37] describes the plantar fascia, or the aponeurosis, and the intrinsic musculature as the force transmitters from one end of the arch to the other. As the metatarsalophalangeal joints are dorsiflexed in push-off, a "windlass effect" tightens the tie rod (Fig. 1-17).[36-38] The plantar fascia is a broad, dense band of longitudinally arranged collagen fibers.[37] Collagen fibers are designed to resist tensile forces. As increased loads are applied the plantar fascia becomes progressively stiffer or more able to resist deformation.[39] Hence, tension at one end of the tie rod is transmitted to the other end, pulling the ends closer together.

The plantar aponeurosis has three components, central, lateral, and medial.[5] The central component originates from the posteromedial calcaneal tuberosity. The lateral or peroneal component originates from the lateral margin of the medial calcaneal tubercle and is connected with the origin of the abductor digiti minimi muscle. Finally, the medial or tibial component fibers originate distally and medially and are continuous with the abductor hallucis muscle.[5] As noted above, the plantar aponeurosis originates predominantly from the medial aspect of the calcaneus. Therefore, tension of the tissue

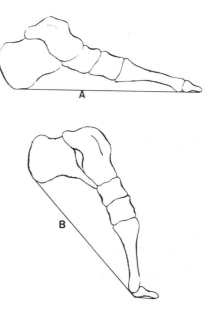

FIGURE 1–17. The windlass effect. (A) Plantar aponeurosis slack position; and (B) tightening of the plantar aponeurosis in pushoff.

promotes inversion of the calcaneus and supination of the subtalar joint. Thus, the windlass mechanism is important in establishing a rigid lever for push-off.

Numerous authors have demonstrated that the longitudinal arches are not supported by muscle.[41-44] Lapidus[45] was one of the first to describe the concept of the foot functioning as a truss. A truss is a triangular structure with two beams connected by a tie rod. The vertical forces transmitted to the foot in weightbearing are attenuated by the truss mechanism. Therefore, intrinsic and extrinsic muscles are not used in static arch support.[4] Mann[46] reports activity of the intrinsic muscles, abductor hallucis brevis, flexor hallucis brevis, flexor digitorum brevis, and abductor digiti minimi in stabilizing the transverse tarsal joint during the stance phase of gait. In normal feet the onset of intrinsic muscle activity is initiated at approximately midstance, or after 35% of stance phase. In contrast, the onset of intrinsic muscle activity in flat-footed subjects was within the first 25% of the stance phase.[46,47] A fallen or flattened arch cannot be raised by exercises.[41]

The transverse arch is formed by the cuneiforms and the cuboid (Fig. 1-18).[5] Support of the forefoot is by means of the heads of the metatarsals. The metatarsals are held together by ligament and muscle. The six elements that prevent splaying the forefoot include; Lisfranc's ligament, the transverse metatarsal ligament, the interosseous muscles, the peroneus longus muscle, the plantar extension of the posterior tibial tendon, and the adductor hallucis muscle (Fig. 1-19).[48]

Cavanagh[49] reported that in a symptom-free population the static peak pressures in the forefoot were 2.5 times lower than the peak pressures under the heel. Thus, about 60% of the weightbearing load is carried by the rearfoot, 8% by the midfoot, and 28% by the heads of the metatarsals. These peak pressures during standing are approximately 30% of those produced during walking and 16% of those during running.[49] The second and third metatarsal heads bear the greatest forefoot pressures.[50] The fact that the first ray does not bear the greatest pressure in standing indicates that it has a more dynamic function during push-off. Earlier studies by Stokes and coworkers[51] indicated that the forces under the first metatarsal during walking were found to be the highest. Hutton and Dhannedran[52] reported that the first ray is the largest and strongest of all. The first metatarsal bone is twice as wide as the second metatarsal and four times as strong.[52] Furthermore, the peroneus longus, posterior tibialis, and anterior tibialis muscles attach to the first ray and function to dynamically stabilize it in the propulsive phase

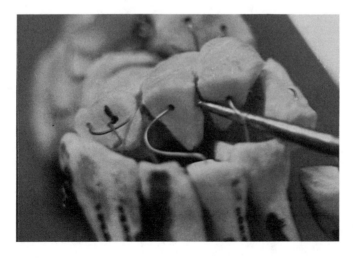

FIGURE 1-18. Transverse arch cuboid and cuneiforms.

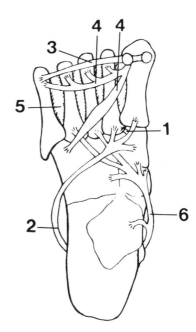

FIGURE 1–19. Structures within the forefoot to prevent "splaying." (1) LisFranc's ligament; (2) peroneus longus tendon; (3) transverse metatarsal ligament; (4) adductor hallucis; and (5) interossous muscle.

of gait. The head of the first metatarsal has a large joint surface and sesamoid bones to give the flexor hallucis longus a mechanical advantage, minimizing joint forces.[51] Finally, the inclination angle of the first metatarsal to the horizontal is greater than that of the other metatarsals, reducing the shearing and bending forces of weightbearing.[51]

TOES

The function of the toes is important to the biomechanics of the forefoot. During walking the toes help to stabilize the longitudinal arch and maintain floor contact until the final phase of push-off.[47] Approximately 40% of the body weight is borne by the toes in the final stages of foot contact.[51] During the stance phase of gait the greatest load is through the first metatarsophalangeal joint.[47] Weightbearing forces to the toes are attenuated by the tension in the toe flexor tendons and tendon sheaths.[51] During standing, the peak pressure to the toes is minimal.[49]

Dorsiflexion of the toes, especially the first MTP joint, is important to the windlass mechanism. Metatarsophalangeal joint movement occurs in two cardinal body planes. The sagittal plane movement of the MTP joint is flexion and extension, and the transverse plane movement is abduction and adduction. Sixty to seventy degrees of dorsiflexion is necessary for tension to develop within the aponeurosis. The instant center of rotation of the first metatarsophalangeal joint is within the head of the metatarsal. Hallux valgus and hallux rigidus deformities, which are subluxations of the first MTP joint, alter the instant center of rotation of the MTP joint. Often with these deformities the center of rotation falls outside the head of the first metatarsal.[53] The mobility of the sesamoid bones is important to the normal mechanics of the first MTP joint. Displacement of the medial and lateral sesamoids during dorsiflexion of the MTP joint was measured to be 10 to 12 mm.[53] Hallux valgus deformities demonstrate significantly less sesamoid displacement than normal joints.[53] Hallux valgus produces lateral subluxation of the sesamoid bones and the flexor hallucis longus muscle. The altered position of the sesamoid bones transforms the flexor hallucis longus and brevis from flexors to adductors, contributing to the severe loss of plantar flexion.[53]

The sesamoid bones are the attachment sites for several important soft tissue structures. Flexor hallucis brevis, oblique head and transverse component of the adductor hallucis, flexor hallucis longus fibrous tunnel, and the deep transverse metatarsal ligament all insert into the borders of the medial and lateral sesamoid bones.[5] The sesamoid bones maintain proper alignment of the flexor hallucis longus tendon and are also responsible for absorbing vertical pressures in push-off. Figure 1-20 shows the first MTP joint with the sesamoid bones in place. The flexor hallucis longus passes between the sesamoids.

The last four toes are attachment sites for the extensor digitorum tendon, the flexor digitorum tendon, the dorsal and plantar interossei, and the lumbrical muscles.[48] The interosseous and lumbrical muscles dynamically stabilize the toes on the floor in the tiptoe position.[48] Failure of the lumbrical and interosseous muscles to function accounts for toe deformities such as claw toes.[48]

Summary of Closed Kinetic Chain Function

The triplanar joints of the foot include the talocrural, subtalar, midtarsal, first ray, and fifth ray. Pronation and supination are the triplanar movements of the foot. Pronation occurs directly after heel strike, for shock absorption, adjustment to the terrain, and torque conversion. Supination occurs during the push-off phase of gait. Supination of the subtalar joint allows the foot to function as a rigid lever for propulsion. A rigid foot during the propulsive phase allows muscle pulleys to be established. The pulleys established by the tarsal bones change the direction of pull of the muscle,

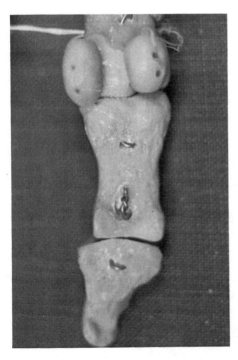

FIGURE 1-20. Sesamoids of the first metatarsophalangeal joint that house the flexor mechanism of the flexor hallucis longus tendon.

TABLE 1–3 Closed Kinetic Chain Mechanics of the Foot and Ankle

1. Heel Contact to Weight Acceptance
Rearfoot
  Talocrural plantar flexion
  Subtalar joint pronation
  Tibial internal rotation
  Talar adduction and plantar flexion
  Calcaneal eversion
Midfoot
  Midtarsal pronation
  Unlocking of cuboid/navicular
  Forward displacement (clockwise rotation) of talus
  Counterclockwise rotation of navicular
Forefoot
  Supination twist-dorsiflexion of the first ray
2. Early Midstance/Midstance/Late Midstance
Rearfoot
  Early—Talocrural: anterior movement of the tibia over the talus; subtalar reversal of
    pronation
  Midstance—Closed kinetic chain dorsiflexion; subtalar: neutral position
  Late—Continued anterior movement of tibia over talus; subtalar: supination abduction
    and dorsiflexion of talus
Midfoot
  Midtarsal reversal of pronation
Forefoot
  Full weightbearing of the metatarsal heads
3. Push-off and Propulsion
Rearfoot
  Talocrural: tibial external rotation
  Subtalar: supination
Midfoot
  Midtarsal supination-cuboid/navicular are rigid-talus counterclockwise rotation-navicular
    clockwise rotation
Forefoot
  Pronation twist-first ray plantar flexion
  Sesamoids weightbearing

increasing the efficiency of muscle function. Table 1-3 summarizes the closed kinetic chain movements of the foot and ankle.

MUSCLE FUNCTION AND NORMAL MECHANICS

During walking, muscle is used to initiate movement, stabilize osseous structures, and decelerate movement.[12] Electromyographic (EMG) studies are commonly used to analyze the function of muscle during the gait cycle. The combined knowledge of EMG activity and foot function during the gait cycle is necessary to give the clinician a complete picture of muscle function. This section describes the functions of the major muscles of the foot and ankle during the different phases of the gait cycle (Table 1-4).

The anterior tibialis is an important muscle during the swing phase. Directly after toe-off, early swing, and midswing, the anterior tibialis assists dorsiflexion of the foot for clearance of the ground. Just prior to heel strike, slight supination of the foot is accomplished by the accelerating or concentric action of the anterior tibialis muscle.[19]

TABLE 1–4 Muscle Function during the Stance Phase of Gait

Muscle	Action
Heel Contact to Weight Acceptance	
Anterior tibialis	*Eccentric* — control pronation of subtalar joint
Extensor hallucis longus	*Eccentric* — decelerate plantar flexion and posterior shear of tibia
Extensor digitorum	on talus
Posterior tibialis	*Eccentric* — decelerate pronation of subtalar joint and internal
Soleus	rotation of tibia
Gastrocnemius	
Midstance	
Posterior tibialis	*Eccentric* — decelerate forward movement of tibia
Soleus	
Flexor hallucis longus	
Flexor digitorum longus	
Posterior tibialis	*Concentric* — supinate subtalar and midtarsal joints
Soleus	
Gastrocnemius	
Push-off and Propulsion	
Peroneus longus	*Concentric* — plantar flex first ray
Abductor hallucis	
Peroneus brevis	*Antagonistic* — to supinators of subtalar and midtarsal joints
Flexor digitorum longus	*Concentric* — stabilize toes against ground
Extensor hallucis longus and brevis	*Concentric* — stabilize first metatarsophalangeal joint
Abductor hallucis	*Concentric* — stabilize midtarsal and forefoot, raise medial arch
Abductor digiti quinti	of foot in push-off
Flexor hallucis brevis	
Flexor digitorum brevis	
Extensor digitorum brevis	
Interossei, lumbricals	

Directly after heel strike, the anterior tibialis and the toe extensors (extensor digitorum longus and extensor hallucis longus) demonstrate maximal electrical activity.[4,12] The decelerating function of these muscles resists plantar flexion of the foot at heel strike and controls pronation of the forefoot during the contact period.[19] The anterior tibialis at heel strike and immediately afterward decelerates the tibia, resisting a posterior shear force.

Immediately after heel strike, there is no activity of the pronators. As previously noted, pronation is a controlled passive movement. As the forefoot makes contact with the ground, the posterior tibialis, soleus, and gastrocnemius muscles further decelerate pronation of the subtalar joint and internal rotation of the lower extremity.[19,54]

During midstance, the soleus, posterior tibialis, flexor hallucis longus, and flexor digitorum longus muscles reduce the forward momentum of the tibia.[19] The activity of the posterior tibialis, soleus, and the gastrocnemius maintain stability of the midtarsal joint by accelerating subtalar joint supination during the midstance and early propulsive phases of gait.[19] External rotation of the lower leg is initiated by swing-through of the countralateral limb and the action of the gastrocnemius rotating the femur externally.[19,55]

As the foot prepares for push-off, supination of the subtalar joint is initiated to establish a rigid lever and pulleys for extrinsic muscles. For example, at heel-off the peroneus longus plantar flexes the first ray. The plantar flexion of the first metatarsal is facilitated by the cuboid pulley. The cuboid changes the direction of pull of the peroneus longus, increasing efficiency of plantar flexion of the first ray. The abductor hallucis muscle also plantar flexes the first metatarsal during propulsion.[19] The peroneus brevis is active in the early propulsive phase as an antagonist to the muscles that supinate the subtalar and midtarsal joints.[19]

The extensor digitorum longus assists the lumbricals in stabilizing the IP joints during propulsion. The flexor digitorum longus stabilizes the toes against the ground during push-off.[19] The extensor hallucis longus and flexor hallucis longus and brevis stabilize the first metatarsal phalangeal joint during propulsion.

The intrinsic muscles include the abductor hallucis, abductor digiti quinti, flexor hallucis brevis, flexor digitorum brevis, extensor digitorum brevis, the interossei, and lumbricals. Several authors have reported that the intrinsic muscles of the foot play a dynamic role in stabilization of the midtarsal joint and forefoot during the push-off phase.[4,46]

SUMMARY

The normal biomechanics of the foot and ankle can be divided into static and dynamic components. The static components include the bones, joint surface congruity, ligaments, and fascia. The dynamic components include the kinetics of the tarsal bones and muscle function.

The combined effects of the static and dynamic structures of the foot and ankle are responsible for force attenuation within the foot and lower limb. The windlass effect of the plantar aponeurosis, the tensile strength of the plantar ligaments, the beam effect of the metatarsals, and the joint congruity of the tarsal and metatarsal bones encompass the static mechanisms for force attenuation.

The triplanar movements of the foot and ankle and the interrelationship of muscle function are the dynamic components of force attenuation. Pronation is initiated at heel strike and is controlled by an eccentric action of muscle and the restraining characteristics of connective tissue. Pronation allows the foot to absorb compressive forces, adjust to uneven terrain, and maintain equilibrium. Supination establishes a rigid lever for push-off and creates pulley systems for several extrinsic foot muscles. Pronation occurs directly after heel strike and reaches its maximum at footflat. Resupination occurs during earlier midstance, allowing the foot to pass through a neutral position at midstance. Supination begins during late midstance and continues until toe-off.

Understanding the functional biomechanics of the foot and ankle has profound implications for clinical applications. The inability of the lower limb to convert transverse rotation at the subtalar joint could have detrimental effects on other joints in the chain such as the knee, midtarsal joint, and forefoot. It is imperative for the clinician treating lower extremity dysfunction to have an understanding of the normal biomechanics of the foot and ankle. Furthermore, the clinician must understand the interdependency of the foot and ankle, and the normal function of the lower kinetic chain.

GLOSSARY

Adduction/Abduction: Movements of the foot and ankle in the transverse plane.

Closed kinetic chain: A series of joints in which the terminal joint is the first joint to meet with resistence during movement.

Closed kinetic chain dorsiflexion: Anterior movement of the tibia on the talus.

Dorsiflexion/Plantar flexion: Movements of the foot and ankle in the sagittal plane.

Inversion/Eversion: Movements of the foot and ankle in the frontal plane.

Kinetic chain: A series of joints interconnected by soft tissue and muscle in which movement of one joint will influence the movements of others in the chain.

Neutral position of the subtalar joint: The position one third of the way through the total range of motion of the subtalar joint from the fully everted position to full inversion. Midposition of the subtalar joint range of motion, zero pronation, and zero supination.

Open kinetic chain: A series of joints in which the terminal joint is non-weightbearing.

Open kinetic chain pronation: Dorsiflexion, abduction, and eversion.

Open kinetic chain supination: Plantar flexion, adduction, and inversion.

Pronation/Supination: The triplanar movements of the foot and ankle.

Subtalar joint closed kinetic chain pronation: Talar adduction and plantar flexion and calcaneal eversion.

Subtalar joint closed kinetic chain supination: Talar abduction and dorsiflexion and calcaneal inversion.

Triplanar joints of the foot and ankle: Talocrural, subtalar, midtarsal, first ray, and fifth ray.

Triplanar movements: Movement in three body planes simultaneously around an oblique axis. The movement is perpendicular to the axis.

REFERENCES

1. Smidt, GL: Biomechanics and physical therapy, a perspective. Phys Ther 64:1807, 1984.
2. Cailliet, R: Foot and Ankle Pain. FA Davis, Philadelphia, 1968.
3. Tachdjian, MO: The Child's Foot. WB Saunders, Philadelphia, 1985.
4. Conroy, GC and Rose, MD: The evolution of the primate foot from the earliest primates to the Miocene hominids. Foot Ankle 3:342, 1983.
5. Sarrafian, SK: Anatomy of the Foot and Ankle. JB Lippincott, Philadelphia, 1983.
6. Brown, LP and Yavorsky, P : Locomotor biomechanics and pathomechanics: a review. J Orthop Sports Phys Ther 9:3, 1987.
7. Hlavac H: Compensated forefoot varus. J Am Podiatr Med Assoc 60:229, 1970.
8. Jaffe, WL and Laitman, JT: The evolution and anatomy of the human foot. In Jahss, MH (ed): Disorders of the Foot, Vol 1. WB Saunders, Philadelphia, 1982, p. 1.
9. McCrea, JD: Pediatric Orthopaedics of the Lower Extremity. Futura, Mt. Kisco, NY, 1985.
10. Inman, VT: The Joints of the Ankle. Williams & Wilkins, Baltimore, 1976.
11. Kotwick, JE: Biomechanics of the foot and ankle. Clin Sports Med 1:19, 1982.
12. Inman, VT, Rolston, HJ, and Todd, F: Human Walking. Williams & Wilkins, Baltimore, 1981.
13. Hicks, JH: The mechanics of the foot. 1. The joints. J Anat 87:345. 1953.
14. Root, ML, Orien, WP, and Weed, JN: Clinical Biomechanics. Vol 11: Normal and Abnormal Function of the Foot. Clinical Biomechanics, Los Angeles, 1977.
15. Gross, CM: Gray's Anatomy. Lea & Febiger, Philadelphia, 1968.
16. Barnett, CH and Napier, JR: The axis of rotation at the ankle joint in man: Its influence upon the form of the talus and the mobility of the fibula. J Anat 86:1, 1952.
17. Close, JR, and Inman, VT: The action of the ankle joint. Prosthetic Devices Research Project, Institute of Engineering Research, University of California, Berkeley. Series 11, Issue 22:5 The Project Berkeley, University of California, Berkeley, 1952.

18. Morris, JM: Biomechanics of the foot and ankle. Clin Orthop 22:10, 1977.
19. Stormont, DM, et al: Stability of the loaded ankle. Am J Sports Med 13:295, 1985.
20. McCullough, CL and Burge, PD: Rotatory stability of the load-bearing ankle. J Bone Joint Surg 62B:460, 1980.
21. Harper, MC: Deltoid ligament: An anatomical evaluation of function. Foot Ankle 8:19, 1987.
22. Frankel, VH and Nordin, M: Basic Biomechanics of the Skeletal System. Lea & Febiger, Philadelphia, 1980.
23. Lambert, KL: The weight-bearing function of the fibula. A strain gauge study. J Bone Joint Surg 53A:567, 1971.
24. Viladot, A, et al: The subtalar joint: Embryology and morphology. Foot Ankle 5:54, 1984.
25. Kapandji, IA: The Physiology of the Joints, Vol II, The Lower Limb. Churchill Livingstone, London, 1970.
26. Harris, R and Beath, T: Hypermobile flat-foot with short tendoachilles. J Bone Joint Surg 30A:116, 1948.
27. Warwick, R and Williams, P (eds): Gray's Anatomy, British ed 35. Philadelphia, WB Saunders, 1973.
28. Manter, JT: Movements of the subtalar joint and transverse tarsal joints. Anat Rec 80:397, 1941.
29. Elftman, H: The transverse tarsal joint and its control. Clin Orthop 16:41, 1960.
30. Phillips, RD, et al: Clinical measurement of the axis of the subtalar joint. J Am Podiatr Med Assoc 75:119, 1985.
31. Subotnick, SI: Biomechanics of the subtalar joint and midtarsal joints. J Am Podiatr Med Assoc 65:756, 1975.
32. Green, DR and Carol, A: Planal dominance. J Am Podiatr Assoc 74:98, 1984.
33. Phillips, RD and Phillips, RL: Quantitative analysis of the locking position of the midtarsal joint. J Am Podiatr Med Assoc 73:518, 1983.
34. Wright, DG, et al: Action of the subtalar and ankle-joint complex during the stance phase of walking. J Bone Joint Surg 46A:361, 1964.
35. Bordelon, LR: Surgical and Conservative Foot Care. Charles B. Slack, Thorofare, NJ, 1988.
36. Hicks, JH: The mechanics of the foot. II. The plantar aponeurosis. J Anat 88:25, 1954.
37. Perry, J: Anatomy and biomechanics of the hindfoot. Clin Orthop 177:9, 1983.
38. Mann, RA: Surgical implications of biomechanics of the foot and ankle. Clin Orthop 146:111, 1980.
39. Wright, DG and Rennels, DC: A study of the elastic properties of plantar fascia. J Bone Joint Surg 46A:482, 1964.
40. Sarrafian, SK: Functional characteristics of the foot and plantar aponeurosis under tibiotalar loading. Foot Ankle 8:4, 1987.
41. Jones, RL: The human foot. An experimental study of its mechanics, and the role of its muscles and ligaments in the support of the arch. Am J Anat 68:1, 1941.
42. Basmajian, JV and Stecko, G: The role of muscles in arch support of the foot. J Bone Joint Surg 45A:1184, 1963.
43. Smith, JW: Muscular control of the arches of the foot in standing: An electromyographic assessment. J Anat 88:152, 1954.
44. Hicks, JH: The mechanics of the foot. IV. The action of muscles on the foot in standing. Acta Anat 27:180, 1956.
45. Lapidus, PW: Kinesiology and mechanical anatomy of the tarsal joints. Clin Orthop 30:20, 1963.
46. Mann, RA and Inman, VT: Phasic activity of intrinsic muscles of the foot. J Bone Joint Surg 46A:469, 1964.
47. Mann, RA and Hagy, JL: The function of the toes in walking, jogging and running. Clin Orthop 142:24, 1979.
48. Viladot, A: The metatarsals. In Jahss, MH (ed): Disorders of the Foot, Vol 1. Philadelphia, WB Saunders, 1982, p 659.
49. Cavanagh, PR: Pressure distribution under symptom-free feet during barefoot standing. Foot Ankle 7:262, 1987.
50. Gieve, DW and Rashi, T: Pressures under normal feet in standing and walking as measured by foil pedobarography. Ann Rheum Dis 43:816, 1984.
51. Stokes, IAF, et al: Forces acting on the metatarsals during normal walking. J Anat 129:579, 1979.
52. Hutton, WC and Dhaneddran M: The mechanics of normal and hallux valgus feet: A quantitative study. Clin Orthop 157:7, 1981.
53. Shereff, ML, et al: Kinematics of the first metatarsophalangeal joint. J Bone Joint Surg 68A:392, 1986.
54. Sutherland, DH, et al: The role of the ankle plantar flexors in normal walking. J Bone Joint Surg 62A:354, 1980.
55. Mann, RA: Biomechanics of running. In Mack, RP (ed): Symposium on the Foot and Leg in Running Sports. St. Louis, CV Mosby, 1982, p 1.

CHAPTER 2

Abnormal Biomechanics

Robert A. Donatelli, MA, RPT

This chapter discusses the etiology, classification, and mechanics of abnormal pronation and supination. Abnormal pronation and supination within the joints of the foot and ankle are nothing more than hypermobilities and hypomobilities, respectively. For example, a flexible flatfoot (abnormal pronation) describes a hypermobile unit unable to produce an effective push-off during the gait cycle. The lack of efficient propulsion is perpetuated by abnormal mechanics of the rearfoot. The poor mechanics of the subtalar joint may result in first ray (first metatarsal/first cuneiform articulation) hypermobility. The term "first ray insufficiency syndrome" is often used to describe this hypermobility. The insufficiency or hypermobility of the first ray refers to dorsiflexion of the first ray that is unable to bear weight effectively during propulsion. As a result of faulty mechanics, the foot is unable to establish an effective lever for push-off. In addition, the abnormal mechanics reduce the ability of the foot to attenuate the excessive forces of weightbearing. Soft tissue breakdown may occur, causing changes in muscle function and osteologic remodeling. These changes can produce a rigid deformity. The foot becomes unable to function as a shock absorber or mobile adapter to the changing ground surfaces. Thus, a hypermobile foot may become hypomobile as a result of pathologic changes within the soft tissue structures.

ABNORMAL PRONATION

There are many terms to describe abnormal pronation. Flatfoot, pes planus, pes valgoplanus, pronated foot, calcaneovalgus foot, valgus foot, and talipes calcaneovalgus are several of the terms found in the literature that describe or identify abnormal pronation.[1-6] In this text, the term "abnormal pronation" is used to describe the flatfoot deformities noted above, and the terms are interchangeable.

The literature classifies the etiology of abnormal pronation into three basic categories: congenital, acquired, and secondary to neuromuscular diseases. However, a discussion of flatfoot associated with neuromuscular disease is beyond the scope of this chapter. The term congenital means "to be born with" or "to have been present at birth."[7] Congenital flatfoot can result from genetic factors or malposition of the fetus in the uterus. Congenital deformities can be further classified as rigid or flexible. The most common rigid flatfoot deformities with possible genetic etiology include: convex pes valgus (congenital vertical talus), tarsal coalition, and congenital metatarsus varus.[5,6] The most common congenital flexible flatfoot deformity is talipes calcaneovalgus.[5,6]

Acquired flatfoot can result from abnormalities which are intrinsic or extrinsic (or both) to the foot and ankle. Intrinsic causes of acquired flatfoot include: trauma, ligament laxity, bony abnormalities of the subtalar joint, forefoot varus, forefoot supinatus, rearfoot varus, and ankle joint equinus. Extrinsic factors causing abnormal pronation include: rotational deformities of the lower extremity and leg length discrepancies.

Abnormal pronation, or flatfoot, can be a deformity present at birth, or an acquired deformity that develops after weightbearing begins. Acquired flatfoot may result from compensation at the subtalar joint. This compensation is an attempt to modify an intrinsic and/or extrinsic foot abnormality.

Congenital Deformites

RIGID DEFORMITIES

Convex pes Valgus

Convex pes valgus, or congenital vertical talus, is a dislocation of the talocalcaneonavicular joint that the fetus develops in the uterus within the first trimester of pregnancy.[5,8-10] The etiology is uncertain, and the deformity may occur either in isolation or in association with central nervous system abnormalities such as spina bifida and arthrogryposis.[8-10] Convex pes valgus may also occur as an isolated primary deformity of unknown etiology.[5]

The most striking characteristic of the convex pes valgus deformity visible on X-ray is plantar rotation of the talus toward a more vertical position (Fig. 2-1). However, the vertical position of the talus is commonly observed in other flatfoot deformities, such as talipes calcaneovalgus. Thus, the distinguishing feature in convex pes valgus is the position of the navicular, which is completely dislocated, articulating with the dorsal surface of the neck of the talus.[9-11] In talipes calcaneovalgus, there is a sag at the talonavicular articulation, and joint congruity is compromised, without complete dislocation. During the first three years of life the navicular bone cannot be accurately visualized roentgenographically.[5,10] Therefore, the clinician must be aware of other differential characteristics, such as a valgus and equinus (plantar flexed) position of the hindfoot. A dorsiflexion force to the foot causes bending at the mid-tarsal joint, producing a convexity along the the foot's plantar aspect. To compensate for the limited dorsiflexion at the ankle joint the forefoot abducts and tilts upward at the midtarsal joint, creating a "rocker-bottom" appearance to the plantar aspect (Fig. 2-2).[9,11]

Tarsal Coalitions

Tarsal coalition may be either a complete or incomplete fusion of the talus, calcaneus, cuboid, navicular, and cuneiforms.[5,12-17] The joint fusion may be fibrous, cartilaginous, or osseous; and can occur during the development of the fetus.[12] Stormont and Hamlet[13] found the most common tarsal coalition to be the calcaneonavicular, followed by the talocalcaneal. The etiology of tarsal coalitions strongly suggests an hereditary component.[13-15,18,19]

Subtalar joint motion becomes progressively more limited with ossification of the

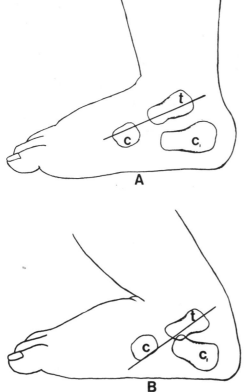

FIGURE 2–1. (*A*) Normal weightbearing. Bisecting line passes through the talus and cuboid. (*B*) Abnormal pronation-talipes calcaneovalgus. Bisecting line passes below the cuboid, indicating a plantar flexed talus which is common in the congenital flatfoot (c, cuboid; t, talus; c_1, calcaneus).

coalition. The fusion can occur at the anterior, middle, or posterior facets of the subtalar joint. Limitations at the subtalar joint may be difficult for the clinician to determine. Limited mobility of the calcaneus may be concealed by movement at the midtarsal joint and tilting of the talus in the mortise or ankle joint.[17] The examiner must grasp the calcaneus firmly and attempt to move it into both eversion and inversion to determine subtalar joint restrictions. Figure 2-3 demonstrates the range of motion of the adult subtalar joint. The calcaneus is forced into a valgus position when talocalcaneal, calcaneonavicular, or talonavicular coalition occurs.[12] This position causes a breakdown of the midtarsal area, and the arch flattens.

Rigid Metatarsal Deformities

The nomenclature for metatarsal deformities is confusing. Most of the literature describes metatarsus varus and metatarsus adductus synonymously. However, for the purposes of this chapter the forefoot deformities are divided into rigid and flexible categories. The rigid metatarsal deformity metatarsus varus, as described by Kite, is a medial subluxation of the tarsometatarsal joints.[20] The hindfoot is in a slightly valgus or neutral position, with the navicular lateral to the head of the talus.[5,20] The term "metatarsus adductovarus" is used to refer to the combination of adduction and inversion of the forefoot and is discussed in the next section.

Congenital rigid metatarsal deformities do not present as flatfoot deformity at birth. In fact, the literature describes metatarsus varus as a "third of clubfoot."[20-22] Kite

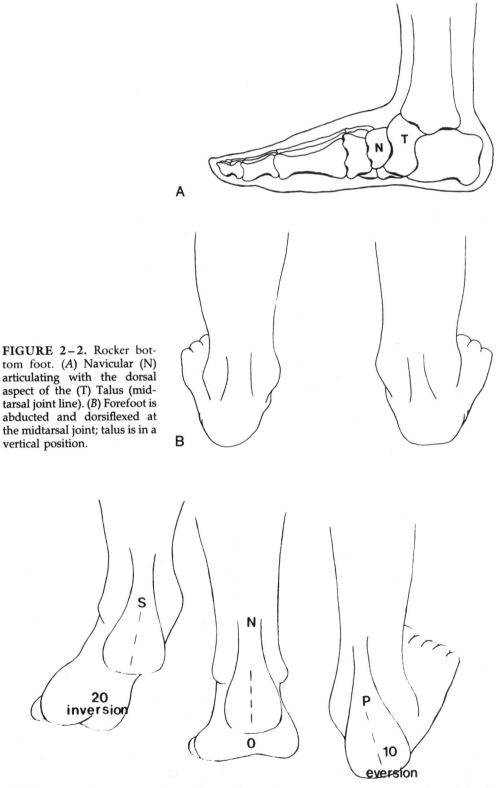

FIGURE 2-2. Rocker bottom foot. (*A*) Navicular (N) articulating with the dorsal aspect of the (T) Talus (midtarsal joint line). (*B*) Forefoot is abducted and dorsiflexed at the midtarsal joint; talus is in a vertical position.

FIGURE 2-3. Range of motion of the subtalar joint is measured by calcaneal inversion and eversion 20/10. Zero is the perpendicular or neutral position of the subtalar joint.

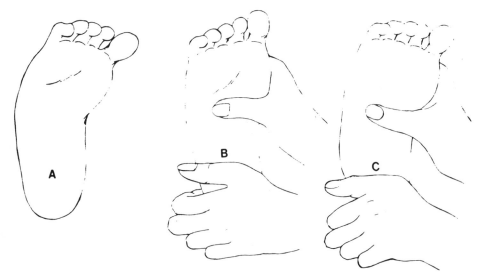

FIGURE 2–4. Range of motion of the forefoot. (*A*) Metatarsus adductus position of the forefoot. (*B*) Passive reduction of the metatarsus adductus deformity to the midline. (*C*) Metatarsus varus. Rigid forefoot deformity unable to abduct the forefoot to the midline.

observed 300 cases of congenital metatarsus varus. In 94% of these, the deformity was present at birth. The average age at which the metatarsus varus deformity was recognized was 2.8 months.[20] According to Kite, because most congenital deformities are fully developed at birth, metatarsus varus is a congenital muscle imbalance, which increases with the lapse of time after birth, similar to the deformities associated with poliomyelitis.[20] The etiology of rigid metatarsus deformities has both genetic and environmental factors.[5] Abnormal pronation secondary to metatarsus adductovarus deformities develops after weightbearing in an attempt to compensate for the deformity.

There are several clinical signs to assist in the diagnosis of a rigid metatarsal deformity. The forefoot cannot be abducted past the midline position (Fig. 2-4). In severe cases, the forefoot cannot passively be reduced from the in-toe position. The clinician must be careful to abduct the forefoot against the resistance of the rearfoot. If the forefoot is abducted against the resistance of the leg, abduction of the foot could occur as a result of external rotation of the leg. Normal dorsiflexion range of motion at the ankle joint is present. Observation of the foot demonstrates a prominent lateral aspect of the foot in the area of the cuboid and the fifth metatarsal.[6,20]

FLEXIBLE DEFORMITIES

Talipes Calcaneovalgus

The most common congenital flexible flatfoot deformity is talipes calcaneovalgus, which occurs in approximately 1 in 1000 births.[5,6,23,24] There is a high correlation between the presence of calcaneovalgus in the newborn and the later development of flatfoot in the older child.[5,15,25]

Tachdjian reports the etiology of talipes calcaneovalgus is a malposition of the fetus in the uterus.[5] As the fetus develops the posture is determined by the development of neuromuscular function. The limbs assume various postures as different muscle groups become active. Between 12 and 26 weeks of fetal development the feet are dorsiflexed and everted. If such a position persists beyond this stage of development the feet could be excessively pronated at birth, either unilaterally or bilaterally.[5]

The appearance of the foot in talipes calcaneovalgus is one of dorsiflexion and eversion. The dorsal surface of the foot is in contact with the anterolateral surface of the lower limb (Fig. 2-5). The calcaneus is in a valgus position and the talus is plantar

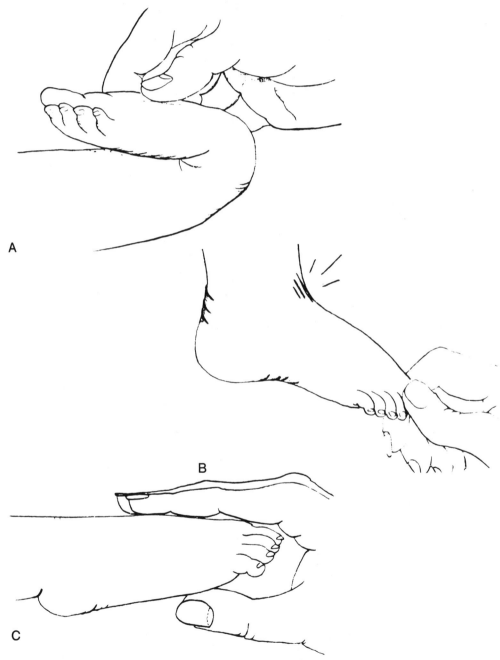

FIGURE 2–5. (*A*) Passive dorsiflexion of the foot. Contact of the forefoot on the anterior aspect of the lower leg. Typical sign found in talipes calcaneovalgus. (*B*) Limited plantar flexion. (*C*) Normal plantar flexion.

flexed.[23,24,26,27] The plantar flexed talus can be observed upon X-ray, and is not to be confused with the convex pes valgus deformity. The latter, as previously mentioned, is associated with central nervous system deformities. In convex pes valgus a dislocated navicular bone is the distinguishing characteristic.

An important clinical observation of talipes calcaneovalgus is the limitation of plantar flexion at the ankle joint. The plantar flexion range is usually limited to 90° or less. Any attempt to move the foot into plantar flexion beyond 90° is met with resistance of the soft tissue. Furthermore, during the neonate's first four to six months, stroking of the plantar aspect of the foot will produce a dorsiflexion and eversion movement.[6]

Ferciot explains that in talipes calcaneovalgus, there is a tendency for the entire lower limb to be positioned in external rotation, and this positioning occurs during fetal development.[24] He believes there is a delay in the development of the limb bud, with incomplete rotation and a positional stretching of the Achilles tendon. Thus, the feet are held in a position of dorsiflexion and eversion before birth.[24]

Flexible Metatarsal Deformities

For the purposes of this chapter, the flexible metatarsal deformities include those deformities present at birth that are secondary to malposition of the fetus in the uterus. McCrea has the most operative classification system of deformities. His system of classification describes the deformity within the body planes. There are four metatarsal deformities: metatarsus adductus, metatarsus varus, metatarsus adductovarus, and forefoot adductus.[6] Metatarsus adductus is a transverse plane deformity, with adduction of all five metatarsals at the tarsometatarsal joint (Fig. 2-6). Metatarsal varus is a frontal plane deformity of subluxation at the tarsometatarsal joint, with all of the metatarsals inverted and little or no adduction present (Fig. 2-7). Metatarsus adductovarus is a combination of the frontal and the transverse plane deformities, with adduction and inversion occurring simultaneously at the tarsometatarsal joint (Fig. 2-8). Metatarsus

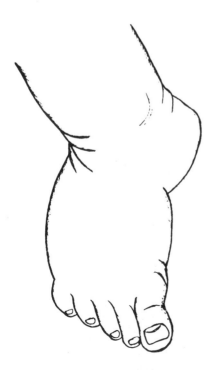

FIGURE 2–6. Metatarsus adductus. Transverse plane deformity with subluxation at the tarsometatarsal joint.

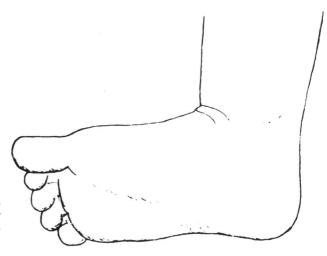

FIGURE 2–7. Metatarsus varus. Frontal plane deformity with subluxation at the tarsometatarsal joint.

adductovarus is the most common deformity. Forefoot adductus is a single or combined deformity occurring at the midtarsal joint (Fig. 2-9).

Clinical examination of the metatarsus adductus deformities usually reveals a convex lateral border and a concave medial border (Fig. 2-10). Passive movement of the forefoot should reduce the deformity, allowing the forefoot to return to the midline. There are no limitations of the ankle joint into dorsiflexion or plantar flexion, and the calcaneus is in a perpendicular or slightly varus position.[6]

At birth, a metatarsus adductus deformity does not present with the characteristics of flatfoot. According to McCrea, the metatarsus adductus deformities may develop into metatarsal in-toeing abnormalities if they are present when the child begins to weight-

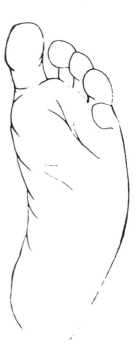

FIGURE 2–8. Metatarsus adductovarus. Combined transverse and frontal plane deformity with subluxation at the tarsometatarsal joint.

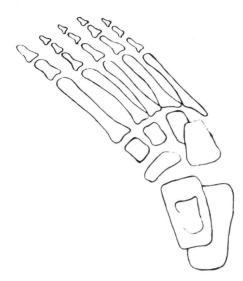

FIGURE 2–9. Forefoot adductus. Subluxation at the midtarsal joint.

bear.[6] In-toeing may cause impaired ambulation in the young child. Often, because of the toe-in position, the child is unable to run without tripping and demonstrates an awkward gait. The body's center of gravity is shifted to the lateral aspect of the foot. Normally, the weightbearing stress line is through the central portion of the foot.[6] If the metatarsus adductus deformity is not corrected, foot mechanics will be altered with weightbearing. Abnormal pronation develops as a compensation for the forefoot deformity. The rearfoot and the midfoot collapse, which results in abduction of the forefoot, adduction and plantar flexion of the talus, and eversion of the calcaneus.[6,28,29] The alterations in the foot mechanics allow the center of gravity of the body to shift from a

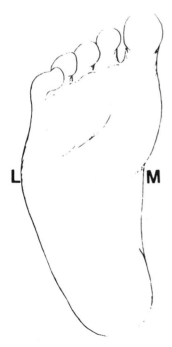

L   M

FIGURE 2–10. Concavity of the medial border (M) and convexity of the lateral border (L) of the foot give the appearance of an infant ("C" shaped) foot in metatarsus adductus deformity.

lateral to a more medial position, producing a more stable and less awkward gait. Therefore, metatarsus adductus deformities do not represent true congenital flatfoot. The abnormal pronation develops as a compensation for the deformity after weightbearing.

Acquired Deformities

The acquired flatfoot deformity can develop after birth as a result of trauma, ligament laxity, or bony abnormality of the subtalar joint. Acquired flatfoot can also be a compensation for an abnormality which is intrinsic and/or extrinsic to the foot.[25, 28-30]

INTRINSIC DEFORMITIES

Traumatic Flatfoot

Trauma to the tibialis posterior tendon is often described as a cause of acquired adult flatfoot.[31,32] The tibialis posterior is a strong supinator of the foot and produces adduction, inversion, and plantar flexion of the ankle.[28] The muscle-tendon unit of the tibialis posterior is an important stabilizer of the rearfoot, preventing valgus (eversion) deformities.[33] Rupture of the tendon imposes an excessive stress to the hindfoot static structures (ligaments and bone) designed to maintain good alignment. The movement of the calcaneus into the valgus position causes collapse of the talocalcaneal articulation. The calcaneus can be described as subluxing under the talus. The talus moves medially as the calcaneus moves laterally. An important clinical sign in posterior tibialis rupture is the "too many toes sign"; that is, four or five toes can be visualized by an observer from the posterior aspect of the foot when the patient stands (Fig. 2-11). In addition, inability of the patient to rise up onto the toes in the weightbearing position is an indication of tibialis posterior weakness.

Ligament Laxity

Ligament laxity is an important consideration in the development of a flatfoot deformity. Ligamentous support is important in maintaining the medial arch.[33-35] If sufficient tensile strength is present within the long and short plantar ligaments, the

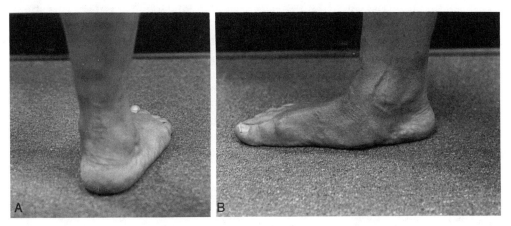

FIGURE 2-11. "Too many toes" sign on the right resulting from a ruptured tibialis posterior tendon. Five toes are visible from the posterior aspect of the foot.

spring ligament, and the plantar fasciae, good joint congruity and alignment will be established. A certain amount of ligament laxity is present in the normal child's foot. Young children have a greater range of joint motion than most adults. As the child matures, the margins of increased ranges of joint motion diminish by about half by early adolescence.[6] A child just beginning to walk demonstrates significant medial and lateral instability of the foot.[6] The appearance of flatfoot at this early age may be attributed to ligament laxity. If the tensile strength of the ligaments does not increase as the child matures, a position of pronation will be maintained. As the child becomes older and gains weight, stress will increase on the ligamentous and muscular structures. The increase in weightbearing forces may produce microtrauma to the weak ligamentous and muscular structures, eventually producing soft tissue destruction and increased possibility of joint collapse. Prolonged pronation in childhood can produce a structurally irreparable adult flatfoot.[36]

Bony Abnormality of Subtalar Joint

Harris and Beath have reported the significance of the bony architecture in maintaining proper joint congruity between the talus and calcaneus.[37] Bony abnormalities between the articular facets of the talus and calcaneus may be significant factors in the development of flatfoot. The stability and congruity of the subtalar joint are dependent on ligamentous, muscular, and bony support. The articular surfaces of the subtalar joint are composed of three facets: anteromedial, anterolateral, and posterior. The anteromedial facet is the most important of the three for support of the head and neck of the talus. The anterior medial facet of the subtalar joint is formed by the anterior aspect of the calcaneus and a bony prominence along the anteromedial aspect of the calcaneus called the sustentaculum tali. In the stance phase of gait, from heel strike to footflat, the vertical body weight is shifted to the medial aspect of the foot as the tibia rotates internally.[28] Pronation at the subtalar joint includes plantar flexion and adduction of the talus as the calcaneus moves into eversion. The anteromedial facet and the posterior facet are important articulations for normal pronation. If the anteromedial facet does not provide good support to the head and neck of the talus, the forces at heel strike could push the talus into excessive plantar flexion and adduction, one component of abnormal pronation (Fig. 2-12).

The manner in which the head of the talus is supported by the anterior aspect of the calcaneus can be classified as strong, mild, or weak.[37] Strong support is indicated by a talar head that is placed solidly on the calcaneus with total joint congruity. This strong osseous support to the talar head permits full weightbearing without changing the talocalcaneal position. Mild osseous support is demonstrated when the head of the talus is partially sustained by the anterior aspect of the calcaneus. Weak osseous support results when the head of the talus is without anterior medial calcaneal contact, with only the sustentaculum tali to support the head. When the osseous support is weak, the head and neck of the talus project over the anteromedial end of the calcaneus. The lack of support may produce excessive medial and plantar movement of the talus during the pronation phase, causing the calcaneus to tilt into eversion. The excessive movements of the talus and calcaneus are important components in the development of abnormal pronation and acquired flatfoot deformity.

Pronation Compensatory Caused by Intrinsic Deformities

The four most common intrinsic abnormalities resulting in compensated abnormal pronation are: forefoot varus, forefoot supinatus, subtalar varus, and ankle joint equinus.[25,28] The compensation for the deformity usually occurs at the subtalar joint.

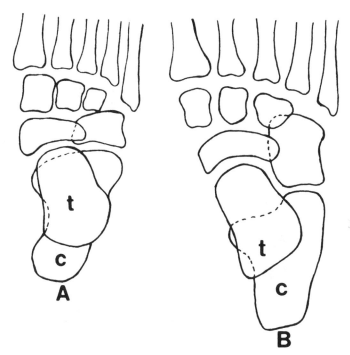

FIGURE 2-12. Anterior calcaneal support of the talus. (*A*) Strong support. (*B*) Weak support which predisposes the foot in weightbearing to abnormal pronation (t, talus; c, calcaneus).

When the subtalar joint compensates for the deformity by pronating, the compensatory pronation occurs in addition to the normal amount of pronation necessary for ambulation. This compensatory pronation occurs every time the foot is placed on the ground. Furthermore, compensatory pronation may occur at the wrong time. For example, pronation may occur during the supination phase of stance. Root, Orien, and Weed[28] reports that pronation is most destructive to the foot when it occurs in the push-off phase of gait.

Maximum pronation is normally reached after approximately 25% of the stance phase is completed.[38] Compensatory pronation usually continues past 50% of the stance phase. The foot never supinates.

In summary, compensatory pronation may be excessive, persistent, and untimely during the stance phase, resulting in destruction of the soft tissue and in foot pathology. Because the subtalar joint is triplanar, it has the ability to move in three body planes: frontal, sagittal, and transverse.[28] The ability of the subtalar joint to move in three planes allows it to compensate for deformities in the body planes.[28,29,39]

Compensated Forefoot Varus. Forefoot varus is the most common intrinsic deformity that results in abnormal compensatory pronation.[28,40-43] Root and associates[28] define forefoot varus as an inversion of the forefoot on the rearfoot, with the subtalar joint held in neutral (Fig. 2-13).[28] Forefoot varus is a frontal plane deformity that is compensated, in weightbearing, by eversion of the calcaneus (Fig. 2-14). The compensatory movement of the calcaneus into eversion is accompanied by talar adduction and plantar flexion.[23]

Compensation for forefoot varus deformity occurs at the subtalar joint. This compensation can be measured by the amount of calcaneal eversion in the standing posi-

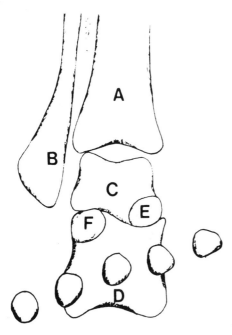

FIGURE 2–13. Forefoot varus. Inversion of the forefoot on the rearfoot with the subtalar joint in neutral. A) tibia B) fibula C) talus D) calcaneus E) talonavicular articulation F) calcaneal-cuboid articulation.

tion. For example, 8° of forefoot varus should result in 8° of calcaneal eversion. The eversion range of motion of the subtalar joint determines the amount of compensation movement available. For example, if the eversion range of the calcaneus is measured at 10°, the subtalar joint is capable of compensating for a forefoot deformity of up to 10°. If the forefoot varus is greater than 10°, additional compensation must be accomplished

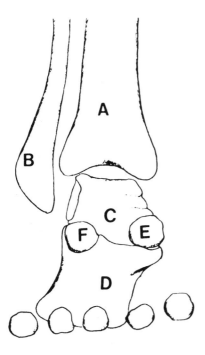

FIGURE 2–14. Compensated forefoot varus in weightbearing. A) tibia B) fibula C) talus D) calcaneus E) talonavicular articulation F) calcaneal-cuboid articulation.

elsewhere. A forefoot varus deformity may be totally compensated, partially compensated, or uncompensated at the subtalar joint.

A forefoot varus deformity alone is not destructive to the foot; however, the method of compensation is detrimental to the normal mechanics of the foot. The subtalar joint must pronate to compensate for the forefoot deformity. In addition, normal pronation must occur to assist the lower kinetic chain to attenuate weightbearing forces such as torque conversion, anterior shear, and compression. The combination of normal pronation and compensatory pronation is excessive and may be destructive to the foot and ankle. Many clinicians have observed that compensation for forefoot varus is a clinically significant factor in the development of mechanical pain and dysfunction within the foot, lower third of the leg, and knee.[42, 44-46]

McCrea,[6] explains that forefoot varus results from prolonged abnormal pronation rather than from a primary cause or result of a flatfoot deformity. As the foot continues to function from a collapsed position of pronation, the forefoot will eventually assume a varus attitude in conjunction with the everted position of the calcaneus. A functional shortening of the muscles attaching to the dorsal medial aspect of the foot maintains this varus position of the forefoot.[6]

DiGiovanni and Smith define forefoot varus as a sagittal plane deformity of the first ray. The dorsal hypermobility of the first ray results from abnormal pronation and is also referred to as "first ray insufficiency."[15] The dorsiflexed hypermobile first ray results from inability of the peroneus longus to stabilize the first ray. The cuboid pulley allows the peroneus longus to plantar flex and abduct the first ray, producing a stable structure from which to push off.[28] The peroneus longus pulley system is reinforced by locking up the midtarsal joint during supination of the subtalar joint.[28,47-49] The cuboid becomes a rigid structure around which the peroneus longus functions. Abnormal pronation reduces the ability of the foot to return to supination. Thus, the midtarsal joint, specifically the cuboid, is in a poor position. The poor position of the cuboid creates an inefficient pulley for the peroneus longus muscle, causing instability of the first ray[28] (Fig. 2-15).

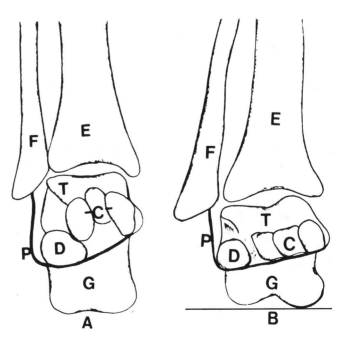

FIGURE 2-15. Cuboid pulley. (A) Normal pulley of cuboid. (B) Abnormal pronation cuboid pulley is less effective. E, tibia; F, fibula; P, peroneus longus tendon; D, cuboid; C, cuneiforms; G, calcaneus; T, talus.

Partially Compensated or Uncompensated Forefoot Varus. Inability of the subtalar joint to pronate, offsetting a forefoot varus deformity, may result in partial or complete compensation at the joints distal to the subtalar joint. Compensations may occur within the joints of the midtarsal or the first ray, or both.

During the stance phase of gait, an uncompensated or partially compensated forefoot varus may manifest itself by an increase in the abduction of the foot from the midline. The abduction of the forefoot occurs around the transverse axis of the midtarsal joint. It is accompanied by eversion. Abduction and eversion are pronation movements occurring at the midtarsal joint. Pronation of the midtarsal joint is in addition to subtalar compensatory pronation, or else replaces it.

Jahss[15] refers to talonavicular and navicular cunieform sag as a collapse of the medial arch. Excessive movement of these joints may occur when the subtalar joint is limited and unable to produce enough compensatory pronation. The excessive mobility of the midfoot and forefoot may cause subluxation of the talonavicular and navicular-cuneiform articulations. These subluxations will produce soft tissue trauma and medial arch pain.

Forefoot Supinatus. Forefoot supinatus is difficult to distinguish from forefoot varus. Forefoot supinatus is a soft tissue deformity that occurs around the longitudinal axis of the midtarsal joint.[28] The forefoot is held in a supinated position secondary to contracture or spasm of the anterior tibialis muscle. In contrast, forefoot varus results from failure of the head and neck of the talus to fully derotate from the infantile position.[28]

Forefoot supinatus and forefoot varus are compensated at the subtalar joint during the stance phase of gait. The compensation is the same for both deformities — the subtalar joint pronates if complete compensation occurs to increase weightbearing of the first ray. Another method of compensation for forefoot varus and forefoot supinatus is plantar flexion of the first ray.[28] In the non-weightbearing position, the first ray is hypermobile and plantar flexed. During the gait cycle, plantar flexion of the first ray is an attempt to correct an uncompensated forefoot varus. This compensation causes instability of the forefoot and rearfoot in the propulsive phase of gait.

Rearfoot Varus. Another intrinsic frontal plane deformity resulting in compensatory pronation is rearfoot varus, not to be confused with the calcaneal varus position as a compensation for forefoot valgus (see Abnormal Supination, below). The rearfoot varus deformity can be described as a varus neutral heel. If the subtalar joint functions from the varus neutral position, the heel will contact the ground in an inverted position. As the heel hits the ground, the rearfoot must be stable. The calcaneus moves from the varus position to a vertical position. The movement of the heel from varus to vertical is a relative eversion or pronation of the subtalar joint. This positioning becomes detrimental to the foot if, in addition to normal pronation, compensatory pronation must also occur.

To protect the ankle from trauma, the subtalar joint must pronate at heel strike. The calcaneal eversion distributes the weight medially, permitting the subtalar joint to function as a shock absorber and to adjust to changing terrain. The inability to pronate causes instability with minimal changes in the contour of the walking or running surface, leaving the patient more vulnerable to ankle sprains.

Many patients demonstrate restricted calcaneal eversion. Patients who complain of repeated ankle sprains may have limited eversion of the calcaneus beyond the vertical position (Fig. 2-16). Limited calcaneal eversion is another example of a rearfoot varus deformity. Limited eversion produces instability of the ankle from heel strike to footflat.

Ankle Joint Equinus. Ankle joint equinus is an intrinsic sagittal plane deformity that causes compensatory pronation.[28,37,43,50-53] Root and coworkers[28] define ankle joint

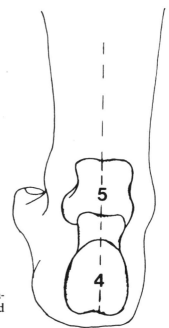

FIGURE 2–16. In the neutral or vertical position of the subtalar joint, a vertical line would bisect both the talus (5) and calcaneus (4).

equinus as the lack of dorsiflexion of the ankle with the subtalar joint in neutral position. The most common cause of ankle joint equinus is limited flexibility of the gastrocnemius and soleus muscle groups.[50,51] Harris and Beath[37] reported a congenital shortening of the gastrocnemius and soleus muscles. Sgarlato was the first to distinguish between the soleus or the gastrocnemius as the limiting agent of dorsiflexion of the ankle joint.[54] He demonstrated that a shortened soleus muscle can be distinguished from a shortened gastrocnemius by flexing the knee and passively dorsiflexing the ankle. A shortened soleus prevents 10° of dorsiflexion at the ankle joint with the knee flexed. The gastrocnemius equinus limits dorsiflexion with the knee extended. A combined limitation in dorsiflexion of the gastrocnemius and soleus muscle groups produces restrictions with the knee extended and flexed.[54] The subtalar joint is held in the neutral position in the above test.

Anopol[52] describes the foot as a two-lever arm mechanism. The short arm of the lever is the length of the Achilles tendon from insertion on the calcaneus to the center of the ankle joint. The long arm runs from the insertion of the Achilles tendon to the metatarsophalangeal (MTP) joint. The short lever arm of the Achilles tendon can manage twice the force of the long lever arm. For example, every time a person weighing 100 kg takes a step, 100 kg of force is placed on the ball of the foot, and 200 kg is exerted on the calf muscles.[52] If the calf muscles (gastrocnemius and soleus) become tight, dorsiflexion of the ankle joint will be limited, increasing the pull of the gastrocnemius. The increased force of the muscle pull may cause the calcaneus to move into eversion to place the lateral aspect of the tendon on slack. Therefore, a tight Achilles tendon may be the cause of excessive pronation of the subtalar joint.

Furthermore, limited dorsiflexion of the ankle joint during the stance phase produces an inability of the tibia to move anterior to the talus from footflat to midstance. This limitation may also be compensated for by pronation of the subtalar joint. A common finding in a flatfoot is the change in the alignment of the midtarsal joint line (Fig. 2-17). The lateral weightbearing x-ray of a normal foot demonstrates a line forming

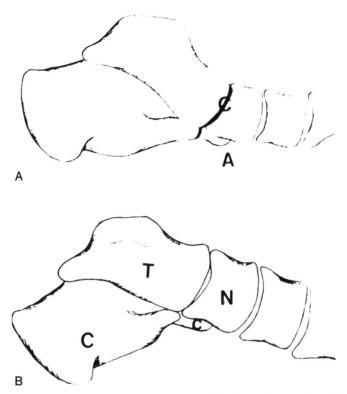

FIGURE 2-17. (A) Abnormal pronation of subtalar joint in weightbearing. Movement of the talus anterior to the calcaneus causes an anterior break in the Cyma (C) line.[6] (B) Normal subtalar joint in weightbearing. Cyma line (or midtarsal joint line) is "S" shaped.

an S, called the Cyma line. This anatomic line passes between the talus and the navicular bones and the cuboid and calcaneus (midtarsal joint line). Excessive pronation of the subtalar joint causes an anterior break in the Cyma line. The anterior movement of the talus that occurs during pronation of the subtalar joint may compensate for the lack of anterior movement of the tibia.

EXTRINSIC DEFORMITIES

Rotational deformities and leg length discrepancies are the two most common extrinsic abnormalities of the lower extremities causing compensatory pronation.

Rotational Deformities

The rotational deformities of the lower extremity can be divided into deformities of the thigh and the lower leg. Rotational deformities of the thigh include femoral anteversion, retroversion, antetorsion, and retrotorsion. The lower leg deformities include internal and external tibial torsion.

The limb buds orginate in a laterally rotated, abducted, and flexed position relative to the pelvis.[55] Early in development, the limb first rotates medially to bring the great toe to the medial side of the foot and to rotate the knee and leg into an anterior position.[55,56] The normal rotational process may be altered by genetic or environmental factors.[56]

Etiology. Considerable confusion exists in the literature regarding the terminology of rotational deformities of the thigh or femur. "Femoral version" and "torsion" are often used synonymously when discussing rotational deformities. Femoral torsion, also called the "angle of declination," is defined (for the purposes of this chapter) as a twist in the femur bone. Femoral version is defined as an altered relationship between the femoral head and neck and the acetabulum.[6] Femoral version may be caused by contractures of the soft tissue structures around the hip. The soft tissue contractures can be precipitated by intrauterine positioning of the lower extremity.[6,56] Malposition in the uterus is also the most common cause of torsional deformities of the femur and tibia.[56] Sitting and sleeping postures may perpetuate or delay resolution of femoral torsion or version deformities of the femur or tibia.[56,57] Rotational variations of the femur and tibia have a genetic factor. Evaluation of the parents rotational profiles can often predict a child's rotational variations.[56] The cause of excessive external tibial torsion can be iatrogenic.[56] The management of clubfoot deformities using long leg cases or Denis Brown splints may create a lateral rotational deformity of the tibia.

In summary, femoral torsion and version and tibial torsion may be caused by soft tissue deformities, malposition in the uterus, sitting postures, sleeping postures, and genetic and iatrogenic factors.

Rotational Deformities of the Thigh. The femoral antetorsion angle is used to describe the relationship of anterior rotation of the proximal head and neck of the femur to the condyles of the distal femur (Fig. 2-18).[56,58] If the femur were placed on the table top with the posterior aspect of the condyles in contact with the table, the head and neck of the femur would be elevated away from the table anteriorly. Therefore, the axis of the head and neck would form an angle with the transcondylar axis of the femur. The angle of declination, or anteversion, is 30°–40° at birth, and between 8°–15° in the adult.[6]

Excessive femoral anteversion or medial femoral torsion can produce an in-toeing gait.[6,56,58] Patients who have significant femoral anteversion or medial femoral torsion deformity will have hip internal rotation of 60°–90° and external rotation of less than 25°.[58] The foot progression angle can help to determine the degree of in-toeing or out-toeing during gait. The foot progression angle can be defined as the angle between the axis of the foot and the line of progression.[56] In-toeing is expressed as a negative value and out-toeing is a positive value. Normally the foot progression angle should be between +8° and +12°, or that of an out-toe foot position.[58] Excessive femoral retro-

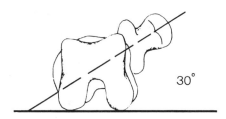

30°

Antetorsion

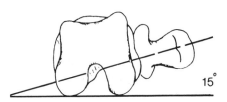

15°

FIGURE 2–18. Antetorsion of 30° (*top*) is abnormal; 15° is normal (*bottom*).

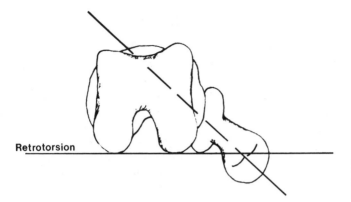

Retrotorsion

FIGURE 2–19. Retrotorsion is rare and can result in out-toeing.

version or lateral femoral torsion deformities are rare (Fig. 2-19).[58] These deformities would cause excessive out-toeing or a foot progression angle of +15° or more.

Clinically, to distinguish between hip anteversion and medial femoral torsion deformities, it is important to evaluate the range of motion of the hip in four positions. Test the patient in a supine posture, with the hip and knee extended; the knee flexed and hip extended; the hip flexed 90° and knees extended; and the hip and knee flexed. If the findings are consistent in all four positions, there is probably osseous torsion.[59] However, if there is an inconsistency in rotational values from one position to another, one must suspect soft tissue contractures. Roentgenographic procedures such as fluoroscopy, axial scans, and computed tomography (CT) are also used to determine the degree of femoral torsion deformities.[58]

Compensations throughout the lower extremity may occur if femoral anteversion or medial femoral torsion deformities persist beyond the age of four or five years.[58] In the case of femoral anteversion or medial femoral torsion, the child develops an awkward gait. Excessive compensatory external tibial torsion (greater than 22°) may develop to reduce clumsiness and occasional stumbling in the child with an excessive in-toe gait. Extreme external tibial torsion increases the stress to the medial aspect of the foot.[55] Increased medial force to the subtalar joint produces calcaneal valgus, plantar flexion, and adduction of the talus (abnormal compensatory pronation).[60] Abnormal foot pronation may precipitate patellar malalignment and knee pain. Furthermore, hip and buttock pain may result from strain to the external rotators in an attempt to walk straight.

Five to fifteen percent of femoral rotational deformities in children are not spontaneously corrected by skeletal maturity.[6,58] The child who continues to demonstrate excessive femoral torsion at the age of eight rarely demonstrates significant spontaneous torsion changes, even with conservative management.[58]

Rotational Deformities of the Lower Leg. Tibial torsion is the transverse plane abnormality that occurs in the lower leg. It results from the axial relationship of the foot to the thigh which is due to rotation or twisting of the tibia along its longitudinal axis.[56] "Malleolar torsion" is a term coined by Dr. Merton Root as the preferred term for tibial torsion.[28] Malleolar torsion presents as an excessive anterior or posterior displacement of the medial malleolus relative to the lateral malleolus. The normal adult external torsion angle is approximately 20° (Fig. 2-20).[61]

Internal tibial (malleolar) torsion is present when the angle of malleolar torsion is less than zero. Internal torsion deformity of the tibia is usually associated with congenital metatarsus adductus, clubfoot, and developmental genu varum (bow legs).[57] Hutter

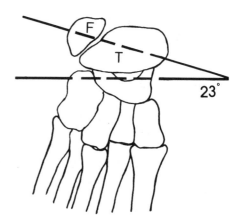

FIGURE 2-20. External torsion of the tibia (or external malleolar torsion) of 23° is within normal limits.

and Scott[61] advocate conservative treatment of internal tibial torsion deformities if they are still present at age three. Correction of tibial torsion is possible during the growth period by application of a night splint, which produces a rotational stress in a direction opposite to that of the deformity (Fig. 2-21). Spontaneous correction of torsion deformities after age 8 is rare. Internal tibial torsion is the most common cause of in-toeing.[56] Metatarsus adductus is also associated with internal tibial torsion and in-toeing.[6,56]

Abnormal external tibial torsion, as previously noted, is usually a result of a compensation for in-toeing. When external tibial torsion is greater than 20°, pronation at the subtalar joint is clinically evident.[28]

Leg Length Discrepancies

Most authors in the podiatric and osteopathic literature divide leg length discrepancies (LLD) into structural and functional leg length differences.[62-64] Structural LLDs are true anatomic differences in the length of the tibia or femur, or both. Functional LLDs are either the shortening or lengthening of a limb, secondary to joint contracture or muscle imbalances.[63]

Structural LLD may be caused by uneven development of the lower extremity in

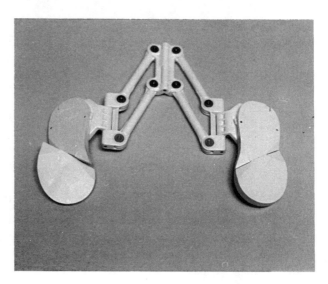

FIGURE 2-21. Derotation brace by Langer Biomechanics Group CRS Counter-rotation system (Langer Biomechanics Group, Deer Park, New York).

utero, fractures, epiphyseal irritation with lengthening, sacral or innominate deformity, or unilateral coxa vara.[65] Functional LLD may be secondary to a tight unilateral psoas muscle, unequal lumbar muscle spasms, hip fascia tightness, shortening or ligamentous laxity, or pronated feet.[65] Botte describes how muscle imbalances may produce a functional LLD.[62] Ipsilateral hip flexor tightness, secondary to muscle guarding or spasm, may cause ipsilateral limb shortening. In the case of the functional LLD, a change in position of the tight muscle may reduce the LLD. The clinician can safely assume that if an LLD is suspected, regardless of the cause, there is always an associated asymmetry to be found. At some point(s) between the head and the foot, the body will attempt to compensate for an unbalanced lower kinetic chain.

In relationship to the foot and ankle, the most important biomechanical compensation for leg length discrepancy is at the subtalar joint.[62-64] On the long–limb side, the subtalar joint pronates in an attempt to reduce the vertical height of the leg, while on the short–limb side the subtalar joint supinates in an attempt to increase the length of the leg (Figs. 2-22 and 2-23). The inclination angle of the calcaneus is increased in the supinated foot and decreased in the pronated foot (Fig. 2-24). Plantar flexion, adduc-

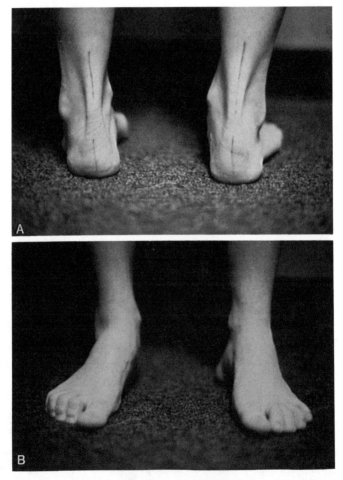

FIGURE 2–22. Posterior (A) and anterior (B) views of the foot in LLD. The right subtalar joint is pronated, reducing the length of the long leg. The left subtalar joint is supinated to increase the length of the short leg.

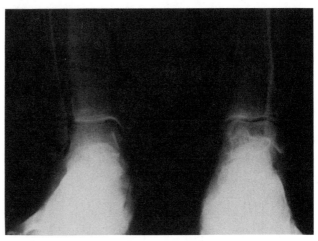

FIGURE 2–23. Anterior x-ray of patient in Figure 2–22. Note the tibia and fibula relationship. In the right ankles the tibia is internally rotated and the talus is adducted. In the left ankle, the tibia is externally rotated. The syndesmosis space is open and visible on the right, and reduced on the left.

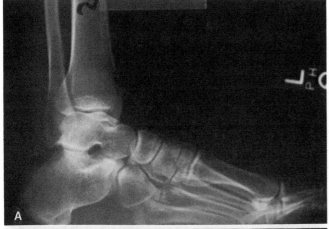

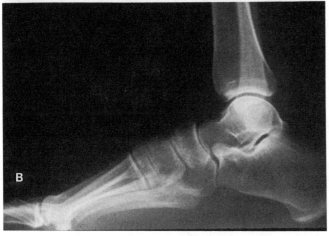

FIGURE 2–24. (*A*) Weight-bearing x-ray of the shorter foot in LLD. Note the increased inclination angle of the calcaneus on the supinated foot. (*B*) Weightbearing x-ray of the longer foot in LLD. Note the decreased inclination angle of the calcaneus on the pronated foot.

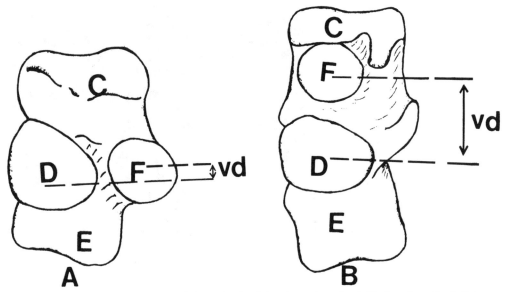

FIGURE 2–25. (A) Pronation of the subtalar joint (anterior view). Reduced vertical distance (vd) reduces the height of the rearfoot. (B) Supination of the subtalar joint (anterior view). Increased vertical distance (vd) increases the height of the rearfoot.

tion, and subsequent calcaneal eversion will actively shorten the long leg by reducing the vertical height of the subtalar and talocrural areas (Fig. 2-25). The subtalar joint on the contralateral lower extremity may reciprocally supinate, "thereby increasing the calcaneal inclination, in an effort to lengthen the shorter limb and balance the pelvis."[64]

These changes in the kinetic chain may not cause any problem for the sedentary individual, but an athlete or runner may suffer from the effects of an abnormal gait cycle. Blustian observed that the longer leg will maintain a prolonged stance phase. As the cadence increases, double support diminishes, subjecting the longer leg to greater stress for longer periods.[64] More complaints of pain and dysfunction are likely to be present on the side with the longer leg and pronated subtalar joint.

Compensations for an LLD do not follow consistent patterns, and the clinician should be aware of various patterns that may exist.[66] Accommodation to a short leg may have any of the following compensation patterns; pelvic tilt, sacral tilt, pelvic side shift, pelvic rotation, and lumbar scoliosis.[65]

Summary

Congenital or acquired abnormal pronation (Table 2-1) changes the alignment of the calcaneus, talus, cuboid, and navicular bones. The change in alignment produces poor articular congruity and alters the arthrokinematics of the ankle, subtalar, and midtarsal joints. The excessive arthrokinematic movements produce excessive forces within the foot and ankle, and throughout the lower kinetic chain. The tibia, talus, and calcaneus move simultaneously, as the foot pronates. The talus and tibia are rotated medially, and the calcaneus rolls laterally into eversion. In abnormal pronation the calcaneus has been described as subluxing under the talus. Such arthrokinematics are abnormal because they are excessive and persistent throughout the stance phase. Nor-

TABLE 2-1 Abnormal Pronation

I. *Congenital Abnormal Pronation*
  A. Rigid deformities
    1. Vertical talus–convex pes valgus
    2. Tarsal coalitions
    3. Rigid metatarsal deformity
  B. Flexible deformities
    1. Talipes calcaneo valgus
    2. Flexible metatarsal deformities
II. *Acquired Abnormal Pronation*
  A. Intrinsic deformities
    1. Traumatic
    2. Ligament laxity
    3. Bony abnormalities of subtalar joint
    4. Compensatory pronation for intrinsic deformities
      a. Compensated forefoot varus
      b. Partially compensated or uncompensated forefoot varus
      c. Forefoot supinatus
      d. Rearfoot varus
      e. Ankle joint equinus
  B. Extrinsic deformities
    1. Rotational deformities of the lower extremity
    2. Leg length discrepancy

---

mal pronation compensation is a temporary condition of the subtalar joint.[28] Normal compensation might occur in response to a change in the terrain.

Changes in the mechanics of the rearfoot and midfoot produce certain anatomic changes typical of flatfoot. These can be observed in the weightbearing, or (in severe cases) in the non-weightbearing, position. The changes include everted position of the calcaneus, medial bulging of the navicular tuberosity, abduction of the forefoot on the rearfoot, and a reduction in the height of the medial arch.[28,67] As a result of the excessive pronation, the soft tissue structures are traumatized over a long period of time, resulting in breakdown and pathology.

ABNORMAL SUPINATION

Abnormal supination is the inability of the foot to pronate effectively during the stance phase of gait. This is commonly referred to as the high-arched foot, or pes cavus. Abnormal supination is a hypomobility of the joints of the foot and ankle that may result from muscle imbalances and soft tissue contractures. Abnormal supination usually is associated with a rigid structure which is unable to function as an efficient shock absorber or an adapter to changing terrain. The abnormal supinator usually does not demonstrate a progressive breakdown in tissue (producing a hypermobile foot), such as occurs in the flexible, pronated foot. Rather it is an inflexible foot that causes tissue inflammation and possible joint destruction.

Terminology in the literature describing a high-arched foot is confusing. A pure pes cavus deformity is plantar flexion of the forefoot on the rearfoot.[5,6,15] The pes cavus deformity is usually associated with other deformities of the rearfoot and forefoot. For example, the calcaneus can be in a varus position, in which case the deformity is referred to as "pes cavovarus." The calcaneus can be in equinus or in plantar flexion thus described as "pes equinocavus." Finally, the calcaneus can be in a dorsiflexed, position, which is referred to as "calcaneocavus." In all pes cavus deformities the forefoot is either completely or partially in plantar flexion. Pes cavovarus is plantar flexion of the medial column or first ray. In the standing position the rearfoot moves into varus to compensate for the forefoot.

Therefore, pes cavus describes deformities of the forefoot and rearfoot in the sagittal and/or frontal plane. Some of the terms used to describe pes cavus include bolt foot, clubfoot, talipes plantaris, hollow foot, contracted foot, and nondeforming clubfoot.[15]

Classification of Pes Cavus

Earlier studies labelled this high-arched foot "hollow claw foot."[68,69] Steindler,[69] clinically described three important aspects of the pes cavus foot: increased height of the longitudinal arch, dropping of the anterior arch with plantar flexion of the forefoot, and some amount of dorsal retraction of the toes, or claw toes (hyperextension of the metatarsophalangeal and flexion of the interphalangeal joints).[69] He reported an interdependency of the toe deformity and the increased height of the medial arch.

Samilson and Dillin classified the pes cavus foot according to the apex of the longitudinal arch.[70] Anterior or forefoot cavus has its apex at the metatarsocuneiform joints. Midfoot cavus has its apex between the metatarsocuneiform joints and the anterior tuberosity of the calcaneus. Hindfoot cavus is characterized by increased vertical height of the calcaneus of 30° or more.[70] The vertical height is measured by the calcaneal pitch (or inclination angle of the calcaneus) on weightbearing roentgenograms of the foot. The angle is formed by the horizontal line and a line along the plantar aspect of the calcaneus from posterior to anterior calcaneal tuberosity (Fig. 2-26).[5,6,70]

McGlamry and Kitting[71] report plantar flexion of the forefoot on the rearfoot or the apex of the cavus at the tarsometatarsal and the midtarsal joints; however, they call these deformities metatarsal equinus and forefoot equinus, respectively.

McCrea classifies cavus deformities into several categories. Anterior cavus manifests plantar flexion of the forefoot on the rearfoot, occurring at the tarsometatarsal or the midtarsal joint.[6] The second major classification is posterior cavus, which causes changes at the subtalar joint. Posterior cavus also causes an increase in the inclination angle of the calcaneus. The third and most frequent type is a combination of the posterior and anterior cavus, referred to as the global type.[6]

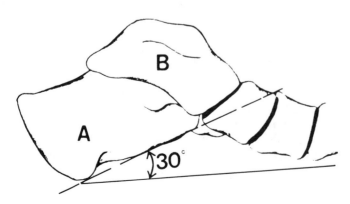

FIGURE 2-26. Inclination angle of the calcaneus is 30°. A, Talus; B, calcaneus.

In simple pes cavus, the plantar flexion deformity of the forefoot is equal on the medial and lateral columns. Therefore, weightbearing is evenly distributed over the first and fifth rays. The heel is usually in neutral position, allowing for equal distribution of weight in the rearfoot. The pes cavus foot is often associated with other deformities, such as equinus and varus.

Combined Pes Cavus Deformities

Tachdjian delineates three combined deformities, pes cavovarus, -calcaneocavus, and -equinocavus.[5] The combined deformities describe forefoot and rearfoot changes in the pes cavus foot.

PES CAVOVARUS (FOREFOOT VALGUS, RIGID PLANTAR FLEXED FIRST RAY)

Pes cavovarus is plantar flexion of the medial column or first ray (first metatarsal, first cuneiform). The position of the first ray is equinus or fixed plantar flexion. Passive testing of the first ray with the patient in the non-weightbearing prone position demonstrates limited movement of the first metatarsocuneiform joint into dorsiflexion.[5,72] Because of the interconnection of the first and second metatarsal bones by the transverse metatarsal ligament, plantar flexion of the second ray is also present.[15,73] Mobility of the plantar flexed second ray is restricted to dorsiflexion to a lesser degree. Observation of the fifth ray demonstrates normal mobility and a neutral position.[5] This "stair-stepped" position of the metatarsals, from plantar flexion of the first ray to neutral position of the fifth, is clinically the same as the description of forefoot valgus given by Root and coworkers.[28] Forefoot valgus is defined as eversion of the forefoot on the rearfoot with the subtalar joint in neutral position (Fig. 2-27). As previously noted, DiGiovanni and Smith[47] do not acknowledge forefoot deformities in the frontal plane,

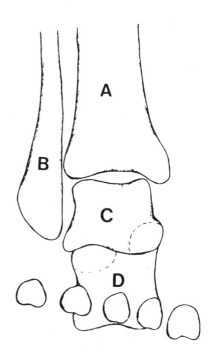

FIGURE 2–27. Uncompensated forefoot valgus. Eversion of the forefoot on the rearfoot with the subtalar joint held in neutral. A, tibia; B, fibula; C, talus; D, calcaneus.

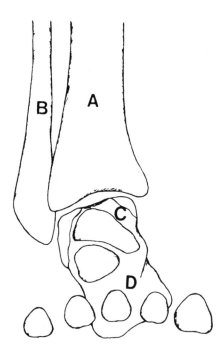

FIGURE 2–28. Compensated forefoot valgus. Inversion of the rearfoot. A, tibia; B, fibula; C, talus; D, calcaneus.

such as forefoot varus or valgus. Rather, they attribute these clinical findings to a sagittal plane deformity of the first ray moving into dorsiflexion and plantar flexion, respectively.

In either case, forefoot valgus or a fixed plantar flexed first ray must be compensated for during the stance phase of gait. In a normal foot, the forefoot strikes the ground directly after heel strike. However, with a fixed plantar flexed first ray, the first metatarsal strikes the ground first. Rapid supination of the subtalar joint occurs, immediately shifting the weight laterally (and onto) the fifth metatarsal head (Fig. 2-28).[5,28] As a result of this compensated supination, the foot does not return to pronation during the stance phase of gait. The lack of pronation reduces the ability of the foot to absorb shock and adapt to changing terrain, causing ankle instability. As the rearfoot inverts or supinates, the cuboid pulley becomes a strong lever for the peroneus longus muscle (see Fig. 2-15). The muscle now has a mechanical advantage exerting a strong plantar flexion force on the first ray.[28] The deformity may become progressively worse, and soft tissue changes may cause an increased rigidity. Therefore, the rearfoot varus may perpetuate and, in some cases, precipitate forefoot valgus.

Another type of pes cavovarus deformity is flexible forefoot valgus. In this condition the foot is very unstable and develops significant forefoot symptomatology.[74] Rearfoot compensation is unnecessary. Flexible forefoot valgus does not promote the locking of the forefoot against the rearfoot, and thus produces an instability in push-off.[75] The valgus position of the forefoot (plantar flexed first ray) can be observed in the non-weightbearing position.

CALCANEOCAVUS

Calcaneocavus deformity describes a dorsiflexion (calcaneus) position of the rearfoot with the forefoot fixed in equinus (plantar flexion).[5] In the weightbearing position, the subtalar joint does not need to compensate for intrinsic deformities. The rearfoot is usually in neutral, or in a position perpendicular to the ground. Calcaneocavus deformity is almost always the result of a neurologic disorder and subsequent weakness or paralysis of the gastrocnemius and soleus muscle groups.[76]

PES EQUINOCAVUS

Pes equinocavus, the third type of pes cavus deformity described by Tachdjian, is an equinus position of the forefoot, hindfoot, and ankle joint. Tachdjian reports that pes equinocavus is secondary to talipes equinovarus or clubfoot.[5]

Etiology of Pes Cavus Deformities

The etiology of pes cavus can be divided into three causes: neurologic, contracture of soft tissue structures, and idiopathic.[77-86] The most clinical and scientifically documented article describing the etiology of pes cavus was presented in 1963 by Brewerton, Sandfier, and Sweetnam.[77] They reported evidence of central nervous system disorders in 66% of 77 patients followed in a pes cavus clinic over a five-year period. The neurologic disorders included Friedrich's ataxia, peroneal muscular atrophy, poliomyelitis, spina bifida, cerebral palsy, spinal cord tumors, myelodysplasia, spastic paraplegia, and spastic monoplegia.[77]

Causes of pes cavus that are appropriate for physical therapy treatment includes muscle imbalances, and weakness of the intrinsic and/or extrinsic muscle groups of the foot and ankle. Several common muscle groups implicated in the mechanism producing pes cavus are:

1. Weakness of the dorsiflexors of the foot and ankle (anterior tibialis and extensor digitorum muscles), resulting in dropping of the forefoot, which causes contracture of the plantar fascia and shortening of the gastrocnemius and soleus muscle groups.[77,80,82]
2. Unopposed activity of the supinators of the foot, producing a plantar flexed, adducted, and inverted foot position that allows rapid contracture of the plantar fasciae.[77,80] Weakness of the peroneal muscles produces overactivity of the posterior tibialis and anterior tibialis, the antagonist muscle groups.
3. Overactivity of the peroneus longus muscle, producing plantar flexion of the first ray and forefoot pronation. The fixed plantar flexion of the first ray must be compensated by subtalar joint supination or inversion of the calcaneus.[6,28,80]
4. Overactivity of the abductor hallucis, flexor digitorum brevis, flexor hallucis brevis, and quadratus plantae has been described as a deforming factor in pes cavus. Garceau and Brahms denervated these muscle groups in 47 cases of pes cavus.[81] Their goal was to stop the progressive increase of pes cavus. The results demonstrated improvement in foot balance, performance, and stability, reducing the pes cavus deformity.
5. Weakness of the gastrocnemius-soleus muscle group, producing a dorsiflexed calcaneus. This weakness may produce a calcaneocavus deformity.[76,77,80] Brockway reports an elongation of the Achilles tendon, with no evidence of weakness in the calcaneocavus deformities.[85]

Contractures of the skin, subtarsal ligaments, and the plantar fascia are common in the pes cavus foot.[80,83] The plantar fascia is a strong support to the longitudinal arch and is designed to prevent excessive calcaneal eversion (valgus).[34,80] The deforming force of the plantar fascia (inversion of the calcaneus) is resisted by the Achilles tendon. Once the calcaneus moves into inversion secondary to supination of the subtalar joint, the Achilles tendon becomes an active supinator of the subtalar joint and perpetuates the deformity.[80]

Congenital Talipes Equinovarus (Clubfoot)

Congenital talipes equinovarus is usually a rigid deformity.[5] The clubfoot deformity does not resemble a typical pes cavus foot, although it has several similar characteristics. Three distinctive clinical observations in clubfoot are inversion (varus) of the hindfoot (heel), inversion and adduction of the forefoot, and equinus of the ankle and subtalar joint.[6] The varus heel position and the equinus (plantar flexed) ankle are also found with the pes cavus foot type. As previously noted, Tachdjian reports pes equinocavus secondary to talipes equinovarus.[5]

The exact cause of the clubfoot deformity is unknown. Genetic factors have been implicated by several studies.[5,87,88] Palmar[89] examined four possible inheritance factors: sex-linked, autosomal-recessive, multiple gene inheritance, and autosomal-dominance. Palmar determined that if there was a family history of the talipes equinovarus deformity, a 10% chance of a recurrence existed.[88]

In addition to the genetic factors, environmental factors may be operational.[5,89] The mechanical theory, or environmental factor, was first advanced by Hippocrates, who proposed that the fetal foot was malpositioned in the uterus, and that the equinovarus posture was produced by external forces. As a result of rapid growth in malposition, the ligaments and muscles developed adaptive shortening, and the tarsal bones, especially the talus, responded by changing contour, producing articular malalignment.[5] More recently, a popular explanation for clubfoot involves pressure of the uterine wall increased by the fetus' kicking against it.[89]

The third causal factor in talipes equinovarus is neuromuscular dysfunction— peroneal nerve lesions, peroneal dysplasia, arthrogryposis, or myelomeningocele.[5,90,91]

BONY DEFORMITIES

The talus is the principal bone affected in talipes equinovarus. The anterior end of the talus is medial and there is plantar deviation.[5,89–94] The long axis of the head and neck of the talus forms an angle with the long axis of the body, called the "declination angle" of the talus.[5] The normal angle in the adult is 150° to 160°. In talipes equinovarus the angle is decreased from 135° to 115°, representing medial and plantar deviation of the head and neck of the talus.[5] Figure 2-29 demonstrates a normal adult declination angle and an abnormal angle characteristic of a clubfoot deformity. The navicular is displaced mediad and plantad, articulating with the medial aspect of the head and neck of the talus. In severe cases, the navicular bone articulates with the medial malleolus of the tibia.[5]

The contour of the calcaneus is normal. In order to maintain its articulation with the talus, it must rotate on its long axis inward and downward beneath the talus.[5] The calcaneocuboid articulation is anterior, medial, and plantar deviated, further accentuating the varus deformity.

Soft tissue changes occur as a result of the bone malalignment. The ligaments, capsules, muscles, tendons, tendon sheaths, vessels, and skin are shortened on the medial and posterior aspects of the foot.[5]

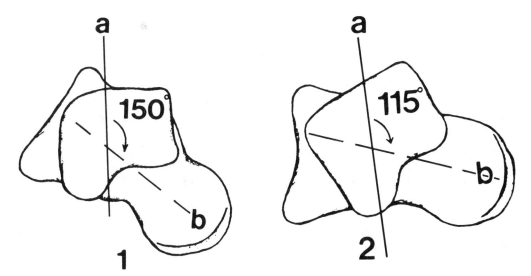

FIGURE 2–29. (1) Long axis of the body of talus, with normal declination angle of the talus from 150° to 160°. (2) Long axis of the head and neck of the talus, with abnormal declination angle of the talus from 115° to 135°. Reduction of the declination angle of the talus is present in the clubfoot deformity.

Summary

Pes cavus is a rigid deformity. It may include several combinations of deformities, such as equinus, varus, adductus, and calcaneus (Table 2-2). Pes cavus can be the result of neurologic disease, muscle imbalance, or contracture of soft tissues.

The biomechanics of the foot in pes cavus are the reverse of those in pes planus. The abnormally supinated foot does not act as an effective shock absorber. The rearfoot is prone to instabilities, secondary to compensatory supination of the subtalar joint, as noted in pes cavovarus or forefoot valgus deformities. A varus heel can be a primary deformity, as described in talipes equinovarus. The primary calcaneal varus deformity can produce ankle instability and precepitate plantar flexion of the first ray or forefoot valgus.

TABLE 2–2 Abnormal Supination

I. Pes cavus
    A. Anterior cavus
    B. Posterior cavus
    C. Global
II. Combined pes cavus deformities
    A. Pes cavovarus-forefoot valgus-rigid plantar flexed first ray
    B. Calcaneocavus
    C. Pes equinocavus
III. Congenital talipes equinovarus (clubfoot)

CONCLUSION

The foot is an important link in the lower kinetic chain. Abnormal pronation (flatfoot) and abnormal supination (high-arched foot, pes cavus) may produce alterations in the arthrokinematics of the foot and ankle.

Congenital abnormal pronation includes deformities present at birth that produce severe alteration between the talus, calcaneus, navicular, and cuboid articulations. Convex pes valgus, tarsal coalitions, and talipes calcaneovalgus are the most common. Abnormal pronation, however, is usually an acquired deformity resulting from an attempt to compensate for deformities intrinsic and/or extrinsic to the foot and ankle. Foot deformities are described in relationship to the body planes. The most common frontal plane deformities resulting in compensatory abnormal pronation are forefoot varus, rearfoot varus, and metatarsus varus. The most common sagittal plane deformity causing abnormal pronation is ankle equinus. The transverse plane deformities resulting in compensatory pronation include rotational deformities of the lower extremity and metatarsus adductus.

Abnormal supination is usually a rigid deformity in which the foot lacks shock absorption capabilities. Pes cavus, plantar flexion of the forefoot on the rearfoot, may be combined with other deformities, such as varus and adductus. Pes cavovarus, hypomobile plantar flexion of the first ray, and forefoot valgus are terms that describe a combined deformity of pes cavus that involves plantar flexion and hypomobility of the first ray (sagittal plane deformity and compensatory rearfoot varus (frontal plane deformity). Although a hypermobile plantar flexed first ray is described as forefoot valgus, it is usually an attempt to compensate for forefoot varus. Calcaneocavus and pes equinocavus are also combined pes cavus deformities. Calcaneocavus is pes cavus with a dorsiflexed calcaneus. Pes equinocavus describes a plantar flexed calcaneus and ankle joint. Both deformities are combined with plantar flexion of the forefoot.

The causes of pes cavus that lend themselves to physical therapy are muscle imbalance and soft tissue contractures. The muscle hyperactivity usually results from neurologic disorders which may be present at birth or may develop as the child matures.

Abnormal foot and ankle mechanics resulting from abnormal pronation or supination deformities may cause increased weightbearing forces throughout the lower kinetic chain. The inability to attenuate the increased stress may result in soft tissue breakdown and damage.

GLOSSARY

Positions of the Foot

Abductus: Abducted position or a fixed deformity in the transverse plane
Adductus: Adducted position or a fixed deformity in the transverse plane
Calcaneus: Dorsiflexed position or a fixed deformity in the sagittal plane
Equinus: Plantar flexed position or a fixed deformity in the sagittal plane
Valgus: Everted position or a fixed deformity in the frontal plane
Varus: Inverted position or a fixed deformity in the frontal plane

Deformities of the Foot

Ankle joint equinus: Limited dorsiflexion of the ankle joint with subtalar joint in neutral position

Calcaneocavus: Dorsiflexed position of the os calcis

Convex pes valgus: Congenital vertical talus, or rocker bottom foot

Forefoot valgus: Eversion of the forefoot on the rearfoot with subtalar joint in neutral position

Forefoot varus: Inversion of the forefoot on the rearfoot with subtalar joint in neutral position

Hallux abductovalgus: Subluxation in the transverse plane of the first metatarsophalangeal joint

Hallux limitus: Subluxation of the first metatarsophalangeal joint in the sagittal plane

Hallux rigidus: The latter stage of hallux limitus, leading to ankylosis of the first metatarsophalangeal joint

Metatarsus adductovarus: Adduction and inversion of the forefoot

Metatarsus adductus: Adduction of the forefoot

Metatarsus varus: Inversion of the forefoot

Pes cavovarus: Plantar flexion of the first ray, or medial column

Pes cavus: Plantar flexion of the forefoot on the rearfoot

Pes equinocavus: Plantar flexion of the forefoot, rearfoot, and ankle joint

Tailor's bunion: Subluxation in the transverse plane of the fifth MTP joint with the toe in varus position.

Talipes calcaneovalgus: Congenital flatfoot, dorsiflexion and eversion of hindfoot

Talipes equinovarus: Clubfoot—inversion and plantar flexion of hindfoot and adduction of forefoot

Tarsal coalition: Congenital union between two or more tarsal bones

References

1. Rose, GK: Correction of the pronated foot. J Bone Joint Surg 44B:642, 1982.
2. Lelievre, J: Current concepts and correction in the valgus foot. Clin Orthop 70:43, 1970.
3. Evans D, Cardiff, and Wales: Calcaneo-valgus deformity. J Bone Joint Surg 57B:270, 1975.
4. Purnell ML, et al: Congenital dislocation of the peroneal tendous in calcaneovalgus foot. J Bone Joint Surg 65B:316, 1983.
5. Tachdjian, MO: The Child's Foot. WB Saunders, Philadelphia, 1985.
6. McCrea, JD: Pediatric Orthopaedics of the Lower Extremity. Futura Publishing, New York, 1985.
7. Thomas, CL (ed): Taber's Cyclopedic Medical Dictionary, ed 16. FA Davis, Philadelphia, 1989.
8. Drennan, JC, et al: The pathological anatomy of convex pes valgus. J Bone Joint Surg 53B:445, 1971.
9. Herdon, CH and Heyman, CH: Problems in the recognition and treatment of congenital convex pes valgus. J Bone Joint Surg 45A:413, 1963.
10. Coleman, SS, et al: Pathomechanics and treatment of congenital vertical talus. Clin Orthop 70:62, 1970.
11. DeRosa, PG: Congenital vertical talus: The Riley experience. Foot Ankle 5:118, 1984.
12. Jayakumar, S and Cowell, HR: rigid flatfoot. Clin Orthop 122:77, 1977.
13. Stormont, DM and Peterson, HA: The relative incidence of tarsal coalition. Clin Orthop 181:24, 1983.
14. Cowell, HR and Elener, V: Rigid painful flatfoot secondary to tarsal coalition. Clin Orthop 177:54, 1983.
15. Jahss, MH: Disorders of the Foot, Vol 1. WB Saunders, Philadelphia, 1982.
16. Turek, SL: Orthopaedics: Principles and Their Application. JB Lippincott, Philadelphia, 1977.
17. Herzenberg, JE et al: Computerized tomography of talocalcaneal tarsal coalition: A clinical and anatomic study. Foot and Ankle 6:273, 1986.
18. Boyd, HB: Congenital talonavicular synostosis. J Bone Joint Surg 26A:682, 1944.
19. Challis, J: Hereditary transmission of talonavicular coalition in association with anomaly of the little finger. J Bone Joint Surg 56A:1273, 1974.
20. Kite, JH: Congenital metatarsus varus. J Bone Joint Surg 332A:500, 1950.
21. Kite, JH: Congenital metatarsus varus. J Bone Joint Surg 49A:388, 1967.
22. Heyman, CH, et al: Mobilization of the tarsometatarsal and intermetatarsal joints for the correction of resistance adduction of the forepart of the foot in congenital clubfoot or congenital metatarsus varus. J Bone Joint Surg 40A:299, 1958.
23. Giannestras, NJ: Recognition and treatment of flatfeet in infancy. Clin Orthop 70:10, 1970.
24. Ferciot, CF: Calcaneovalgus foot in the newborn and its relation to developmental flatfoot. Clin Orthop 1:22, 1953.
25. Kolker, LD: A biomechanical analysis of flatfoot surgery. J Am Podiatr Med Assoc 63:217, 1973.

26. Bleck, EE and Berzins, UJ: Conservative management of pes valgus with plantar flexed talus flexible. Clin Orthop 122:85, 1977.
27. Barry, RJ and Scranton, PC: Flat feet in children. Clin Orthop 181:68, 1983.
28. Root, ML, Orien, WP, and Weed, JN: Clinical Biomechanics, Vol 2, Normal and Abnormal Function of the Foot. Clinical Biomechanics, Los Angeles, 1977.
29. Mereday, C, Dolan, C, and Lusskin, R: Evaluation of the University of California Biomechanics Laboratory shoe insert in "flexible" pes planus. Clin Orthop 82:45, 1972.
30. Gould, N: Evaluation of hyperpronation and pes planus in adults. Clin Orthop 181:37, 1983.
31. Johnson, KA: Tibial posterior tendon rupture. Clin Orthop 177:140, 1983.
32. Funk, DA, Cass, JC, and Johnson, JA: Acquired adult flatfoot secondary to posterior tibial-tendon pathology. J Bone Joint Surg 68A:95, 1986.
33. Basmajian, JV and Stecko, O: The role of muscles in arch support of the foot: An electromyographic study. J Bone Joint Surg 45A:1184, 1963.
34. Hicks, JH: The mechanics of the foot. II. The plantar aponeurosis. J Anat 88:25, 1954.
35. Hicks, JH: The mechanics of the foot. IV. The action of muscles on the foot in standing. Acta Anat 27:180, 1955.
36. Jones, BS: Flatfoot: A preliminary report of an operation for severe cases. J Bone Joint Surg 57B:279, 1975.
37. Harris, RL and Beath, T: Hypermobile flatfoot with short tendo Achilles. J Bone Joint Surg 30A:116, 1948.
38. Inman, VT, Rolston, HJ, and Todd, F: Human Walking. Williams & Wilkins, Baltimore, 1981.
39. Green, RD: Planal dominance. J Am Podiatr Med Assoc 74:98, 1984.
40. Bordelon, RL: Hypermobile flatfoot in children: Comprehension, evaluation, and treatment. Clin Orthop 181:7, 1983.
41. Duckworth, T: The hindfoot and its relation to rotational deformities of the forefoot. Clin Orthop 177:39, 1983.
42. Taunton, JE, et al: A triplanar electrogoniometer investigation of running mechanics in runners with compensatory overpronation. Can J Appl Sports Sci 10:104, 1985.
43. Perkins, G: Pes planus or instability of the longitudinal arch. Proc Roy Soc Med 41:31, 1847.
44. Hughes, LY: Biomechanical analysis of the foot and ankle for predisposition to developing stress fractures. J Orthop Sports Phys Ther 7:96, 1985.
45. Vetter, LW, Helfet, DL, et al: Aerobic dance injuries. Phys Sports Med 13:114, 1985.
46. Micheal, R and Holder, L: The soleus syndrome: A cause of medial tibial stress (shin splints). Am J Sports Med 13:87, 1985.
47. DiGiovanni, JE and Smith, SD: Normal biomechanics of the adult rearfoot. J Am Podiatr Med Assoc 66:812, 1976.
48. Phillips, RD and Phillips, RL: Quantitative analysis of the locking position of the midtarsal joint. J Am Podiatr Med Assoc 73:518, 1983.
49. Subotnick, S: Biomechanics of the subtalar and midtarsal joints. J Am Podiatr Med Assoc 49:756, 1975.
50. Subotnick, SI: Equinus deformity as it affects the forefoot. J Am Podiatr Med Assoc 61:423, 1971.
51. Melilla, TV: Gastrocnemius equinus: Its diagnosis and treatment. Arch Podiatr Med Foot Surg 2:159, 1975.
52. Anopol, G: Mechanics in weak and flat feet. Am J Surg 7:256, 1929.
53. Bordelon, LR: Hypermobile flatfoot in children. Clin Orthop 181:7, 1981.
54. Sgarlato, TE: Compendium of Podiatric Biomechanics. California College of Podiatric Medicine, San Francisco, 1971.
55. Sarrafian, SK: Anatomy of the Foot and Ankle: Descriptive, Topographic, Functional. JB Lippincott, Philadelphia, 1983.
56. Staehli, LT: Rotational problems of the lower extremities. Orthop Clin North Am 18:503, 1987.
57. Knight, RA: Developmental deformities of the lower extremities. J Bone Joint Surg 36A:521, 1954.
58. Bleck, EE: Developmental orthopaedics III: Toddlers. Develop Med Child Neurol 24:533, 1982.
59. Mittleman, G: Transverse plane abnormalities of the lower extremities: Intoe and outtoe gait. J Am Podiatr Med Assoc 61:1, 1971.
60. James, SL: Chondromalacia of the patella in the adolescent. In Kennedy (ed): The Injured Adolescent Knee. Williams & Wilkins, Baltimore, 1979.
61. Hutter, CG and Scott, W: Tibial torsion. J Bone Joint Surg 31A:511, 1949.
62. Botte, RR: An interpretation of the pronation syndrome and foot types of patients with low back pain. J Am Podiatr Med Assoc 72:595, 1982.
63. Okun, SJ, Morgan, JW, and Burns, MJ: Limb length discrepancy: A new method of measurement and its clinical significance. J Am Podiatr Med Assoc 72:595, 1982.
64. Blustein, SM and D'Amico, JC: Leg length discrepancy: Identification, clinical signs, and management. J Am Podiatr Assoc 75:200, 1985.
65. Beal, MC: The short leg problem. J Am Osteopath Assoc 76:745, 1977.
66. Subotnick, S: Case history of unilateral short leg with athletic overuse injury. J Am Podiatr Med Assoc 70:255, 1980.
67. Anderson, AFA and Fowler, SB: Anterior calcaneal osteotomy for symptomatic juvenile pes planus. Foot Ankle 4:274, 1984.
68. Jones, RA: Discussion of the treatment of pes cavus, section orthopaedics. Proc Roy Soc Med 20:1126, 1927.

69. Steindler, A: The treatment of pes cavus (hollow claw foot). Arch Surg 11:325, 1921.
70. Samilson, RL and Dillin, W: Cavus, Cavovarus, calcaneocavus: An update. Clin Orthop 177:133, 1983.
71. McGlamry, DE and Kitting, RW: Equinus foot, an analysis of the etiology, pathology, and treatment techniques. J Am Podiatr Med Assoc 63:165, 1973.
72. Root, ML, Orien, WP, and Weed, JH: Biomechanical Examination of the Foot, Vol 1. Clinical Biomechanics, Los Angles, 1971.
73. Bossely, CL and Cairney, PC: The intermetatarsophalangeal bursa: Its significance in Morton's metatarsalgia. J Bone Joint Surg 62A:184, 1980.
74. Schoenhaus, HD and Jay, RM: Cavus deformities: Conservative management. J Am Podiatr Med Assoc 70:235, 1980.
75. Green, DR, Sgarlato, TE, and Wittenburg, M: Clinical biomechanical evaluation of the foot. J Am Podiatr Med Assoc 65:732, 1975.
76. Bradley, GW and Coleman, SS: Treatment of the calcaneocavus foot deformity. J Bone Joint Surg 63A:1159, 1981.
77. Brewerton, DA, Sandifer, PH, and Sweetnam, DR: "Idiopathic" pes cavus. Br Med J 2:659, 1963.
78. Todd, AH: Treatment of pes cavus. Proc Roy Soc Med 28:117, 1934.
79. Cole, WH: The treatment of claw-foot. J Bone Joint Surg 22:895, 1940.
80. Dwyer, FC: The present status of the problem of pes cavus. Clin Orthop 106:254, 1975.
81. Garceau, GJ and Brahms, MA: A preliminary study of selective plantarmuscle denervation for pes cavus. J Bone Joint Surg 38A:553, 1956.
82. Hughes, KW: Talipes cavus. Br Med J 2:902, 1940.
83. Rugh, TJ: The plantar fascia: Study of its anatomy and of its pathology in talipes cavus: New operation for its correction. Am J Surg 2:307, 1927.
84. Barenfeld, PA, Wedely, MS, and Shea, JM: The congenital cavus foot. Clin Orthop 79:119, 1971.
85. Brockway, A: Surgical correction of talipes cavus deformities. J Bone Joint Surg 22:81, 1940.
86. Jahss, MH: Evaluation of the cavus foot for orthopedic treatment. Clin Orthop 181:52, 1983.
87. Preston, ET and Fell, WT: Congenital idiopathic clubfoot. Clin Orthop 122:102, 1977.
88. Palmar, RM: The genetics of talipes equinovarus. J Bone Joint Surg 46A:542, 1964.
89. Irani, RN and Sherman, MS: The pathological anatomy of clubfoot. J Bone Joint Surg 45A:45, 1963.
90. Kaplan, EB: Comparative anatomy of the talus in relation to idiopathic clubfoot. Clin Orthop 85:32, 1972.
91. Ponseti, IV and Smoley, EN: Congenital club foot: The results of treatment. J Bone Joint Surg 45A:261, 1963.
92. Ghali, NN, et al: The results of plantar reduction in the management of congenital talipes equinovarus. J Bone Joint Surg 65A:1, 1983.
93. Lovell, WW and Hancock, CI: Treatment of congenital talipes equinovarus. Clin Orthop 70:79, 1970.
94. Kite, JH: Conservative treatment of the resistant recurrent clubfoot. Clin Orthop 70:93, 1970.

CHAPTER 3

Normal Development of Gait

Deborah Corradi-Scalise, MA, PT
Wen Ling, PhD, PT

Independent ambulation is the highest form of human locomotion. As clinicians, we are constantly evaluating both the potential for, and the quality of, ambulation. In order to evaluate and treat pathologic gait patterns, it is first necessary to understand the normal development of gait and its components.

Walking (or normal gait) is not an independent occurrence. It is rather, the ultimate product of a series of developmental changes that begin at birth. Since a typical adult walking pattern does not become evident until age seven,[1-3] one cannot expect the usual components of adult walking to be clinically present before that age. Therefore descriptions of the gait characteristics of normal children at various ages are presented here as a basis for the effective treatment of children in similar age groups with pathologic gait patterns (Figs. 3–1 to 3–3).

Typically, independent standing occurs at 9½ months and at about 13 months,[4] the child is able to utilize independent walking as a primary means of locomotion. The gait pattern utilized is an immature (or toddler) form of walking. Initially, the toddler maintains a wide base of support, excessive hip and knee flexion as seen during wide-range stepping movements, ankle joint pronation, toe curling, and upper extremity abduction with elbow flexion.[2,5] Progression is in a waddling manner, shifting the weight from side to side, rather than stepping forward. Within several months maturational changes have already begun to take place. The child now ambulates with a more narrow base of support, better balance, and forward progression using a rhythmic heel-toe pattern with reciprocal arm swing. A mature form of walking eventually develops. The attainment of independent ambulation by the child is the culmination of many complex musculoskeletal and neurophysiologic maturational changes that have been occurring since the neonatal period.

Internal factors that affect maturation of the central nervous system include the completion of central nervous system myelinization by age two, and the rapid rate of body and brain growth during the first three years. The musculoskeletal system undergoes dramatic changes during the first year of life. The reflexive neonate transforms into a purposeful, independent walker within a 13 to 15 month period.[4] Muscular control

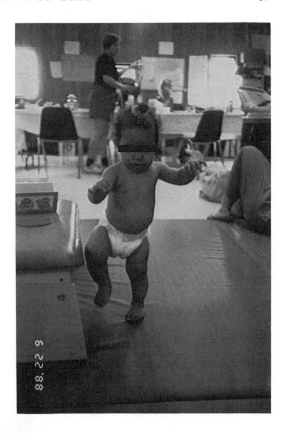

FIGURE 3–1. Toddler gait of a typical 11-month-old. Child began independent ambulation two weeks prior to photograph.

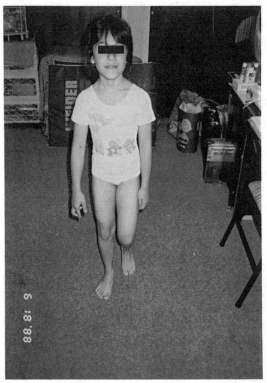

FIGURE 3–2. Mature gait of a typical eight-year-old.

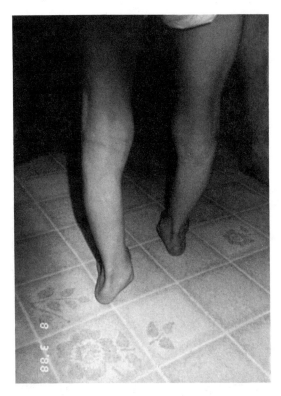

FIGURE 3–3. Pathological gait pattern of a 4-year-old with cerebral palsy.

develops in a cephalocaudad, proximodistal direction. Many other factors influence the development of a mature gait, including sensation, perception, motivation, and proprioception. As the neuromuscular and musculoskeletal systems develop, motor changes occur in response to environmental needs. The change and variability within the environment require adaptation (and therefore, maturation) of the human system. The series of events that change the immature form of walking to the rhythmic heel-toe progression of the adult depend primarily on three developmental processes within the child: the changes that reflect central nervous system maturation; the progression of motor learning; and the increase in physical growth and control of the musculoskeletal apparatus.

COMPONENTS OF GAIT DEVELOPMENT

Neurophysiologic Component

During the first 15 months of life, many changes take place in the nervous and musculoskeletal systems that allow for purposeful, independent walking. These systems develop concurrently and are responsible for the development of a mature gait pattern by the age of seven years.[1–3]

As postulated by Bobath,[6] the maturation of the central nervous system is a reflection of the integration of primitive reflexes by higher cortical structures. At birth, the neonate displays a host of reflexive movements in response to sensory stimuli. These reflexes directly related to standing and walking are the neonatal placing response of the lower extremity, the positive supporting reflex, and the spontaneous stepping reflex. Movement is therefore said to be a sensorimotor experience. These three reflexes serve as the motor pattern for standing and walking, but are modified by the hierarchical control of the central nervous system. The modification of primitive reflexes occurs via the development of the righting and equilibrium reactions. According to Bobath, these reactions are the basis of all functional movements:

> "Willed movements are only partly voluntary as they are based and supported by automatic movements and tonal changes. Normal postural reactions are the background of all human basic motor patterns that children acquire during the first 3 years of life. The automatic changes in posture are represented through the normal postural reflex mechanism (NPRM). The NPRM consists of 2 types of automatic reactions, the righting and the equilibrium reactions. Both types develop in a definite sequence of events, however the righting reactions are active from birth onwards. The more complex equilibrium reactions appear around the 6th month, overlapping with the former. The equilibrium reactions and the child's volitional activities serve to modify the pattern of the righting reactions which become partially inhibited, or disappear altogether between 3–5 years of age."[7]

The righting reactions allow humans to stand erect. They are responsible for maintaining the head and trunk in proper spatial alignment in relation to the ground, with the eyes horizontal. Their major function is to overcome the effects of gravity by moving and stabilizing body parts toward the upright position. Righting reactions are what drive the baby to move, and to eventually maintain an upright posture.[8] The delayed achievement of independent standing and walking in the blind child is a direct result of the absence of the optical righting reaction. As reported by Adelson and Fraiberg,[9] the achievement of gross motor milestones by blind infants was delayed beyond the normal range. They state that blindness has less of an impact on postural achievements than it does on mobility achievements. The average age for standing alone is 11 months for a blind child as compared with 9.5 months for a sighted child.[4] The average age for independent ambulation is 19.25 months for a blind child compared with 13 months for a sighted child.[4]

The equilibrium reactions, in addition, serve to keep the body's center of gravity balanced within the base of support. In children, during initial independent standing and walking, the base of support is very wide. Biomechanically, this allows for stability where muscular and neuromuscular control is lacking. As the body compensates for inefficient muscle activity, the body also increases its energy consumption. As the equilibrium system of the child matures, the walking base narrows and upright balance is preserved. Functional ambulation can be viewed as the body's ability to maintain an upright position and to respond to a series of rises and drops in the center of gravity by utilization of the righting and equilibrium reactions.[10] The precise use of the righting and equilibrium reactions to catch and balance the center of gravity during forward progression allows a minimum expenditure of energy, and therefore an efficient, mature walking pattern.

Children with cerebral palsy display a less than mature gait pattern, due to disturbances in righting and equilibrium. Without central nervous system dysfunction, the ankle-foot complex naturally responds to a posterior displacement of the center of gravity with ankle dorsiflexion and toe extension. A lateral displacement of the center of gravity elicits ankle inversion. Typically, the foot of a child with cerebral palsy serves as a stable, fixed support, but is inefficient for balancing.[11] Gunsolus et al[11] evaluated the dynamic foot responses of 50 children, 20 normal subjects and 30 subjects with cerebral palsy. In the normal group, they found that some beginning walkers used toe clawing in response to posterior displacement, but that more than half used medial arch reactions. Advanced walkers demonstrated mature dynamic foot responses. The children with cerebral palsy were more similar to the normal, beginning walkers, as none of the subjects utilized dorsiflexion during posterior displacement. Additionally, however, none of the dysfunctional subjects utilized medial arch reactions in response to a lateral displacement. These findings demonstrate the need for efficient equilibrium reactions in order for the development of mature standing and walking to occur.

Motor Learning Component

Righting reactions allow man to be upright, and equilibrium reactions maintain balance and control in the upright posture of bipeds. The initiation of gait can be attributed to the central nervous system's generation of a motor program. Motor programs are "stored sets of motor commands both innate and learned that are synthesized into a desired movement."[12] Of the many theories on motor control, two help to explain the initiation of movement: they are the closed-loop theory and the open-loop theory of motor control.

The closed-loop theory of motor control is based on the system's ability to learn and perform skilled movements via peripheral feedback. The sensorimotor feedback loop is responsible for modifications or adaptations of the motor program. Stelmach[13] states that this theory is supported by the research of Mott and Sherrington. The researchers completely eliminated afferent pathways to the limbs of monkeys in an attempt to examine the role of sensation in movement. The destruction of the afferent pathways produced a limb that was essentially paralyzed. Functional grasp was lost, thus emphasizes the importance of an intact sensory system for movement.

The open-loop theory emphasizes a central control mechanism that continuously monitors the peripheral feedback and determines both the spatial and temporal components of a movement. When the desired performance is achieved, an internal model is established, probably in the neocerebellum, and the feedforward mechanism becomes the dominating force in performing the movement; however, when new stimuli are encountered (e.g., performing the movement in a novel environment such as walking on uneven terrain) both feedback and feedforward mechanisms are important components in performing the movement.[13] Initially, a change in motor control occurs via a response to peripheral feedback; however, "once the peripheral mechanisms are adjusted for, and stored, the system may allow for adjustments in advance of the movement by incorporating the peripheral effects into the motor plan. The central nervous system can then act to correct errors even before they become expressed through the motor act."[14] This allows for the automation seen in a mature walking pattern.

In physical therapy, after central nervous system insult with subsequent disruption of the ability to walk, the goal of treatment is functional ambulation. Various physical therapy activities and exercises are utilized to regain motor control, including gait training in health care facilities. These indoor activities are insufficient to allow the individual to regain functional ambulation. Practice for walking should include real-world environments such as a crowded city street, supermarket, or train station. Due to the variability between environments, problem solving must occur to develop the appropriate motor programs necessary for successful walking within different settings. Motor learning occurs in response to a specific need or desire for a skill. Peripheral feedback is necessary, and ongoing problem solving and adjustment must be made to adapt to the variability of each task within different environments. Only with repetition can the variability in the environment be anticipated. And it is only by repetition in a variable and functional environment (streets, escalators, train stations) that we can hope to enable patients to problem solve (and thus modify) the motor program to adapt to variable situations and to function independently.

Brooks[15] has described the neurobehavioral analysis of motor skill learning by stating that intended motor acts are based on perceptions of what is to be done at a particular time, based on sensory information both past and present. The environmental demands placed on the individual motivate the motor act, but it is the combination of cognitive abilities that guide and execute the musculoskeletal system's response. This theory may explain, in part, why mentally retarded children and adults without primary physical disabilities tend to be awkward or clumsy, and tend to display a less than normal pattern of ambulation. Although motor acts (such as walking) are attempted, the cognitive portion of the brain which drives the musculoskeletal system may not be able to acknowledge the most efficient movement pattern for the task. We may see less than optimal balance in walking due to the inability to activate an efficient motor program.

Biomechanical Component

Initially, the acquisition of independent standing and walking is characterized by inefficient, exaggerated postures and positions that provide stability within the system. "The neural structures that act to control movement must be adapted to the constraints imposed by the structure of the musculoskeletal system (flexibility of muscles) and the physical laws governing movement (gravity, friction)."[16] Therefore, due to the biomechanical alignment of the infant's lower extremities (anterior pelvic tilt, hip flexion, abduction, and external rotation) and to the structure of the infant's body (short legs, high center of gravity), initial ambulation occurs in a "staccato" manner. The motor program is working within the constraints of the physical structure of the toddler (Fig. 3–4). In order to ambulate at all, the motor program must adapt to the physical structure of the child.

As the child's physical structure matures, mechanical and kinesiologic changes occur within the muscles and joints, with a subsequent lowering of the body's center of gravity (Fig. 3–5). Thus in the more physically mature child, the functional purpose of the motor task remains the same, but the means of attaining the goal changes to a more precise execution, in relation to the body structure. For the infant to progress to independent standing and walking, the musculoskeletal system must possess enough strength and dynamic control to move against the external forces, especially gravity.

Maturation of the musculoskeletal system is an important determinant of the development of a typical adult gait pattern. The soft tissue limitations imposed by the anterior pelvic tilt and hip flexion (seen in a toddler) must resolve, upon maturation, to allow for the appropriate proximal and distal joint alignment and muscular function.

Physiologically, the neonate displays increased flexion of all joints with a relatively high center of gravity located "at the base of the lower level of the thoracic spine."[17] The wide base of structural support maintained by lower extremity flexion, abduction, and external rotation in the infant allows for the stability upon which movement can be initiated. The development of control and movement occurs in a cephalocaudal direction. Head control develops first, followed by trunk control, hip control, and finally leg and foot control. The stabilization pattern of the lower extremities (into hip flexion, abduction, and external rotation) appears initially in all developmental patterns. In the neonate, this posture is primarily due to the intrauterine position and to a physiologic

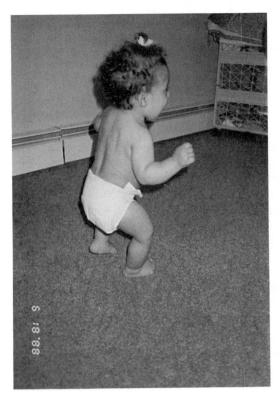

FIGURE 3–4. Sagittal alignment characteristics of toddler. Note arm posturing, anterior pelvic tilt, wide base of support and ankle plantar flexion at toe strike.

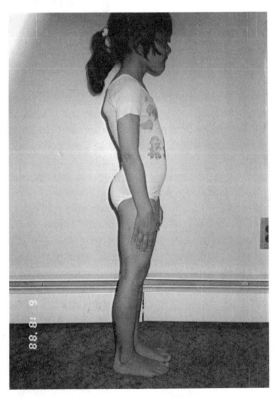

FIGURE 3–5. Typical standing alignment of an eight-year-old child, sagittal view.

increase in flexor tonus. The lower extremity characteristics of the neonate are a 2:1 ratio of external to internal rotation of the hip range of motion, coxa valga of approximately 150°, and the femoral condylar axis facing outward to about 30° to 40°.[18] Once the infant begins to gain control of the musculoskeletal apparatus, the base of support gradually narrows and is replaced by dynamic muscular control.

Initially during independent standing and walking, the child displays limited ability to combine different muscle actions at various joints. Basically, movements are in the "all or none" range, with wide range steps and little availability of various degrees of freedom of combined joint movements. Rather than smooth reciprocal muscle action, much cocontraction is seen around the joints, for stability.[19] The wide base of support for positional stability is exemplified in initial walking. Characteristically, to compensate for a high center of gravity in standing, the toddler widens the base of support so that the center of gravity remains within the base of support, as wide range stepping occurs in conjunction with inefficient pelvic control and coordination. This allows the infant to remain erect and mobile. As the child grows and the physical structure changes, there is a decrease in the anterior pelvic tilt and subsequent hip flexion. The trunk becomes straighter and the lower extremities grow longer. We therefore see a lowering of the center of gravity (Figs. 3–6 and 3–7). The wide range lower extremity propulsive movements become smoother and are now counterbalanced by eccentric muscle contractions, which act to decelerate the body against gravity. Specifically, the foot drop of the one-year-old child disappears as the ankle dorsiflexors develop eccentric muscle control in order to lower the foot to the ground prior to midstance. Graded knee control develops during midstance as the hip moves over the supporting foot with the gastroc-

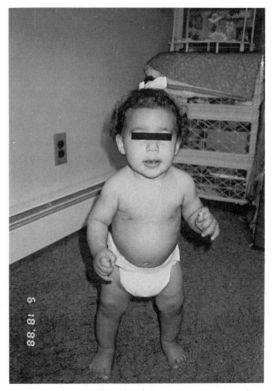

FIGURE 3–6. Typical standing posture of a toddler, frontal view.

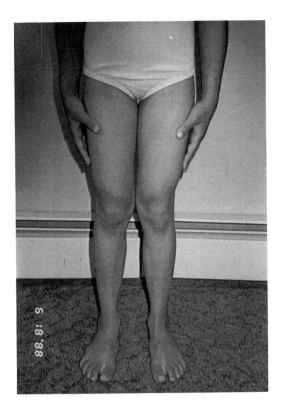

FIGURE 3-7. Typical standing alignment of an eight-year-old, frontal view.

soleus muscle group impeding (decelerating) the forward movement of the tibia over the supporting foot.

The importance of musculoskeletal maturation in the development of mature gait was reported by Sutherland et al[20] in 1980. The gait patterns of 186 normal children between the ages of one and seven years were analyzed utilizing high speed movies, a digitizer, a computer, and electromyograms (EMGs). The results indicate that subjects less than two years old have greater knee flexion and ankle dorsiflexion during the stance phase, and that their knee flexion wave (stance phase knee flexion after foot strike, and subsequent knee extension prior to toe off) is diminished. Sutherland observed that, as the child matures, cadence decreases, while walking velocity and step length increases. Important factors in the development of a mature pattern of these determinants are increasing limb length and greater limb stability, manifested by the longer duration of single-limb stance.

The increase in muscle strength and dynamic muscle control allows the infant to move in and out of a variety of postures. Muscles experience full elongation, concentric contractions, and eccentric contractions in supported positions (such as prone and supine) before the child attempts them while sitting or standing.

"Walking is initiated by inclining the body forward and placing it ahead of its center of gravity. To regain balance, one leg must be brought forward ahead of the shifting center of gravity. Man attempts to minimize the forces that tend to impede effortless motion by attempting to keep his center of gravity on a straight horizontal line during walking."[21] Inman[22] discussed the six determinants of gait that are utilized by the adult to minimize the vertical displacement of the center of gravity during walking. Pelvic rotation forward and backward minimizes the drop in the center of gravity during heel strike. Pelvic tilt laterally minimizes the excessive rise of the center of gravity by dropping the pelvis about 5° during midstance. Knee flexion and the concurrent foot and ankle movement each aid in minimizing the excessive rise and fall of the center of gravity by lengthening and shortening the leg during the stance phase of gait. Lateral motion of the pelvis, which causes the relative adduction of the femur, also aids in minimizing the excessive rise of the center of gravity.

Children gradually learn through muscle functioning to efficiently control the center of gravity. Biomechanical alignment in standing and walking varies with age.

GAIT CHARACTERISTICS BY AGE

The work of Sutherland[2,20] details following the gait characteristics of children.

The one-year-old independent walker is unable to efficiently control the displacement of the center of gravity due to immature musculoskeletal alignment and functioning. Characteristically, the pelvis is tilted anteriorly with a subsequent increase in lumbar lordosis; the base of support is wide; and the upper and lower extremities are flexed, abducted, and externally rotated. During walking the one-year-old child displays increased knee and ankle flexion in stance, footflat, mild foot-drop, decreased duration of single limb stance with the stance leg supporting the body, and the swing leg accelerating the body by rotating the hips. Knee flexion is present during stance, and ankle plantar flexion occurs at foot strike. During the swing phase, there is increased hip flexion, abduction, and external rotation. Hip external rotation is present throughout the entire gait cycle. The typical cadence is rapid (180 steps/minute), step length is short a (20 cm), and walking velocity is slow (60 cm/sec). The duration of single limb stance is 32% of the gait cycle.

The two-year-old child characteristically displays a decrease in hip abduction, external rotation, and pelvic tilt. The knee moves into flexion after foot strike, and then begins to extend before toe-off. Heel strike is present upon initial contact, and during swing ankle dorsiflexion is evident. Reciprocal arm swing is present, as well as a heel-toe gait pattern. At age two, the child's cadence has decreased, and step length and walking velocity have both increased.

By the age of three, the child displays an adult pattern of joint rotation and has achieved an adult pattern of walking, with the exception of a decreased step length and abnormally high cadence. In comparison to a three-year-old child, a seven-year-old child has a decreased cadence, increased walking velocity, and the duration of single limb stance has increased to 38% of the gait cycle (which is close to that of adult at 39%).

To review, the gait characteristics of neophyte walkers are immature, as evidenced by the wide base of support in response to a high center of gravity. As the child develops, the walking velocity and step length increase, as the cadence decreases. It has been postulated by Sutherland[20] that "step length increases in a linear manner with leg length." As the child's leg length increases, so does the child's height. As height is increased, the center of gravity lowers, eventually eliminating the need for wide base of support seen in the younger child. In combination with more controlled muscle function this results in the maturation of the gait cycle.

When the physical structure is less than optimal, as in cerebral palsy, mature gait is sacrificed. The child with cerebral palsy who has spastic hamstring muscles (and subsequent limitation of active knee extension) will display a shortened step length. Tightness and shortening of the Achilles tendon will elicit either toe-walking, foot-flat gait with

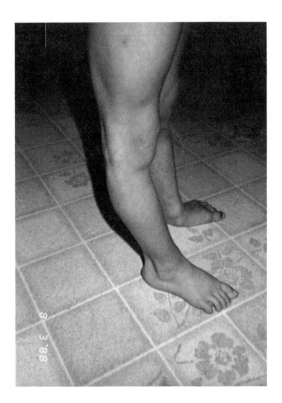

FIGURE 3–8. Pathological gait, four-year-old child, sagittal view. Note knee hyperextension, ankle pronation, plantar flexion, and eversion.

calcaneal eversion, or toe-heel gait (Fig. 3–8). Strotzky[23] in 1983 documented the gait patterns of 39 normal and 6 cerebral palsied children, using high speed cinematography. She found that all of the cerebral palsied children walked more slowly than the normal children. She concluded that the slower gait was due to restricted stride length rather than to decreased cadence. The child with cerebral palsy cannot activate the proper motor program for ambulation due to alignment problems and poor righting and equilibrium reactions.

RESEARCH

There is much controversy in current literature regarding the age at which children display a mature gait pattern similar to normal adults (Table 3–1). This is primarily due to the investigation by researchers of different characteristics of the gait cycle utilizing many methods of gait analysis. Sutherland and associates[20] suggest that a mature gait pattern is well established by age three with only minor changes occurring between ages three and seven. They identified five important determinants of a mature gait pattern: duration of single-limb stance, walking velocity, cadence, step length, and the ratio of pelvic to ankle spread. These characteristics were analyzed throughout the walking cycle using high-speed movies, a Graf-Pen sonic digitizer, a computer and a plotter, as well as electromyograms. Burnett and Johnson[24] state that mature gait (described by heel strike and synchronous arm movements) is constant 22 weeks after the beginning of independent walking, as observed through film analysis. Hip flexion at midstance and a mature foot and knee mechanism appeared within 40 to 55 weeks following the

TABLE 3-1 Age of Acquisition of Mature Gait

Author(s)	Date of Publication	Gait Parameter(s) Studied	Age of Gait Maturation
Okamoto and Kumamoto[1]	1972	Phasic muscle activity	7 years
Berger et al[3]	1984	Phasic muscle activity Knee and ankle joint angles	6-7 years
Sutherland et al[20]	1980	Walking velocity Cadence Step length Duration of single limb stance Ratio of pelvic to ankle spread	3 years
Burnett & Johnson[24]	1971	Heel strike Flexion at midstance Mature foot and knee mechanism	40-50 weeks after the initiation of independent ambulation
Norlin et al[26]	1981	Velocity Stride length Cadence	8-10 years
Corradi-Scalise & Ling[25]	1987	Phasic muscle activity	At least by 8-10 years

initiation of independent gait. Okamoto and Kumamoto[1] studied the learning process of walking and the process of ambulation as it developed with age, utilizing electromyography, foot switches, and observational records. They conclude that by the end of the second year, the arm swing, push-off motion of the foot, and decrease of forward body sway (which are found in the adult) could be recognized. From this point, the ambulation began to lose the characteristics of infant walking and began to acquire adult walking patterns. The adult walking form was nearly accomplished by seven years of age. Corradi-Scalise and Ling[25] described the gait characteristics of eight to ten-year-old children by analyzing phasic muscle activity via EMG telemetry and ground reaction forces on the sole of the foot. They concluded that children ages eight to ten years clearly display a typical gait pattern similar to that of adults. In addition, Norlin, Odennik, and Sandlund[26] studied the gait patterns of 230 children with the use of foot switches. The parameters studied were velocity, stride length, cadence, and the temporal phases of the stride, as well as leg length of the subjects. Their results stated that the gait characteristics change with age and that the changes are most pronounced up to eight to ten years. Thereafter, only minor changes take place, and leg length becomes the dominant factor. Such discrepancies lead to difficulty in assessing and comparing gait in childhood. In order to make relevant comparisons between pathologic gait and normal gait, it is necessary to know more about the development of gait in childhood.

The literature reports that many changes occur within the gait pattern between the inception of walking and age three. After that, only minor changes occur in refinement of movement and in the characteristics of step length, cadence, and walking velocity, which seem to be somewhat dependent on leg length. The consensus in the literature seems to be that by age seven[1-3] a mature gait pattern has developed that is similar to the adult pattern.

A definitive statement regarding the maturation of gait in childhood is imperative if relevant comparisons between pathologic gait and normal gait are to be made. If children in the age range of eight to ten years display a mature gait pattern, then their gait studies can be compared to adult studies of normal gait. If the gait patterns of children younger than eight years old vary with age, then children ages one through seven should be compared to children their own age. This is an important concept when children with pathologic gait or developmental delays, or both, are to be compared with the gait of normal children.

NORMAL VERSUS TYPICAL

Throughout the literature on gait analysis, "normal" joint angles and biomechanical alignments are given. It is important to remember, however, that normal alignment may not, in fact, be typical of the alignment seen in the population. Although there are accepted alignment characteristics of adult walking, because of the innate variability of human beings, typical alignment characteristics should be documented as well as optimal alignment or normal patterns. The quality of walking that achieves the goal of bipedal locomotion can vary widely. Terms such as normal, optimal, and typical must be defined clearly and applied consistently in order to accurately identify and qualify pathology (Figs. 3-9 to 3-11).

We examined 20 normal, healthy eight- to ten-year-old children to determine whether children in that age range display a gait pattern similar to that of adults. A lower extremity examination was performed on each child. Of the 20 children, only 25% displayed no musculoskeletal abnormalities, 50% displayed subtalar joint pronation on weightbearing, 40% displayed genu valgum (either unilateral or bilateral) and 10% displayed genu recurvatum. This clearly adds controversy to the term "normal" as it is applied to the musculoskeletal system of children in this age group. Although 75% of these children did not display "normal" biomechanical alignment, all are considered normal children. Based on comparison with normal walking patterns, 75% never achieved a biomechanically mature gait pattern. Although all these children are functional walkers, and to the untrained eye possess "normal" ambulation patterns, clinically it is useful to describe these typical gait characteristics and to apply them to clients who have so-called pathologic gait.

Typically, in the literature, gait studies have focused on alignment and phasic muscle activities, two very important characteristics of gait. Our study attempted to address the maturation of gait in children utilizing these parameters and through

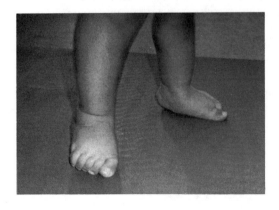

FIGURE 3-9. Subtalar joint pronation upon weight bearing, observed in an 11 month old child, as a reflection of immaturity.

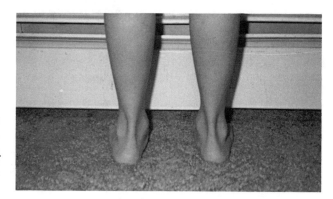

FIGURE 3-10. Ankle joint pronation upon weightbearing, noted in a typical eight-year-old. This typifies the variability of biomechanical alignment in normal children.

theories of motor learning.

Motor control is dependent on central nervous system maturation and musculoskeletal development. The parameter most suited to address maturation of the human gait pattern is muscle activity. Mature gait can be described through the characteristics of phasic muscle activity corresponding to designated phases of the gait cycle, namely stance, swing, and double stance. We studied 20 normal, healthy children, 11 boys and 9 girls in the eight to ten-year age range. A developmental questionnaire was administered to the parents concerning birth history, developmental history, and pertinent medical and surgical history. The short form of the Bruininks-Oseretsky Test of Motor Proficiency (American Guidance Service, Circle Pines, MN 55014) was administered to each child to ensure developmental normalcy. A descriptive study was conducted to analyze phasic muscle activity about the ankle joint and the ground reaction forces on the sole of the foot. An eight channel electromyography telemetry unit (EMG) was utilized to measure phasic muscle activity about the ankle joint. The muscle groups utilized were the ankle dorsiflexors (including the tibialis anterior), extensor digitorum longus, peroneus tertius, extensor hallucis longus, and the ankle plantar flexors (including the gastrocnemius, soleus, flexor hallucis longus, peroneus longus, tibialis posterior, flexor digitorum longus, and peroneus brevis muscles). An electrodynography system (The Langer Biomechanics Group, 21 East Industry Ct, Deer Park, NY 11729) was interfaced with the EMG for the data collection on double stance, stance, and swing phases of gait.

The results of the study indicated that children in the eight- to ten-year age range

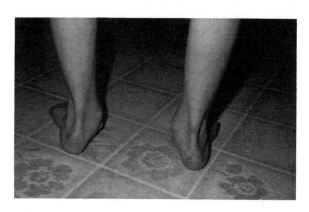

FIGURE 3-11. Severe ankle joint pronation upon weightbearing in a four-year-old child with cerebral palsy.

did display a mature gait pattern similar to that of adults. The skilled coordination of muscle groups about the ankle joint, necessary to perform both the mobility phase of gait (swing) and the stability phases of gait (stance and double stance) were evident. During the stance phase of gait, the left lower extremity demonstrated greater firing of the ankle plantar flexors compared to the ankle dorsiflexors. "The inhibition of one set of muscles, while opposing muscles are in excitation, is a condition for effective movement."[27] The right lower extremity in stance demonstrated no variability between firing of the ankle plantar flexors and dorsiflexors, demonstrating cocontraction. Co-contraction is a more primitive pattern than skilled muscle movement. The left lower extremity was therefore more skilled than the right for the stance phase of gait.

During the swing phase of gait, the reverse was observed. The right lower extremity demonstrated reciprocal inhibition, and the left lower extremity demonstrated co-contraction of agonist and antagonist. The right lower extremity was therefore more skilled during the swing phase of gait than the left.

Analysis of the above findings is of great interest. The screening evaluation of the short form of the Bruininks-Oseretsky Test of Motor Proficiency revealed 90% of the subjects to be right-dominant, as determined by preference of throwing and kicking a ball. The conclusion that can be drawn is that the subjects possessed greater coordination and skill of the right versus the left extremities. This statement in itself is misleading. In 95% of the subjects, during the activity of kicking a ball, which is similar to the swing phase of gait, the right lower extremity performed the mobility activity of kicking the ball, while the left lower extremity performed the stabilizing activity of weightbearing to support the body. These results are consistent with the functions of the lower extremities during gait. The left leg displayed greater skill during the stance phase (skill in weightbearing) and the right leg displayed more skill during the swing phase of gait (skill in kicking). Although the subjects were termed right-footed, foot dominance can be further classified as that lower extremity best coordinated for the specific activity by describing the mobility and stability characteristics of the task.

During double stance, there was no variability between agonist and antagonist of either leg. Co-contraction occurred bilaterally. The balance of muscle activity around the ankle joint provides the stable base seen in the double stance phase of gait.

The results of this study demonstrate that children in the eight to ten-year age range display a mature gait pattern similar to that of adults. The skilled coordination of muscle groups about the ankle joint necessary to efficiently perform both stance and swing phases of gait was observed. Right versus left preference of the lower extremities has also been established in this age group.

The results of our study indicate that children in the age range of eight to ten years display a mature gait pattern. In analyzing this information, the authors conclude that the motor program specific for ambulation was intact in all 20 subjects. Specifically, the differences obtained between skill of right and left lower extremities, regarding efficiency of mobility and stability tasks were evident. This pre-programming of specificity within the leg movements allows intended movements to be performed efficiently with each leg being pre-programmed for specific functions.

SUMMARY

Many factors influence the development of gait in children. The maturation of the neuromuscular system provides the posture and balance necessary to walk. The development of learning and problem solving provides the motivation for the initiation of gait. The maturation of the physical structure of the bones and muscles allows for the optimal interaction of the body with the outside environment, including the force of gravity.

Initially, the gait pattern of the beginning walker is characterized by a wide base of support, anterior pelvic tilt, hip flexion, external rotation and abduction, wide-range stepping movements, ankle joint pronation, toe curling, and upper extremity abduction with elbow flexion. With central nervous system and musculoskeletal maturation, the motor program innate to humans is activated efficiently for functional ambulation. If there is a deficit in biomechanical alignment, postural control, or motor control, the motor program specific for efficient ambulation is not expressed and the pattern of walking is less than typical.

Typical adult gait usually develops by age seven. However, in a certain percentage of the population, mature gait patterns of biomechanical alignment never develop. Therefore, although functional ambulation exists in this population, a normal gait pattern is never really achieved as determined by optimal or normal standards.

REFERENCES

1. Okamoto, T and Kumamoto, M: Electromyographic study of the learning process of walking in infants. Electromyogr Clin Neurophysiol 12:149, 1972.
2. Sutherland, DH: Gait disorders in childhood and adolescence. Williams & Wilkins, Baltimore, 1984, p 10.
3. Berger, W, Altenmueller, E and Dietz, V: Normal and impaired development of children's gait. Human Neurobiol 3:163, 1984.
4. Furno, H et al: Help Checklist. VORT Corporation, Palo Alto, CA, 1984.
5. McGraw, MB: Neuromuscular development of the human infant as exemplified in the achievment of erect locomotion. J Pediatr 17:747, 1940.
6. Bobath, B: Abnormal Postural Reflex Activity Caused by Brain Lesions, ed 3. Rockville, MD, Aspen, 1985, pp 1, 54.
7. Alon, Z: Unpublished material, 1986.
8. Adelson, E and Fraiberg, S: Gross motor development in infants blind from birth. Child Dev 45:114, 1974.
9. Plack, M: Personal Communication, May, 1984.
10. Gunsolus, P, Welsh, C, and Houser, C: Equilibrium reactions in the feet of children with spastic cerebral palsy and normal children. Dev Med Child Neurol 17:580, 1975.
12. Stelmach, GE (ed): Motor Control Issues and Trends. Academic Press, New York, 1976, p 202.
13. Stelmach, GE (ed): Motor Control Issues and Trends. Academic Press, New York, 1976, pp 2-3.
14. Carr, JH, et al: Movement Science Foundations for Physical Therapy in Rehabilitation. Rockville, MD, Aspen, 1987, p 131.
15. Brooks, VB: Brain functions in motor skill learning. Conference on the Neurobehavioral Analysis of Motor Skill Learning. Teacher's College, Columbia University, New York, November 1987.
16. Carr, JH, et al: Movement Science Foundations for Physical Therapy in Rehabilitation. Rockville, MD, Aspen, 1987, p 25.
17. Palmer, CE: Studies of the center of gravity in the human body. Child Dev 15:99, 1944.
18. Resseque, B: Personal communication, Dec, 1984.
19. Carr, JH, et al: Movement Science Foundations for Physical Therapy in Rehabilitation. Rockville, MD, Aspen, 1987, pp 93-154.
20. Sutherland, DH, et al: The development of mature gait. J Bone Joint Surg 62A:336, 1980.
21. Cailliet, R: Foot and Ankle Pain. Philadelphia, FA Davis, 1968, p 45.
22. Inman, VT, Ralston, HJ, and Todd, F: Human Walking. In Lieberman, JC (ed): Human Walking. Williams & Wilkins, Baltimore, 1981, pp 1-28.
23. Strotzky, K: Gait analysis in cerebral palsied and nonhandicapped children. Arch Phys Med Rehabil 64:291, 1983.
24. Burnett, CN and Johnson, EW: Development of gait in childhood. Dev Med Child Neurol 13:207, 1971.
25. Corradi-Scalise, D and Ling, W: Gait patterns of normal school-aged children. Unpublished material.
26. Norlin, R, Odenrick, P, and Sandlund, B: Development of gait in the normal child. J Pediatr Orthop 1:261, 1981.
27. Payton, OD, Hirt, S, and Newton, RA: Scientific Basis for Neurophysiologic Approaches to Therapeutic Exercise: An Anthology. FA Davis, Philadelphia, 1978, p 105.

Biomechanical Evaluation

CHAPTER 4

Clinical Assessment of the Foot

R. Luke Bordelon, MD

INTRODUCTION

This chapter addresses assessment of the foot from a clinical standpoint. It will deal with the foot as a functional unit. The importance of the foot as a functional unit is obvious when one realizes that its function is what has allowed man to walk upright on two feet. [1-5] Laitman and Jaffe observe that the three things that distinguish man from other primates are the cerebral cortex, the vocal cords, and the lower extremity and foot.[3] As clinicians we need to understand that the foot is a special organ.

During the early part of the stance phase, the foot is supple enough to allow adaptation to the contour of the ground and to maintain balance. During the latter part of stance phase, it converts to a rigid lever for push-off (Fig. 4-1). This motion is obligatory during the gait cycle, being initiated by changes in position of the talocalcaneal and the midtarsal joints of the foot, but it is not dependent on muscle action. Rather, changes in the position of the foot occurring during the gait cycle dictate this motion. Support of the foot and conversion of the foot from a supple to a rigid structure for push-off are dependent on the axes of motion of the joints of the foot and ankle, the shapes of bones, and the tension of the ligaments. When theses structures are normal, the foot supports the body and allows bipedal gait with conversion of the foot from the supple to the rigid position at a proper time during the gait cycle.[2,7-9]

THE NORMAL FOOT

The normal foot is defined as one that is supple during the early stance phase and converts to a rigid lever during push-off, in accordance with the obligatory motions of unrestrained gait.[2,7-9] The foot functions in two modes. The first is nonweightbearing, during which the muscles of the foot move it freely in space. The second is the weightbearing mode, when the foot is fixed to the floor by the ground reaction and the

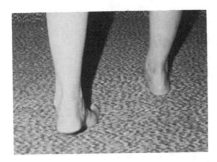

FIGURE 4–1. Demonstration of the changes that occur in the foot during the act of walking. The foot everts to become supple during the early part of stance phase in order to adapt to the ground (as shown by the right foot), and converts to a rigid lever for push-off by the end of stance phase (as shown by the left foot).

body moves over the foot.[5,20] To understand the function of the foot, one must understand the normal components of the foot and their motions. This section discusses the clinical evaluation of the foot in both the nonweightbearing and weightbearing modes.

Clinical Evaluation: Nonweightbearing

The foot examination is performed initially with the foot bearing no weight (Fig. 4-2). The neutral position of the subtalar joint is identified as the position in which the talus and the navicular are congruous, and it is the midpoint of function of the talonavicular joint.[5,10,11] The neutral position is identified by palpating the talonavicular and moving the loaded foot into adduction and inversion and abduction and eversion while applying ample pressure against the fourth and fifth metatarsal bones (Fig. 4-3). The point at which the talus and the navicular bones are congruous is the midpoint of function of the foot, or the neutral position.[2,5,7,8,10,11]

All examinations and measurements of the foot and ankle are performed with the neutral position as the initial reference point (Table 4-1). The foot components are examined first in passive motion, then in active motion.

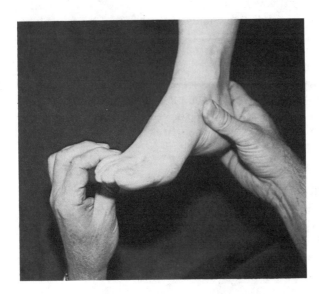

FIGURE 4–2. Examination of placement of the foot in the neutral position by palpating the talonavicular joint with the right thumb and grasping the fourth and fifth metatarsal heads to load and move the foot to ascertain the mid point of function of the talonavicular joint.

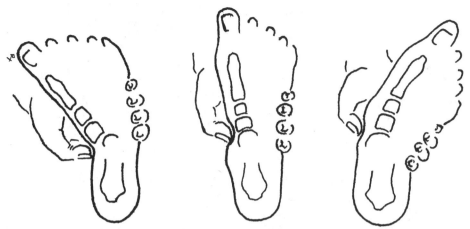

FIGURE 4–3. Demonstration of neutral position of talonavicular joint determined by palpating the relationship of the navicular and the talus. Middle drawing shows a foot with the talonavicular joint congruous, indicating that this is the midposition of function of the subtalar joint complex. (Reprinted with permission from Clinical Orthopedics)

PASSIVE RANGE OF MOTION

With the foot in the neutral position, passive motion of the foot reveals that, in the transverse plane, the foot can be moved into adduction and abduction. The range of adduction is generally twice that of abduction, approximately 30° and 15°, respectively (Fig. 4-4). The forefoot is moved passively through inversion and eversion into varus and valgus positions. This motion generally ranges from 25° of inversion into varus position of 25° of eversion into valgus position.[2,7]

The heel is then grasped and moved in eversion and inversion. The motion of inversion is generally twice that of eversion, about 20° of inversion and 10° of eversion, and a definite soft tissue end-point at the extreme of eversion.[2,5,7]

The position of the first metatarsal bone is then evaluated. This metatarsal should be evaluated first because the motion of the medial segment (the first metatarsal and first cuneiform) has a different range of motion than the lateral four metatarsal bones.[2,7,5,10] The first metatarsal is examined by placing a thumb beneath the metatarsal head and the other thumb beneath the lateral four metatarsal heads (Fig. 4-5). Passive motion of the first metatarsal bone is assessed by pushing the metatarsal bones up and

TABLE 4–1 Elements of Nonweightbearing Assessment

1. Neutral position subtalar joint: congruous position of talus and navicular which is determined by palpation of talus
2. Forefoot transverse plane movement: abduction 30°, adduction 15°
3. Forefoot frontal plane movement: inversion 25°, eversion 25°
4. Rearfoot frontal plane movement: inversion 20°, eversion 10°
5. Position of the first metatarsal in relationship to the lateral four metatarsals
6. First metatarsal mobility in sagittal plane: dorsiflexion 20°, plantar flexion 20°
7. Open kinetic chain supination, pronation, adduction, abduction, inversion, eversion, plantar flexion, dorsiflexion
8. Ankle joint sagittal joint: dorsiflexion 20°, plantar flexion 50° with the knee flexed and extended

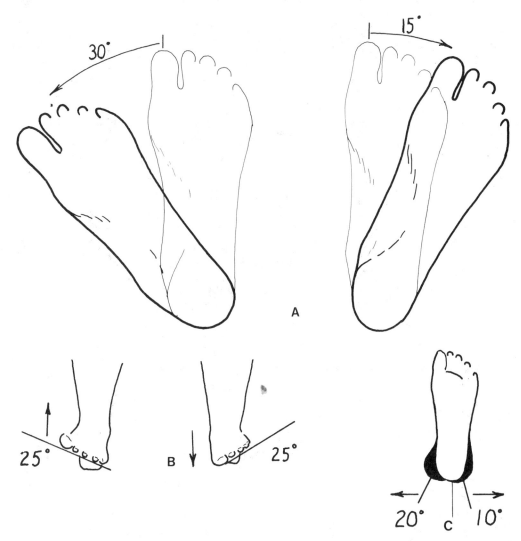

FIGURE 4–4. Passive motion of the normal foot. A) Passive motion in the transverse plane of abduction and adduction usually demonstrates twice as much adduction as abduction with about 30° of adduction and 15° of abduction. B) Passive motion of the forefoot in the frontal plane demonstrates 25° of inversion and 25° of eversion to position of maximum varus and valgus of the forefoot. C) Passive motion of the heel generally demonstrates 20° of inversion and 10° of eversion with a definite end point at the end of eversion.

then down. Passive motion should produce equal movement of the first metatarsal bone in dorsiflexion and plantar flexion (Fig. 4-6). Twenty degrees of first metatarsal dorsiflexion and 20° of plantarflexion are considered to be within normal limits.

ACTIVE RANGE OF MOTION

Active motion of the foot and ankle in the nonweightbearing position is then performed (Fig. 4-7). The motions of the subtalar joint in supination are abduction, inversion, and plantar flexion. The motion of the subtalar joint in pronation is adduc-

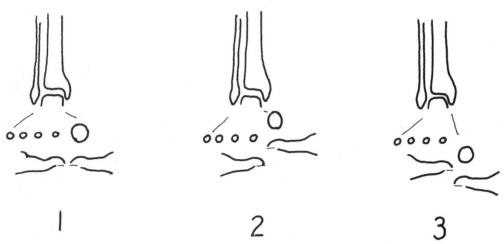

FIGURE 4-5. Position of the first metatarsal is determined by placing thumb under first metatarsal and lateral four metatarsals and observing level: 1) normal position; 2) dorsiflexed position; 3) plantar flexed position.

tion, eversion, and dorsiflexion. The supination and pronation movements are triplanar because of the axes of motion (See Fig. 4-7).[2,5,7,10] Active range of motion of the ankle joint is determined next. Normal motion is from 20° of dorsiflexion to 50° of plantar flexion, measured with the knee flexed or extended.[12]

The muscles are then examined with the foot in the nonweightbearing position. They are tested to determine the muscle strength and the motion produced by the individual contraction of each muscle group.[13] Muscle testing of the extrinsic foot muscles can be divided into anterior, posterior, medial, and lateral compartments. In testing the muscles it is especially important to determine whether there is normal flexibility of the triceps sural muscle group or whether there is limitation of motion by the gastrocnemius-soleus musculotendinous unit.

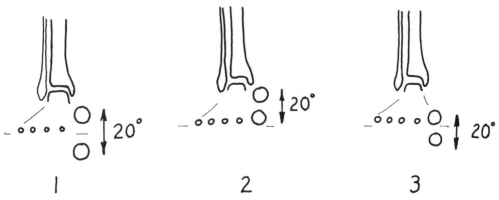

FIGURE 4-6. Passive motion of the first metatarsal: 1) normal passive motion; 2) increased dorsal motion with decreased plantar motion; 3) increased plantar motion with decreased dorsal motion.

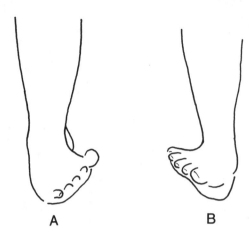

A   B

FIGURE 4–7. Active motion of the subtalar joint, nonweightbearing, is a triplanar motion. A) Supination is active triplanar motion of the subtalar joint complex with the foot moving into adduction, inversion, and plantar flexion. B) Pronation is an active triplanar motion of the subtalar joint with the foot moving into abduction, eversion, and dorsiflexion.

Clinical Evaluation: Weightbearing

With the patient standing, the clinician ascertains the relationship of the foot and ankle to the remainder of the lower extremity and the body by assessing the position of the leg, knee, and thigh along with motions of the hip and knee (Table 4-2). Leg lengths should be measured through clinical assessment or by x-rays. When the normal foot is examined while standing in the neutral position, the weightbearing line passing through the superior iliac spine of the pelvis and the patella also passes through the second metatarsal bone. The forefoot is perpendicular to the tibia in the frontal plane. The heel is in line with the tibia in the frontal plane (Fig. 4-8). The patient's gait is observed next (Table 4-3). With a normal foot and gait the heel everts during the early part of stance phase and the foot becomes supple. Then the foot then converts to a rigid lever for push-off in the later part of stance phase (see Fig. 4-1). Evaluation of gait is discussed in detail in Chapter 6.

The position of the components of the foot, as well as their motion and structure, is the most important consideration in the biomechanical changes of the foot from the supple to the rigid position during gait. However, one must certainly consider the associated effects of the muscles as in Chapter 1 and should also assess the muscle function in both the weightbearing and nonweightbearing modes to ascertain whether there is any specific abnormal muscle function that has produced an aberration of gait. For the purpose of this discussion it will be assumed that the muscles are functioning within normal limits, as is generally the clinical situation, except for gastrocnemius-soleus muscle tightness, which should have been ascertained during the physical examination and testing of the ankle motion.

TABLE 4–2 Weightbearing Assessment

1. Subtalar joint neutral position
2. Weightbearing line through superior iliac spine of the pelvis, patella, and second metatarsal
3. Forefoot perpendicular to the tibia in the frontal plane
4. Heel in line with the tibia in the frontal plane which can be observed from a posterior view

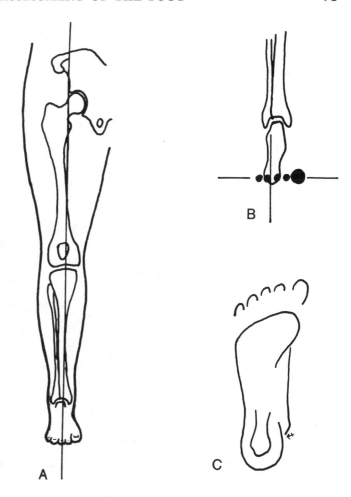

FIGURE 4–8. The position of the components of the normal foot with the foot in the neutral position: A) Weightbearing line through the anterior superior iliac spine and patella passes through the second metatarsal. B) The forefoot is perpendicular to the leg. C) The heel is in line with the tibia.

THE ABNORMAL FOOT

The abnormal foot is defined as a foot presenting some aberration that does not have the position, motion, or function of the normal foot described previously. The two types of abnormal foot are pes planus and pes cavus (Fig. 4-9). Flatfoot, or pes planus, is an abnormality that usually tends to make the foot supple (or to collapse) because it lacks supination sufficient to form a rigid lever during push-off in gait. Conversely, pes cavus is an abnormality in which the foot is rigid and does not become supple upon weightbearing.[2,7–9]

TABLE 4–3 Gait Assessment during Stance Phase

---

1. Heel contact to weight acceptance (early midstance): pronation, shock absorption, torque conversion, balance maintenance, adjust to terrain
2. Midstance or neutral position of subtalar joint
3. Late midstance to push-off: supination, rigid lever, propulsion, pulleys established for extrinsic muscles of the foot and ankle

---

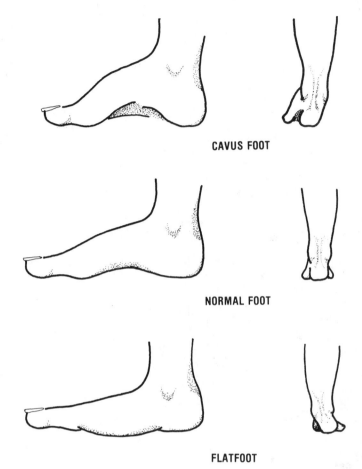

CAVUS FOOT

NORMAL FOOT

FLATFOOT

FIGURE 4-9. The normal foot everts to become supple and inverts to become stable for push-off. The cavus foot is rigid and will not evert to become supple. The flatfoot is excessively supple and does not resupinate to form a rigid lever for push-off.

Flatfoot Deformity

Examination of a flatfoot with the talonavicular joint in the neutral position generally reveals that the positions of the foot components are (1) abduction of the forefoot in relation to the weightbearing line in the transverse plane; (2) varus, or inversion, of the forefoot in the frontal plane; and (3) valgus, or eversion, of the heel in the frontal plane (Fig. 4-10).[2,7,9]

Any one of these abnormalities may produce a flatfoot deformity with ambulation, but generally (and especially if the flatfoot deformity is severe) all three are present; that is, forefoot abduction in weightbearing, forefoot varus in nonweightbearing, and heel valgus in standing.

Upon examination of a flatfoot for motion abduction of the forefoot, forefoot inversion, and heel eversion are generally all increased and the opposite motions are decreased (Fig. 4-11). In a person with flatfoot, the first metatarsal bone is generally dorsiflexed or has an unusually wide range of dorsiflexion motion.

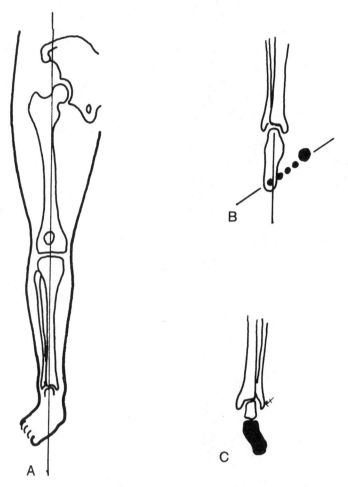

FIGURE 4–10. The abnormal position of the components of the foot usually seen with the flatfoot deformity: (A) abduction of the forefoot lateral to the weightbearing line in the transverse plane; (B) inversion of the forefoot to the varus position in the frontal plane; (C) eversion of the heel to the valgus position in the frontal plane. (Reprinted from Gould, J: The Foot Book. Williams & Wilkins, Baltimore, 1988, with permission.)

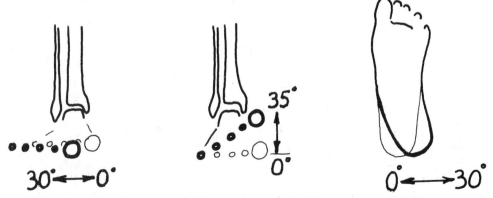

FIGURE 4–11. Depiction of usual motion with flatfoot deformity: (*left*) Increased abduction motion of the forefoot in the transverse plane; (*middle*) increased inversion motion of the forefoot in the frontal plane; (*right*) increased eversion of the heel in the frontal plane.

Pes Cavus

Examination of the cavus foot with the talonavicular joint in the neutral position generally reveals three components: (1) adduction of the forefoot relative to the weight-bearing line in the transverse plane; (2) forefoot valgus in the frontal plane; and (3) heel varus in the frontal plane (Fig. 4-12). The first metatarsal bone is generally plantar flexed and has an increased range of plantar flexion.[2,7,9]

Generally movement in the cavus foot is characterized by increased forefoot adduction in the transverse plane, increased forefoot eversion, and increased heel inversion. Relative to these deformities the opposite movements are decreased (Fig. 4-13). The more severe the condition, the greater the degree of deformity. It is important to understand that only one of these structural deficits may produce foot cavus when walking, but generally in a severely abnormal foot all of these deformities are present. With ambulation the cavus foot is rigid because it does not pronate to unlock the midfoot and subtalar joint, so they may become supple. Therefore, the foot cannot adapt to the ground and cushion the impact.

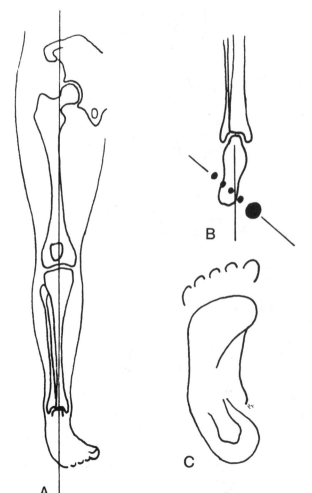

FIGURE 4-12. Position of the components of the foot usually seen with a cavus deformity. A) Forefoot is adducted in the transverse plane relative to the weightbearing line. B) The forefoot is everted to the valgus position in the frontal plane. C) The heel is inverted to the varus position in the frontal plane.

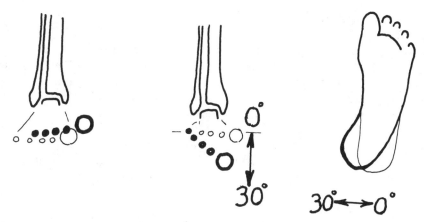

FIGURE 4–13. Depiction of usual motion of cavus foot: (*left*) Increased adduction of the forefoot in the transverse plane; (*middle*) the forefoot in the frontal plane; (*right*) increased inversion motion of the heel.

ORTHOTICS AND SURGICAL CONSIDERATIONS

If the physical examination reveals normal position and motion of the components of the foot, and normal muscle function, the foot should function in a normal manner because there is no structural or gait aberration. If pain is present in a foot of this type, the examiner should search for an intrinsic cause such as primary tendinitis or interdigital neuroma. Alternatively, something extrinsic may produce an abnormality of the foot: either through the loss of muscle function or through secondary deformities resulting from loss of muscle function. Such a situation occurs with the rupture of the posterior tibial tendon: the foot cannot supinate. Ultimately the foot develops secondary fixed deformities of general forefoot abduction in the transverse plane, varus in the frontal plane, and heel valgus in the frontal plane. In a situation where the pain is caused by an arthritic joint, such as the first metatarsal cuneiform or talonavicular, pain may limit the joint range of motion. Limitations of joint motion and gait abnormalities will depend on how that joint functions during the gait cycle.[2]

Orthotic Devices

An orthotic device is defined as a device that assists the foot to function in a more normal manner.[14,15] Following the clinical classification and considering the types of orthotics used, one can see that the normal foot with normal motion does not need an orthotic device. For flatfoot that is supple and does not invert to become rigid during the late phase of weightbearing, a rigid orthotic is used to support the foot and allow it to resupinate.[6] A cavus foot that is rigid and does not evert to become supple during the early phase of weightbearing requires an orthotic that is soft and will absorb shock while increasing the weightbearing area.[2] A more detailed biomechanical evaluation of the foot and ankle and biomechanical orthotic prescriptions are discussed in Chapters 6 and 9.

Surgical Treatment of Flatfoot Deformity

In flatfoot that has a single causal component, the treatment may be directed toward correcting that component. For example, flatfoot produced solely by heel valgus can be corrected by performing osteotomy of the os calcis to bring it into the proper position so that the normal subtalar passive motion of the heel is 10° of eversion to 20° of inversion. If the first metatarsal bone is dorsiflexed, a plantar flexion osteotomy may be performed. If the foot is abducted and the forefoot is in varus, the surgeon can bring the forefoot out of abduction or shorten the medial column (or both) to correct these deformities. The surgery involves an opening wedge osteotomy of the cuboid bone with shortening of the navicular bone; closing wedge osteotomy and fusion of the navicular cuneiform joint; or lengthening of the anterior portion of the os calcis between the anterior and middle facets.[6]

All foot components must be assessed prior to performing surgery for flatfoot if correction of the deformity is to be approached properly. For instance, if the problem is uncompensated forefoot varus with inability of the heel to evert and a varus osteotomy of the heel is performed, the patient may have even greater difficulty because of increased uncompensated forefoot varus.

Surgical Treatment of Pes Cavus

The pes cavus foot is evaluated to see if there is a single specific deformity. If there is, it is corrected. If the first metatarsal is plantar flexed, producing the cavus deformity as well as abnormal gait, a dorsiflexion osteotomy of the first metatarsal bone, soft tissue release, or both are required to correct the problem. If the cavus deformity is the result of heel varus, a closing wedge osteotomy is necessary, which brings the motion of the subtalar joint to as close to normal as possible (20° of inversion and 10° of eversion). If the deformity is associated with or caused by adduction and valgus deformity of the forefoot, the lateral column is generally shortened by a closing wedge osteotomy of the cuboid, the anterior portion of the os calcis, or both. It is more difficult to correct the problem components of the rigid cavus foot than it is to correct the loose hypermobile flatfoot; however, the surgeon attempts to correct either the deformity to produce as structurally normal a foot as possible without fusing any major joints. The mobility of the subtalar joint complex, which includes the subtalar and the midtarsal joints, must be maintained.[6]

SUMMARY

This chapter has covered the assessment of the foot from a clinical standpoint, looking at the foot as a functional organ that developed to allow man to walk with a bipedal gait. The normal foot converts from the supple position during the early part of stance phase to a rigid position during the latter part.

The appearance and motion of the foot with normal parameters for function have been presented. Use of orthotics and surgical considerations based upon these parameters are presented, to allow the clinical practitioner to produce a more normally functional foot.

The components of the flatfoot deformity are abduction of the forefoot; varus or inversion of the forefoot; and valgus or eversion of the heel. The first metatarsal bone is dorsiflexed and generally limited in plantar flexion.

The components of the pes cavus deformity are adduction of the forefoot; valgus or eversion of the forefoot; and varus or inversion of the heel. The position of the first metatarsal bone is generally plantar flexed and rigid.

REFERENCES

1. Bordelon, RL: Foot first: Evolution of man. Foot Ankle 8:, 1987.
2. Bordelon, RL: Surgical and Conservative Foot Care. Charles B. Slack, Thorofare, NJ, 1988.
3. Laitman, JT and Jaffe WL: A review of current concepts on the evolution of the human foot. Foot Ankle 2:284, 1982.
4. Leakey, M: Footprints in the ashes of time. National Geographic 446,: 1979.
5. Root, M, et al: Biomechanical Examination of the Foot, Vol I. Clinical Biomechanics Corporation, 1971.
6. Weaver, K: The search for our ancestors. National Geographic 561, 1985.
7. Gould, J: The Foot Book. Williams & Wilkins, Baltimore, 1988.
8. Bordelon, RL: Hypermobile flatfoot in children: Comprehension, evaluation and treatment. Clin Orthop 181:7, 1983.
9. Bordelon, RL: Management of disorders of the forefoot and toenails associated with running. Clin Sports Med 4:4, 1985.
10. Sgarlato, T: A Compendium of Podiatric Biomechanics. California College of Podiatric Medicine, 1971.
11. Bordelon, RL: Correction of hypermobile flatfoot in children by molded inserts. Foot Ankle 1:143, 1980.
12. American Academy of Orthopaedic Surgeons: Joint Motion-Method of Measuring and Recording. 1965.
13. Goss, CM: Gray's Anatomy. American ed 29. Lea & Febiger, Philadelphia, 1972.
14. Jahss, MH: Atlas of Orthotics: Biomechanical Principles and Applications. CV Mosby, Philadelphia, 1975.
15. Jahss, M: Disorders of the Foot. Vol I. WB Saunders, Philadelphia, 1982, pp 1–36.

CHAPTER 5

Biomechanical Radiographic Evaluation

George Vito, DPM
Stanley Kalish, DPM

This chapter presents basic radiographic techniques used to evaluate foot deformities and injuries. It does not include all radiographic techniques. Rather it is a short synopsis of basic views, commonly performed angular measurements, and the deformities revealed by the described measurements.

It must be remembered that radiographs are never the sole means of making a diagnosis but are instead just one type of finding that must be intergrated with many others in order to arrive at a pertinent clinical assessment or diagnosis.

The most common clinical views of a foot include the dorsoplantar, lateral, medial, lateral oblique, medial oblique, and the axial sesamoidal.[1-3] Radiographs can either be termed projections or views. Projections refer to the way in which the x-ray generator "sees" the body part to be exposed. The views described are the way in which the film "sees" the part to be exposed.[1] For example, a medial oblique *view* can be the same as a lateral oblique *projection*. However, to avoid confusion, all descriptions in this chapter are presented as projections.

PROJECTIONS

The *dorsoplantar projection* is usually taken with the patient in a weightbearing or (if the patient is injured) recumbent position. In a weightbearing position, both feet may be radiographed together, or individually. The generator is positioned 15° from the vertical to ensure proper visualization of the tarsal joints without the generators being in the patient's abdomen (Fig. 5-1). With the patient recumbent, the foot is placed flat on the film, and the knee is flexed 45° with the generator placed perpendicular to the film (Fig. 5-2). With these projections, we are able to examine the transverse plane relationships of the midfoot area, the metatarsals, and the entire forefoot area. The anterior portion of the greater tarsus, Lisfranc's joint, all of the metatarsophalangeal joints, and the inter-

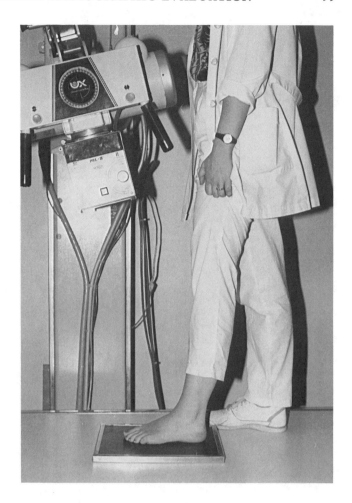

FIGURE 5–1. The generator is positioned 15° from the vertical.

phalangeal joints can be viewed (Fig. 5-3). The articulations and shapes of the navicular, the cuboid, the medial cuneiform bones, and (to a lesser extent) the middle and lateral cuneiform bones can also be evaluated from this projection.

The *lateral projection* is taken with the generator at a 90° angle to the foot.[1] The foot is positioned so that the medial side of the first metatarsal head and the medial side of the calcaneus are against the film. This projection can either be taken weightbearing (Fig. 5-4) or nonweightbearing and gives a proper demonstration of the talus and calcaneus (Fig. 5-5). Most of the cuboid can be seen, and less clearly, visualization of the navicular and the medial cuneiform is also possible. Figure 5-6 clearly identifies the first and fifth metatarsals, and the second through fourth metatarsals overlapping each other. The first digit is relatively visable also.

The *lateral oblique projection* is the most popular oblique projection used in podiatry, giving a slightly distorted and slightly magnified representation of most of the bones of the foot.[2] The patient stands on the film, which is angulated 45° from the central beam (Fig. 5-7). The digits, lesser tarsus, cuboid, fourth and fifth metatarsal articulations with the cuboid, and the metatarsals are clearly seen (Fig. 5-8).

The *medial oblique projection* is exactly the opposite of the lateral oblique projection. The patient stands on the film with the central beam angulated 25° from the vertical

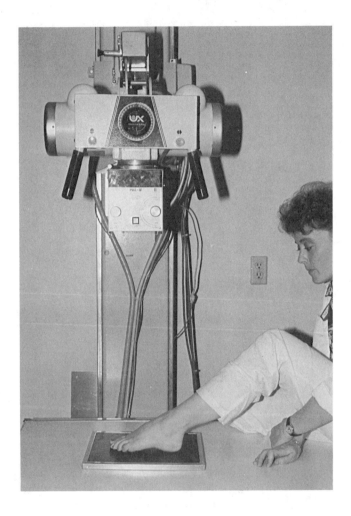

FIGURE 5–2. With the patient in a recumbent position, the knee is flexed at 45°, with the generator perpendicular to the film.

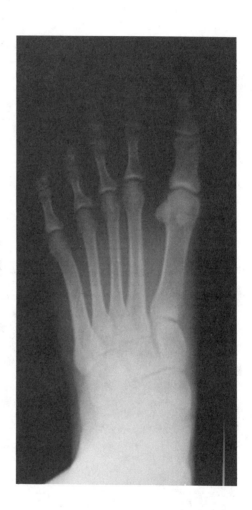

FIGURE 5-3. The dorsoplantar projection.

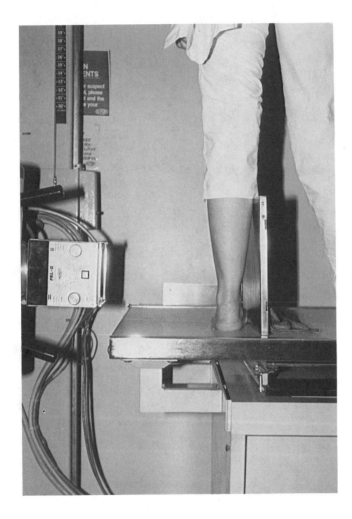

FIGURE 5–4. Weightbearing lateral projection

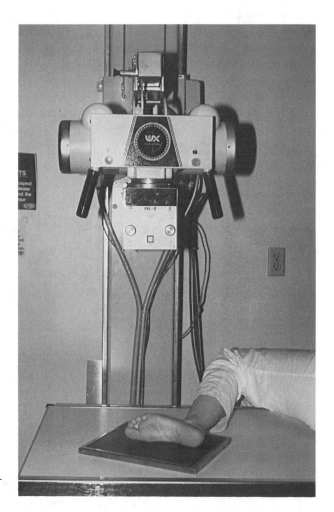

FIGURE 5–5. Nonweightbearing lateral projection.

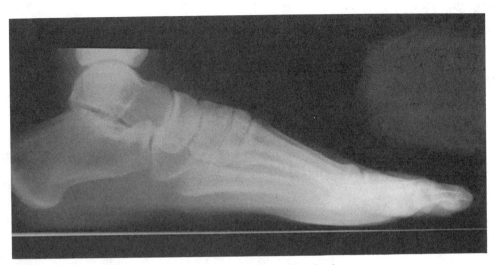

FIGURE 5–6. The lateral projection.

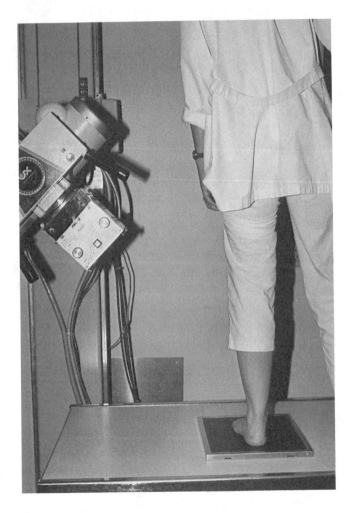

FIGURE 5–7. The lateral oblique projection.

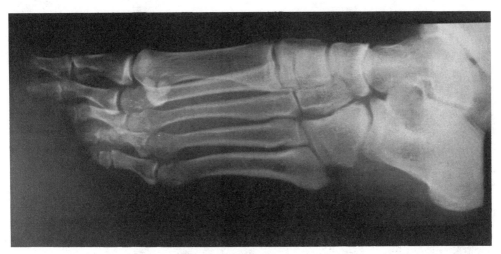

FIGURE 5–8. The lateral oblique projection.

(Fig. 5-9). The digits, tibial sesamoid, first metatarsal, first cuneiform, navicular tuberosity, and the medial calcaneus are seen (Fig. 5-10).

In the *axial sesamoid projection*, the patient stands with the digits against the film. The film holds the digits in extension. The patient first puts weight on the ball of the foot and then, keeping the digits against the film raises the heel enough so that the central ray clears it (Fig. 5-11). The sesamoids, the cristae of the first metatarsal head, and the inferior aspect of the lesser metatarsals are visualized (Fig. 5-12).

ANGULAR AND AXIAL RELATIONSHIPS OF THE DORSOPLANTAR PROJECTION

Longitudinal Axis of the Rearfoot

The longitudinal axis of the rearfoot bissects the posterior surface of the calcaneus and the distal anteromedial corner of the calcaneus. If the posterior surface of the calcaneus cannot be visualized, a line parallel to the lateral border of the calcaneus is constructed to represent the longitudinal axis of the rearfoot (Fig. 5-13).[1]

Longitudinal Axis of the Lesser Tarsus

The longitudinal axis of the lesser tarsus (talus, calcaneus, navicular, cuboid) is used to compare the position of the lesser tarsus to that of both the metatarsus and the greater tarsus. First, one must transect the lesser tarsus by locating the medial aspect of the talonavicular joint and the medial aspect of the joint between the first metatarsal and the first cuneiform.[1] The line that connects them is then bisected. Second, the lateral aspect of the calcaneocuboid articulation and the lateral aspect of the base of the fifth metatarsal are identified. The line connecting them is bisected (Fig. 5-14). The two bisections should then be connected. A line perpendicular to this transection constructs the longitudinal axis of the lesser tarsus.

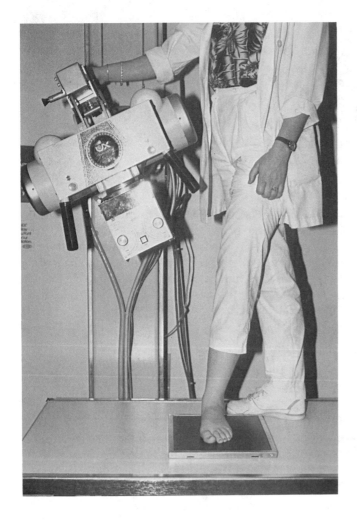

FIGURE 5–9. Medial oblique projection.

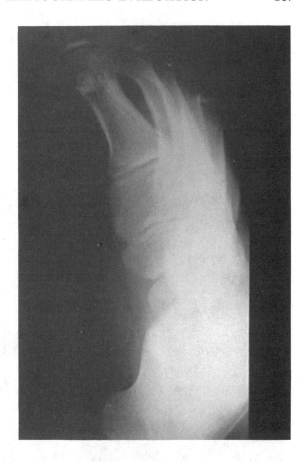

FIGURE 5–10. Medial oblique projection.

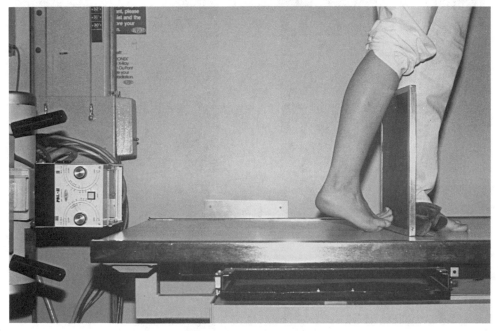

FIGURE 5–11. Axial sesamoid projection.

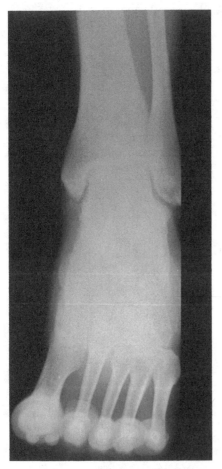

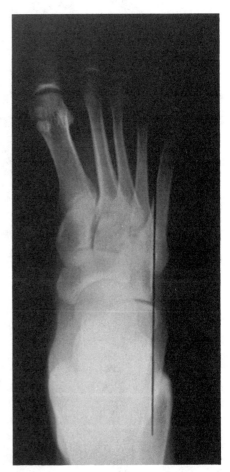

FIGURE 5–12. Axial sesamoid projection.

FIGURE 5–13. The longitudinal axis of the rearfoot.

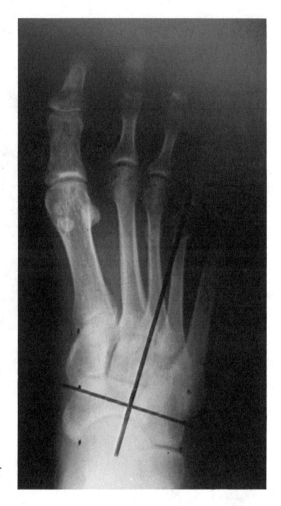

FIGURE 5-14. The longitudinal axis of the lesser tarsus.

Longitudinal Axis of the Metatarsal Bones

The longitudinal axis of the metatarsal is constructed by bisecting the neck of the second metatarsal and the base end of the shaft of the second metatarsal. Connecting these two points gives the longitudinal axis of the metatarsals (Fig. 5-15).

Longitudinal Axis of the Digits

The longitudinal axis of the digits is constructed by bisecting the neck of the proximal phalanx of the second toe and the bisection of its base. Connecting these two points will produce the longitudinal axis of the digits (Fig. 5-16).

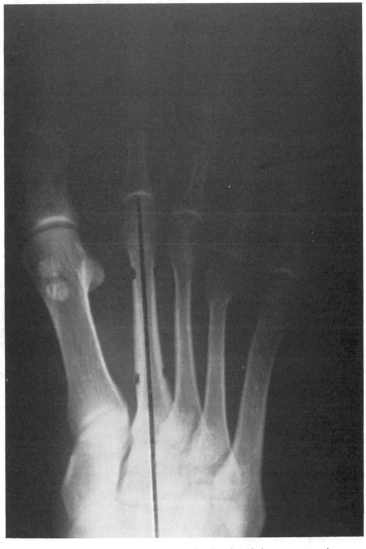

FIGURE 5–15. The longitudinal axis of the metatarsals.

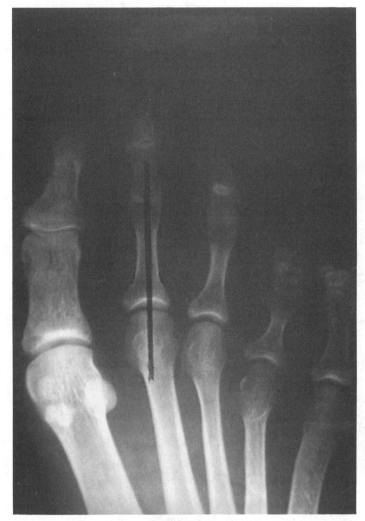

FIGURE 5–16. The longitudinal axis of the digits.

Talocalcaneal Angle

The talocalcaneal angle (Kite's angle) has long been used as an index of relative foot pronation and supination. This angle is formed by a line bisecting the head and neck of the talus (collum tali axis) and the longitudinal axis of the rearfoot (Fig. 5-17). The normal range of this angle is approximately 17°–21°. The articular relationship between the navicular and the talus must also be visualized. Approximately 75% of the head of the talus should articulate with the navicular. Along with this relationship, the axis of the talus should run through the center of the first metatarsal (Fig. 5-18). On pronation, the axis runs medial to the first metatarsal, and on supination, it projects laterally.[1]

The talocalcaneal angle compares the pronation-supination of the rearfoot to that of the forefoot. If the rearfoot is maximally pronated, the forefoot will compensate.

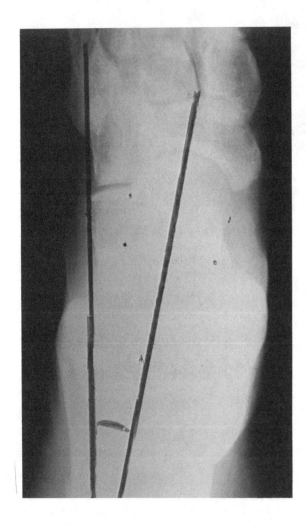

FIGURE 5–17. The talocalcaneal angle.

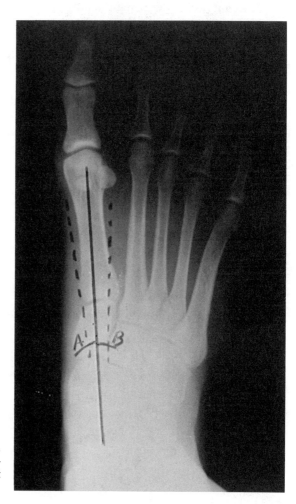

FIGURE 5–18. The talonavicular axis. With pronation, the axis will project medially (A); with supination, it will project laterally (B).

Therefore symptoms of overpronation will be present in the forefoot; the same is true for supination. However, in cases of partial pronation of the rearfoot, if more pronation is needed, the rearfoot will accommodate. This deformity in the rearfoot can be corrected, either by posting the rearfoot with an orthotic or by surgery of the rearfoot. Further discussion of biomechanical orthotics appears in Chapter 9.

Cuboid Abduction Angle

The cuboid abduction angle is formed by a line representing the lateral aspect of the cuboid and the longitudinal axis of the rearfoot (Fig. 5-19). The normal range of this angle is 0°–5°. When the angle is greater than 5°, pronation of the foot has occurred; however, when supination and adduction of the forefoot are seen, this angle may be less than 0°, as a negative value.[6] The angle is a reflection of the rearfoot. When the rearfoot is maximally pronated, the cuboid will be abducted because of the forces exerted through the talonavicular and calcaneaocuboid joints. When the foot is maximally supinated, the cuboid may be adducted. Therefore, correction of this deformity in the rearfoot is accomplished either with orthotic posting or by surgical intervention.

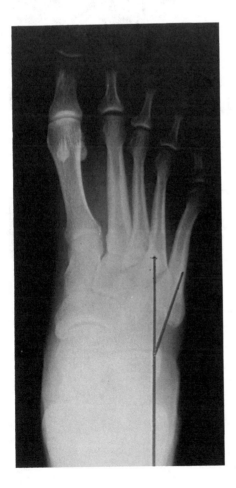

FIGURE 5–19. The cuboid abduction angle.

Talonavicular Angle

The talonavicular angle is constructed by using the collum tali axis and the transection of the lesser tarsus. The normal angular relationship should be between 60° and 80° (Fig. 5-20). An angle of less than 60° represents pronation, while an angle greater than 60° represents supination.[1] Once again, this relationship reflects rearfoot to midfoot accommodation; however, correction of the deformity will occur with forefoot posting of an orthotic to allow limited motion of the talonavicular articulation. If correction cannot be accomplished with an orthotic, fusion of the talonavicular joint may be considered.

Metatarsus Adductus Angle

The metatarsus adductus angle is formed by the intersection of the longitudinal axis of the metatarsus and the longitudinal axis of the lesser tarsus (Fig. 5-21). The normal range is between 6° and 10°.[1] If the rearfoot is in a maximally supinated position, without midfoot and forefoot compensation, the forefoot will be in an adducted position, depending up on the age of the patient. If there is mild adductus in a child, an orthotic with a medial flare can be used to allow the foot to rotate laterally at the tarsometatarsal joint, thus permitting the metatarsal to abduct. However, if the metatarsals are completely ossified and the epiphyseal plates are closed (after age 8–10 years), surgical correction with osteotomies of the first through the fifth metatarsals may be considered. If the deformity can be recognized early in life, this problem can also be treated, with orthotics and through serial casting to lengthen both the medial capsule and the ligamentous attachments of the tarsometatarsal joints.

Metatarsus Primus Adductus Angle (Intermetatarsal Angle)

The intermetatarsal angle is formed by the transverse plane, angular relationship between the first and second metatarsals (Fig. 5-22). The ideal intermetatarsal angle is 8°.[1,2] This angular relationship is a principal consideration in determining treatment for bunion deformities. If the forefoot and the metatarsals are adducted, the intermetatarsal angle can be up to 12° and still be considered normal. If there is a high intermetatarsal angle (over 8°) causing a hallux abductus deformity, surgical correction will be directed toward the base of the first metatarsal. If the intermetatarsal angle is less than 8°, surgical correction will be directed toward the head of the first metatarsal.

Hallux Abductus Angle

The hallus abductus angle is formed by the intersection of the longitudinal axis of the first metatarsal and the longitudinal axis of the proximal phalanx of the hallux. Normal angulation does not exceed 15° (Fig. 5-23).[1,5] If the angle is greater than 15°, a hallux abductus deformity should be considered. If the angle is negative, hallux varus is considered. The angular relationship will determine whether a soft tissue release will be performed at the metatarsophalangeal joint of the first metatarsal or if an osteotomy of the distal aspect of the metatarsophalangeal joint should be undertaken. If there is extreme hallux abductus (25°–30°) osteotomy of either the distal third of the first

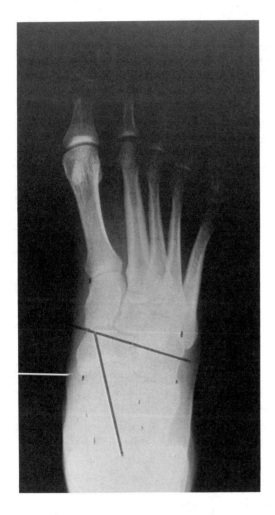

FIGURE 5-20. Talonavicular angle.

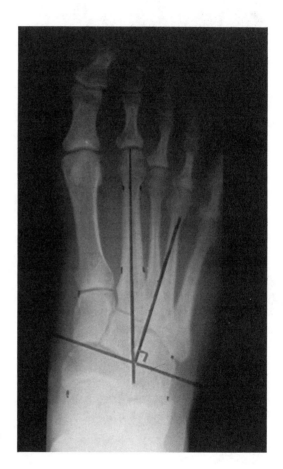

FIGURE 5–21. Metatarsal adductus angle.

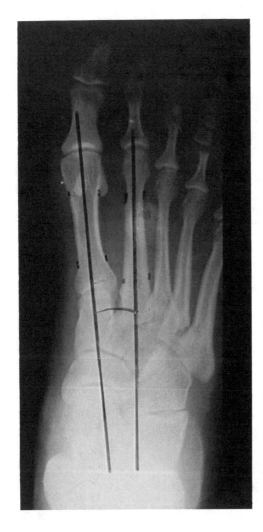

FIGURE 5–22. The intermetatarsal angle.

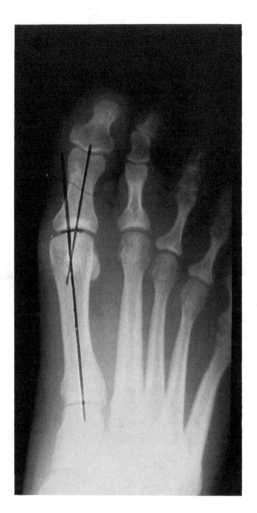

FIGURE 5–23. Hallux abductus angle.

metatarsal or of the proximal phalanx is considered. If the angle is less than 25°, a soft tissue release of the metatarsophalangeal joint may be all that is needed to reduce the deformity.

Hallux Interphalangeal Angle

The interphalangeal angle of the hallux is formed by the intersection of the longitudinal axis of the proximal and distal phalanges of the hallux (Fig. 5-24). The normal angle is 8°–10°. When the angle is greater than 10°, the distal portion of the hallux will be directed in the lateral position against the second digit. This may cause a retrograde force on the metatarsophalangeal joint, resulting in hallux abductovalgus deformity. Therefore, with a large hallux interphalangeal angle (greater than 10°), surgical correction with osteotomies of the distal aspect of the proximal phalanx or of the proximal aspect of the distal phalanx will be needed to reduce this angle.

Proximal Articular Set Angle

The proximal articular set angle is formed by a line perpendicular to the effective articular surface of the first metatarsal head and its intersection with the longitudinal axis of the first metatarsal (Fig. 5-25). This value is then subtracted from 90°. The normal range is 0°–8°. With a hallux abductovalgus deformity, this angle may be considerably greater. The effective articular surface of the metatarsal head is determined by using the most lateral aspect of the articular surface of the first metatarsal head and the most medial aspect of the functioning articular cartilage on the head of the first metatarsal. If the proximal articular set angle is greater than 8°, the deformity (hallux valgus) is with the head of the first metatarsal; therefore any correction to be performed will be undertaken at this location.

Distal Articular Set Angle

The distal articular set angle is formed by a line perpendicular to the effective articular surface of the base of the proximal phalanx of the hallux and its intersection with the longitudinal axis of the proximal phalanx (Fig. 5-26). Again this value is subtracted from 90° and is normally 0°–8°. If the deformity (hallux valgus) is with the proximal phalanx, surgical correction is performed at this level.

Metatarsal Break Angle

The metatarsal break angle is an obtuse, proximal angle formed by points located at the distal centers of the first, second, and fifth metatarsal heads (Fig. 5-27). The average metatarsal break angle is 142.5°.[1,4,5] This value demonstrates that all the metatarsophalangeal joints are aligned and functioning as a fulcrum over which the body weight is raised.[4,5] When a metatarsal is elongated, excessive stress is exerted through the second metatarsal, causing localized pain. Surgical intervention to the lesser metatarsals should be undertaken with caution. There is a failure rate of 57% when metatarsal osteotomies are performed.[3] Orthotic posting of the forefoot is the procedure of choice at this level to

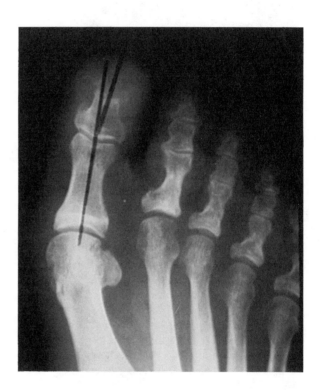

FIGURE 5–24. Hallux interphalangeal angle.

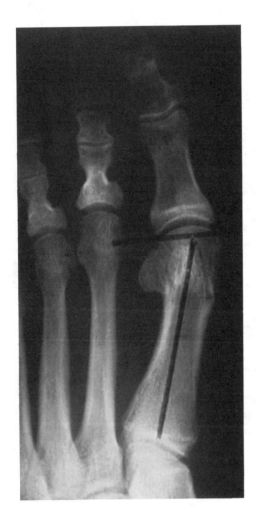

FIGURE 5–25. Proximal articular set angle.

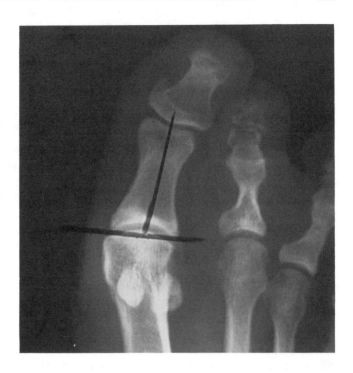

FIGURE 5–26. Distal articular set angle.

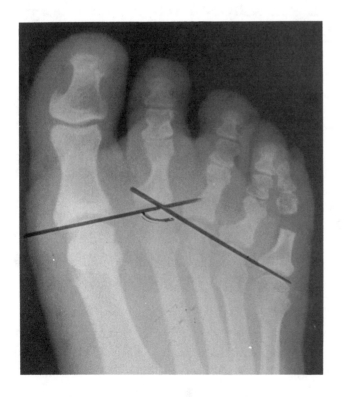

FIGURE 5–27. Metatarsal break angle.

accommodate possible plantar flexion of the second metatarsal or the dorsiflexed attitude of the first and third metatarsals.

Tibial Sesamoid Position

The tibial sesamoid position (TSP) is determined by the relative apposition of the sesamoid to the first metatarsal axis (Fig. 5-28) Seven positions are identified:

TSP 1: Tibial sesamoid lies medially, clear of the first metatarsal axis.
TSP 2: Tibial sesamoid laterally abuts the first metatarsal axis.
TSP 3: Tibial sesamoid laterally overlaps the first metatarsal axis.
TSP 4: Tibial sesamoid is bisected by the first metatarsal axis.
TSP 5: Tibial sesamoid medially overlaps the first metatarsal axis.
TSP 6: Tibial sesamoid medially abuts the first metatarsal axis.
TSP 7: Tibial sesamoid lies laterally, clear of the first metatarsal axis.

Patients who have a tibial sesamoid position greater than TSP 3 usually show abnormalities in the crista.[1] The crista makes up the medial wall for the fibular sesamoid articulation, and the lateral wall for the tibial sesamoid articulation. With a hallux abductus valgus deformity, the surgeon always considers the position of the tibial sesamoid. In most procedures to correct hallux abductus valgus, the conjoined tendons of the transverse and oblique hallux adductor are released from their insertions into the fibular sesamoid and the proximal phalanx of the first metatarsophalangeal joint, respectively. This procedure relieves the tension forces of the adductor tendon on the joint.

ANGULAR AND AXIAL RELATIONSHIPS OF THE LATERAL PROJECTION

Cyma Line

The Cyma line is the articulation between the talonavicular and the calcaneocuboid, Chopart's joint. In the normal foot, these two articulations form a continuous S-shaped curve (Fig. 5-29A). With pronation, the talus slides anteriorly, creating an anterior break in the Cyma line, with the talonavicular joint being distal to the calcaneocuboid joint (Fig. 5-29B). In supination, the talus moves posteriorly into the ankle mortise, and the Cyma line will have a posterior break.[1,5] The talonavicular joint will be proximal to that of the calcaneocuboid joint (Fig. 5-29C).

Collum Tali Axis

The collum tali axis is a longitudinal bisector of the neck of the talus. Because of its variable shape, the radiographic plotting of the axis may be difficult (Fig. 5-30).

Plane of Support

The plane of support is determined by the most plantar aspect of the calcaneal tuberosity and the most plantar aspect of the head of the fifth metatarsal (Fig. 5-31).

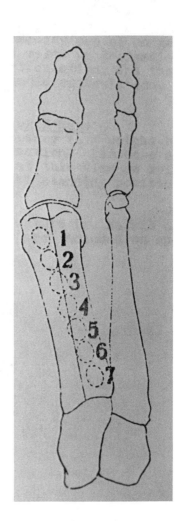

FIGURE 5-28. Tibial sesamoid position.

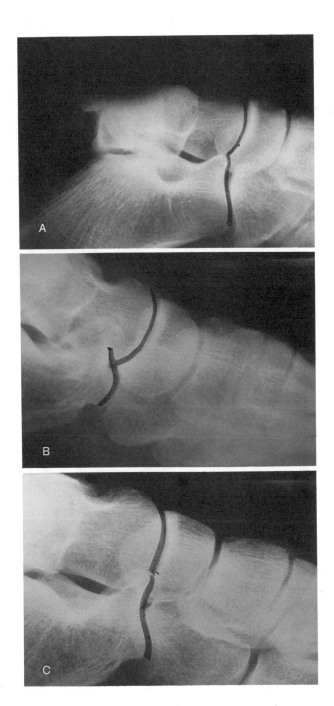

FIGURE 5–29. Cyma line: normal (A), pronated (B), and supinated (C).

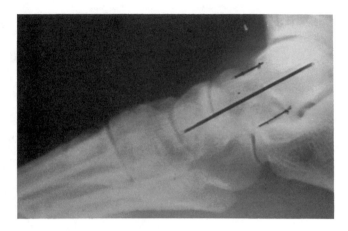

FIGURE 5–30. Collum tali axis.

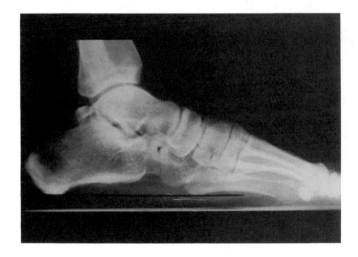

FIGURE 5–31. Plane of support.

Calcaneal Axis

The calcaneal axis is determined by connecting a point representing the most plantar aspect of the tuberosity of the calcaneus with the most distal plantar aspect of the calcaneus (Fig. 5-32).

First Metatarsal Declination Axis

The first metatarsal declination axis is determined by bisecting the neck and the base of the first metatarsal and connecting these points. (Fig. 5-33).

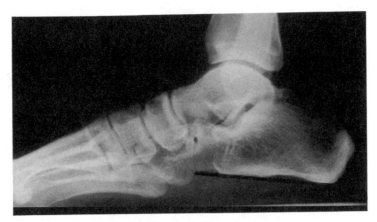

FIGURE 5–32. Calcaneal axis.

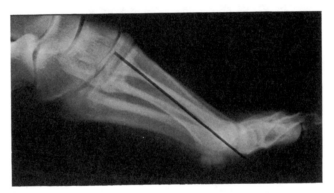

FIGURE 5–33. First metatarsal axis.

Calcaneal Inclination Angle

The calcaneal inclination angle is a determination of relative arch height, and is formed by the intersection of the plane of support and the calcaneal inclination axis (Fig. 5-34). This angle is very useful in evaluating a pronated or supinated foot. The more pronated the foot type, the smaller the angle, with an increased angle in a supinated foot type. The average value is 15°; however, abnormalties of pronation and supination will be expressed well beyond or well below the average measurement.[1] With a greater angle the midfoot may compensate, causing midfoot symptoms; therefore, orthotic control may be used. However if the deformity is not compensated, lateral ankle sprains may occur, potentially necessitating surgical correction. With a small angle, orthotic control may be used if midfoot symptoms occur. With a true uncompensated flatfoot, however, a midfoot arch reconstruction with a calcaneal osteotomy may be performed.

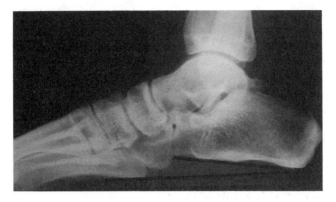

FIGURE 5–34. Calcaneal inclination angle.

Talar Declination Angle

The talar declination angle is constructed by the plane of support and the collum tali axis (Fig. 5-35). This angle averages about 21°.[1,4,5] The collum tali axis should be colinear with the first metatarsal declination axis. Hypermobility in this joint is reflected by symptoms of pain on increased activity. A talar declination angle (greater than 21°) allows for greater pronation, while an angle less than 21° allows for supination. With pronation, an orthotic usually controls the pronation if the deformity is flexible. If the deformity is not flexible, a medial arch suspension may be indicated to raise the arch to a functional level. If supination is the problem, calcaneal osteotomies are indicated on the lateral aspect to reduce the amount of supination.

SUMMARY

One must remember that radiographs do not make the diagnosis, the clinician does. Not one, but many of the angles of axes described in this chapter contribute to making a diagnosis of pertinent foot pathology. The discussion in this chapter was designed to inform clinicians about how radiographs of the foot and ankle are made and interpreted. An understanding of these interpretations permits clarification if the decisions that underlie conservative or surgical intervention for successful podiatric management.

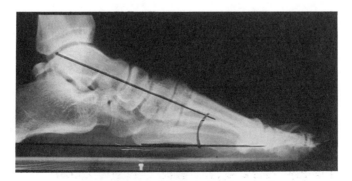

FIGURE 5–35. Talar declination angle.

REFERENCES

1. Weissman, S: Radiology of the Foot. Williams & Wilkins, Baltimore, 1984.
2. Whitney, AK: Radiographic Charting Technique. Philadelphia College of Podiatric Medicine, Philadelphia, 1978.
3. Montagne, J, Chevrot, A, and Galmiche, JM: Atlas of Foot Radiology. Year Book Medical Publishers, Chicago, 1981.
4. Gamble, and Yale,: Clinical Foot Roentgenology, Williams & Wilkins, Baltimore, 1957.
5. Gamble, and Felton,: Applied Foot Roentgenology. Williams & Wilkins, Baltimore, 1966.
6. Bloom, W and Hollenbach, J: Medical Radiographic Technique. Charles C Thomas, Springfield, MO, 1965.

CHAPTER 6

Biomechanical Evaluation for Functional Orthotics

Michael J. Wooden, MS, PT

This chapter describes a step-by-step process of biomechanical evaluation of the foot and ankle complex. Using static and gait analysis methods, a system of problem solving for orthotic therapy is provided.

In many clinics, orthotics are made from plaster impressions of feet, sometimes by minimally trained personnel and often without benefit of measurements and gait analysis. The system described in this chapter utilizes specific observations and measurements that provide many clinical advantages. First, the ideal subtalar joint neutral position is determined, so that deviations from neutral can be observed. Second, limitations and deformities causing these deviations from neutral can be evaluated. Third, measurement reliability can be increased with proper methods and repetition. Fourth, objective data can be obtained. From these data, the clinician can establish a baseline, follow progress, communicate with other clinicians, and determine the appropriate amount of "treatment" to be built in to the orthotic.

Before proceeding with this chapter, the reader is urged to review Chapters 1 and 2, which provide details of normal and abnormal mechanics. Note especially the causes of compensation at the subtalar joint and other joints leading to abnormal pronation and supination. A better understanding of these conditions enhances the ability to evaluate them.

The reader must also realize that this chapter is taken somewhat out of context; that is, only a part of the entire lower quarter screening process is provided. A history must also be obtained, especially if there is evidence of an overuse syndrome related to weightbearing activities. Evaluation of the spine and lower limb for alignment, range of motion, muscle imbalance, and mobility problems is essential, particularly if the pain complaint is extrinsic to the foot. In some cases x-rays and evaluation for neurological and vascular status are needed, as described in other chapters in this book.

This chapter is divided into sections that deal with static and dynamic evaluation procedures. Measurement examples are provided, and a case presentation is offered as a summary. This format will be followed in Chapter 9, when biomechanical orthotics are discussed, and more cases are presented, utilizing the measurement techniques and problem-solving process discussed in this chapter.

STATIC EVALUATION

Observation

With the patient standing, relaxed, and with equal weight on each foot, the examiner observes for postural deviations or for signs of lower extremity deviations (Fig. 6–1). These could include:

1. **Transverse Plane Deviations:** rotation or torsion of the hip, femurs, knees, or tibias, observed from the front or from behind.
2. **Frontal Plane Deviations:** varus or valgus of femurs or tibias, viewed from behind.
3. **Sagittal Plane Deviations:** hip flexor tightness or genu recurvatum, viewed laterally.

The examiner also observes for extremes of foot abduction or adduction and for obvious increases in the concavities under the medial and lateral malleoli. Last, the clinician looks for toe abnormalities such as bunions, clawing, or hammering. Visualization of these abnormalities could be indicative of abnormal mechanics, particularly when there is a history of overuse syndrome or pain secondary to repetitive trauma.

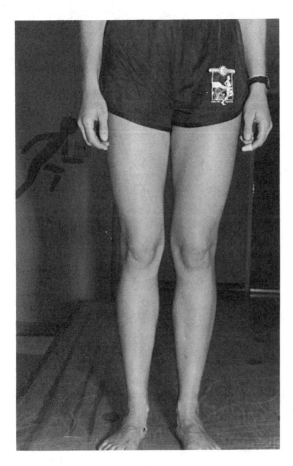

FIGURE 6–1. Observation of the patient in standing, anterior view.

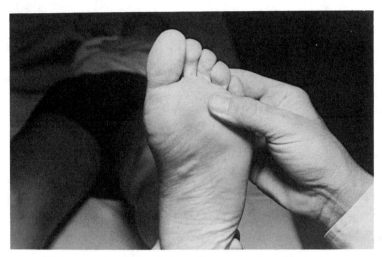

FIGURE 6-2. Check for calluses, or other skin lesions.

Next, with the patient sitting or supine, inspect the plantar aspect of the feet for calluses, keratoses, and other skin lesions (Fig. 6-2). These indicate abnormal weight-bearing and shearing forces. Calluses under the second, third, or fourth metatarsal heads are associated with abnormal pronation because of the lack of push-off provided by the first ray.[1,2] A callus on the medial aspect of the great toe is a sign that push-off is occurring from that part of the toe rather than the plantar aspect and is usually seen in hallux abductovalgus. Calluses under the first and fifth metatarsal heads, as well as along the lateral border of the foot, are usually found in abnormally supinated or cavus feet.[1]

Again, these are observations that show tendencies and relationships. The next several measurements will help to identify and quantify abnormalities and various compensations.

Lines of Bisection

In this method of static evaluation, many of the measurements employ goniometry. A clear plastic goniometer with a rounded edge and 2° increments is best. Lines of bisection are drawn on the lower third of the leg and on the calcaneus.[3] Drawn correctly, these lines provide the examiner with reference lines for goniometry, and later will be used to observe movement during gait. Without x-rays it is impossible to ensure clinically that the lines actually follow the shape of the tibia, talus, and calcaneus. The best that can be achieved are lines visualizing the long axis of the mass of the segments. To reduce but not, unfortunately, totally eliminate the chance of measurement error the lines must be (1) straight, (2) in the midline of the segments, (3) on the posterior aspect of the segments, and (4) able to be lined up continuously in space. This may require moving the calcaneus a few degrees into inversion or eversion, since the foot will not necessarily rest with the lines aligned.

PROCEDURE

The patient is prone with the foot to be measured hanging six to eight inches off the table. The leg is rotated so that the foot is perpendicular to the floor, which will help the examiner mark the back of the leg and the heel. The foot and leg can easily be stabilized by flexing and rotating the opposite limb into the "figure four" position (Fig. 6–3).

When visualizing or measuring for the midline, a series of dots is placed on the lower leg and calcaneus (Fig. 6–4A) using a straightedge and, if necessary, moving the calcaneus into a few degrees of inversion or eversion. The dots are checked to see if they will provide lines that are continuous in space (Fig. 6–4B). The leg and calcaneus lines are then drawn. To avoid soft tissue distortion, especially in standing, the lines are not connected to each other (Fig. 6–4C). Two reference lines are now available for goniometry.

Subtalar Joint Range of Motion: The Neutral Position

The two most popular methods of finding the neutral position of the subtalar joint are palpation[4] and calculation based on range of motion measurements.[3]

PROCEDURE FOR PALPATING

In the palpation technique the head of the talus anterior to the ankle joint is palpated with the thumb and the forefinger while the patient is prone (Fig. 6–5). The other hand grasps the lateral aspect of the foot at the fourth and fifth metatarsals. The foot is maximally pronated (everted), then maximally supinated (inverted). The subtalar joint neutral position is thought to be at the point in the range at which the head of the talus is felt equally on the lateral and medial sides.

Questions regarding reliability and validity arise from this technique. Palpation is dependent on individual sensitivity to condition, position, and mobility and, thus, is difficult to reproduce, particularly between examiners. Bony abnormalities of the talus may make it difficult to palpate equally the medial and lateral aspects. Additionally, the palpation is of the superior aspect of the talus (that is, close to the ankle joint), yet the techniques supposedly test movement of the subtalar joint. Last, using the palpation method makes it difficult to keep the joint in its neutral position while taking subsequent measurements. A recent study of the palpation technique showed fair intratester reliability, but poor intertester reliability.[5]

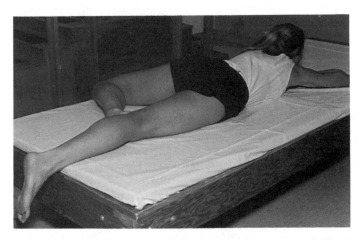

FIGURE 6–3. The prone, "figure 4 position" for static measurements; the foot is perpendicular to the floor and the opposite limb helps stabilize against the medial aspect of the knee.

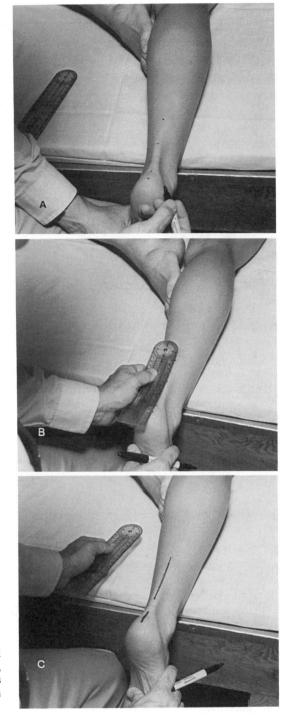

FIGURE 6–4. Midline dots are placed on the lower leg and calcaneus (A), checked to insure that they are continuous in space (B), and then connected to form two lines of bisection (C).

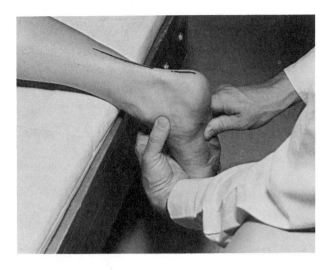

FIGURE 6–5. Palpation for the neutral position of the subtalar joint.

PROCEDURE FOR CALCULATING

An alternative to palpation is calculation of the neutral position based on subtalar range of motion.[3] By using the bisection lines previously described, range of motion is divided into a ⅓ to ⅔ ratio to determine neutral. The arms of a goniometer are placed over the lines drawn, with the axis at about the insertion of the Achilles tendon. Starting at 0° (Fig. 6–6A) the calcaneus is passively inverted (Fig. 6–6B) and the measurement is recorded. This procedure is repeated for eversion (Fig. 6–6C). Since the neutral position lies one third of the way from full eversion, it is calculated by dividing the total range by 3 and subtracting this amount from the end-range eversion (Fig. 6–7). Recent studies have shown this method to have good intertester and intratester reliability.[6,7] Because goniometry is involved, this method is more objective than palpation and provides the clinician with baseline data for future comparison.

Forefoot/Rearfoot Relationship

As discussed in detail in Chapter 2, abnormal alignment of the forefoot can influence the weightbearing position of the subtalar joint.[7] Forefoot varus is a position of inversion of the forefoot on the rearfoot, with the subtalar joint in neutral.[1,2,8] To bring the medial aspect of the foot in contact with the ground during weightbearing, the subtalar joint pronates (the calcaneus everts). Conversely, forefoot valgus, a position of eversion of the forefoot on the rearfoot with the subtalar joint in neutral, will result in subtalar supination (calcaneus inverting).[1,2,9]

These forefoot deformities should be visualized and measured in the uncompensated or non-weightbearing position. Later on, orthotic therapy based on these measurements will be designed to keep the subtalar joint from compensating into either abnormal pronation or abnormal supination.

PROCEDURE

To measure forefoot varus (Fig. 6–8), the right hand grasps the foot at the base of the fifth metatarsal. The subtalar joint is held in its predetermined neutral position with excessive ankle plantar flexion removed. One arm of the goniometer rests against the

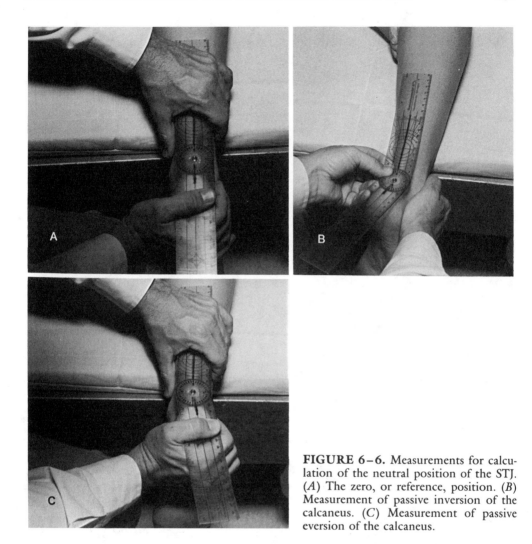

FIGURE 6–6. Measurements for calculation of the neutral position of the STJ. (*A*) The zero, or reference, position. (*B*) Measurement of passive inversion of the calcaneus. (*C*) Measurement of passive eversion of the calcaneus.

26°	Inversion
10°	Eversion
36°	Total ROM
2° Inversion	Neutral
————	FF/RF
————	KE
————	KF
————	1st MTP
————	Tibia
————	Calc

FIGURE 6–7. An example of calculating the neutral position of the subtalar joint.

EV   0°   INV

2°

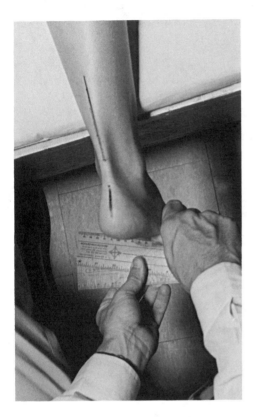

FIGURE 6–8. Measurement of forefoot varus.

metatarsal heads, while the other arm is perpendicular to the heel bisection line. Note that the axis is held laterally. The angle described by the metatarsal heads and the imaginary line perpendicular to the heel line is read and recorded. To measure forefoot valgus, the goniometer axis is held medially, but the rest of the procedure is the same.

With practice, this procedure has shown very good reliability.[6,7] However, care must be taken to reduce the chance of measurement error. Since the lines describing the forefoot/rearfoot angle are several inches apart (from the heel to the metatarsal heads), the foot must be held carefully and viewed along its long axis. This procedure is aided by gently dorsiflexing the ankle to the point of resistance. Avoid dorsiflexing the foot too forcefully, which may momentarily distort the forefoot/rearfoot relationship being measured.

Ankle Joint Dorsiflexion

Ankle joint equinus is a limitation of dorsiflexion at the ankle joint, which can cause the subtalar joint to compensate in weightbearing by pronating abnormally.[1,2,9] The limitation can be caused by tightness of the gastrocnemius/soleus muscle group, bony abnormality at the ankle, or periarticular connective tissue restrictions brought on by trauma or immobilization. Regardless of its cause, equinus must be determined, because it may be a reason for abnormal subtalar joint compensation.

PROCEDURE

With the patient still prone, ankle dorsiflexion is measured by placing the rounded edge of a goniometer at the contour of the heel, while the arms are aligned with the long axes of the fibula and the fifth metatarsal, respectively (Fig. 6–9A). The foot is passively dorsiflexed, and the measurement is recorded (plus or minus 90°). The clinician should try to reduce the possibility of measurement error by:

1. Holding the subtalar joint in neutral position and observing the bisection lines; allowing the foot to pronate may give a false positive recording of dorsiflexion.
2. Pushing dorsally at the midfoot; pushing too far distally on the foot can also give a false positive recording if the midfoot area is hypermobile, as in talipes equinus.

This measurement can be repeated with the knee in flexion (Fig. 6–9B) to help differentiate between soleus and gastrocnemius tightness.

Standing Tibial Measurement

In addition to compensating for forefoot and ankle abnormalities, the subtalar joint can also respond in weightbearing to the position of the tibia. For example, excessive

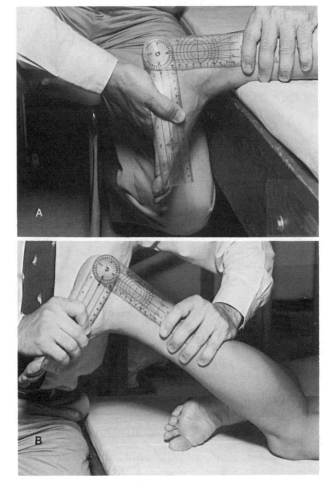

FIGURE 6–9. Measurement of ankle dorsiflexion with the knee extended (*A*) and flexed (*B*).

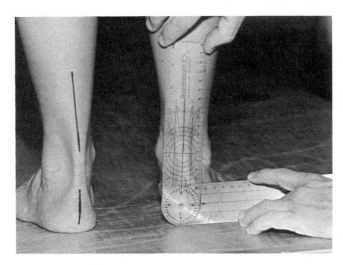

FIGURE 6-10. Standing tibial measurement showing tibial varum.

tibial varus can cause the subtalar joint to pronate to bring the medial aspect of the foot to the floor.[1] While there is no normative data with respect to tibial position, it should be measured, especially in cases where excessive calcaneal valgus does not seem to be caused solely by forefoot varus or ankle joint equinus. Additionally, if tibial position is thought to be an important factor in the calcaneal response, the rearfoot post will be an important part of the eventual orthotic prescription.

PROCEDURE

The leg bisection line is measured in relation to the horizontal surface. One arm of the goniometer rests on the standing surface, while the other arm is placed on the leg bisection line (Fig. 6-10). The measurement is recorded as 0° (vertical) or in degrees of varus or valgus.

Standing Calcaneal Measurement

This measurement assumes that the subtalar joint should be at or near its neutral position in relaxed bipedal standing. The calcaneal bisection line is measured in relation to the horizontal surface.

PROCEDURE

With the patient in a relaxed, balanced stance, one arm of the goniometer rests on the firm level surface, and the other arm is placed on the calcaneal bisection line (Fig. 6-11). The measurement is then recorded as 0° (vertical), or as a deviation in degrees into inversion or eversion. At this point the clinician must ask two questions:

1. How many degrees away from predicted neutral is the calcaneus?
2. In what direction is the calcaneus oriented?

For example, if the predicted subtalar joint neutral position is 2° of inversion, and the standing calcaneal measurement is 8° of eversion, the subtalar joint is actually in 10° of

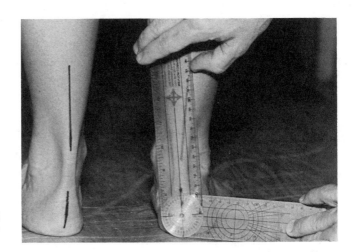

FIGURE 6–11. Standing calcaneal measurement showing 8° of eversion.

eversion (Fig. 6–12). It is also pronated 10° from neutral, perhaps because of forefoot varus, Achilles tendon tightness, or other reasons.

Now that the pathomechanical, compensated position has been determined, gait can be analyzed to observe for abnormal responses of the subtalar joint.

First Ray Position and Mobility

While the patient remains prone, the position of the distal aspect of the first ray is noted. Specifically, the clinician looks for a plantar flexed first ray; that is, when the subtalar joint is held in neutral, the head of the first metatarsal is now in a plantar flexed position relative to the other four.[1]

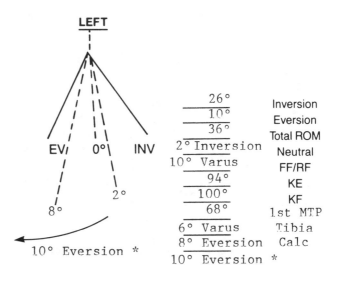

FIGURE 6–12. An example of subtalar joint pronation.

PROCEDURE

Mobility of the first ray is checked by moving it in dorsal and plantar directions while stabilizing metatarsal heads two through five (Fig. 6–13). If it is fixed or hypomobile, the subtalar joint will have to invert (supinate) to bring the lateral aspect of the foot into contact with the ground.[1] A fixed, plantar flexed first ray is measured similarly to forefoot valgus (see forefoot/rearfoot measurement).

First Metatarsophalangeal Joint Range of Motion

A limitation of first metatarsophalangeal (MTP) joint mobility, especially dorsiflexion, can result in gait deviations that promote excessive pronation.[1] Sixty to sixty-five degrees of dorsiflexion is sufficient to prevent these deviations at push-off.[1]

PROCEDURE

The foot is stabilized with one hand as the arms of the goniometer are placed on the long axes of the first ray and the first proximal phalanx. The hallux is dorsiflexed passively and the measurement is recorded as shown in Figure 6–14.

Table 6–1 presents a summary of the static evaluation procedures, listed according to patient position.

DYNAMIC EVALUATION: GAIT ANALYSIS

Gait analysis is used to determine deviations from the normal, or at least ideal, gait pattern. The clinician is looking for signs of abnormal mechanics: pronation or supination occurring at the wrong time during the stance phase of gait.

Gait analysis is best accomplished with the patient on a treadmill, so that repeated cycles can be watched easily. However, the patient should also be observed walking on the floor, since gait patterns used on a treadmill are often different. Gait should be analyzed when the patient is barefoot, in shoes, and eventually, in shoes with orthotics. To assist in specific observations, additional marks are placed on the medial aspect of

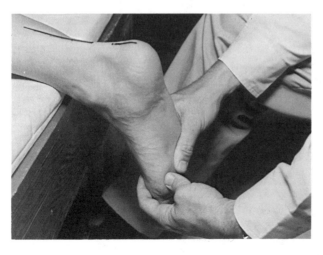

FIGURE 6–13. Checking mobility of the first ray.

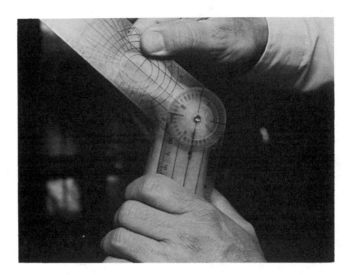

FIGURE 6–14. Measuring dorsiflexion of the first metatarsophalangeal joint.

the foot at the medial malleolus, the navicular tuberosity, and the first MTP joint. All are easily palpable and can be marked as shown in Figure 6–15. The X on the navicular tubercle is observed from the side in relation to the other marks. This observation demonstrates how the medial longitudinal arch rises and falls during various aspects of gait and how the navicular tubercle protrudes to and from the midline. The calcaneal bisection line is used to observe from behind for calcaneal movement, which is primarily in the frontal plane.

Normal Gait

The following discussion briefly summarizes the major characteristics of normal gait:[1,9,10]

TABLE 6–1 Summary of Static Measurements

Procedure	Patient Position
Observation	Standing
Check for calluses	Sitting or supine
Bisection lines	
Subtalar inversion	
Subtalar eversion	
Subtalar neutral	
Forefoot/rearfoot relationship	Prone
Ankle dorsiflexion	
First ray position	
First ray mobility	
Tibia	
Calcaneus	Standing

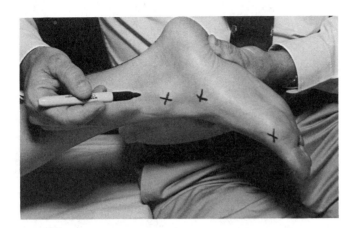

FIGURE 6–15. Placing marks on the medial aspect of the foot: the medial malleolus, the navicular tubercle, and the medial aspect of the first MTP joint.

HEEL STRIKE

The calcaneus is in a neutral to inverted (supinated) position; the navicular is in an upward position along with the medial longitudinal arch; the tibia is externally rotated.

HEEL STRIKE TO FOOTFLAT (NORMAL PRONATION)

The calcaneus everts as the midtarsal joint "unlocks," causing the talus to move medially; the tibia rotates internally. As noted in Chapter 1, these provide shock absorption, accommodation to the walking surface, and attenuation of lower extremity internal rotation. The foot reaches maximum pronation at footflat.

MIDSTANCE

The foot has reached maximal pronation. The navicular and medial longitudinal arch are down and protrude medially; the tibia is rotated internally. In early midstance, a reversal of pronation begins as the tibia is moving anterior to the talus and the subtalar joint passes through neutral. In late midstance, the subtalar joint is supinating.

HEEL-OFF TO TOE-OFF (NORMAL SUPINATION)

The calcaneus inverts from the fully everted position; the midtarsal joint "locks," moving the talus in a lateral direction; the tibia rotates externally; the foot is abducted no more than 10°–15°. The foot and lower limb are now rigid levers for propulsion.

SWING

The ankle is dorsiflexed to clear the floor; the foot is inverted to prepare for the next heel strike. With a knowledge of what should occur during stance in a normal gait, various types of abnormal pronation and supination can be analyzed.

Abnormal Pronation

Three types of abnormal pronation are seen clinically:

1. **Failure to Resupinate.** Normal pronation occurs from heel strike to footflat. During push-off, from heel-off to toe-off, the subtalar and midtarsal joints stay in their pronated positions; therefore there is a loss of a rigid lever.
2. **Late Pronation during Push-Off.** From heel strike to midstance there is little or no pronatory movement of the subtalar or midtarsal joints. From heel-off to toe-off the calcaneus suddenly everts, the navicular falls, and the foot whips into excessive abduction; therefore there is little shock absorption and, again, loss of a rigid lever.
3. **Early Excessive Pronation.** The subtalar and midtarsal joints are pronated throughout the entire stance phase. Because they are fully pronated at heel strike there is no range of motion left for normal pronation. The foot does not supinate in push-off or in swing; therefore, both shock absorption and the rigid lever are lost.

Abnormal Supination

The supinated or high-arched foot can be classified as pes cavus, pes equinocavus, or pes cavovarus.[11] In any case, gait analysis reveals a somewhat inverted calcaneus and an elevated navicular and medial longitudinal arch throughout stance. A rigid lever will be maintained at push-off, but with no normal pronation after heel strike, there is reduced shock absorption. Table 6–2 is a summary of typical observations noted during gait analysis for normal, pronated, and supinated feet.

CASE STUDY

Now that all static and dynamic evaluation procedures have been described, a case study is provided as an example. A 37-year-old factory assembly line inspector presented with a one-year history of pain on the plantar aspect of the second metatarsophalangeal joint aggravated by walking. This was especially true at work where he walks eight to ten hours a day on a concrete surface. X-rays and an examination by an orthopaedist were negative. The diagnosis was capsulitis of the second MTP joint.

Static biomechanical evaluation findings are shown in Figure 6–16. Gait analysis revealed pronation throughout the stance phase of gait, especially on the right. Specifically, the calcaneus was everted, and a collapse of the medial arch was noted at heel strike. The pronated position of the foot was maintained throughout the stance phase of gait. The instability of the foot during push-off caused excessive abduction of the forefoot. These findings indicated early, excessive pronation. Specifically, there was abnormal pronation from heel strike to footflat, which caused a decrease in shock absorption. Additionally, there was no supination during the push-off phase of stance. Therefore the patient was pushing off from a less than rigid lever. In this case, the first ray was hypermobile because of the pronation and was unable to adequately resist ground reaction force during push-off. Therefore, the second metatarsal joint progressively became more weightbearing. Additionally, the second metatarsal head was rotating and shearing against the ground because of the sudden abduction at push-off. At this point,

TABLE 6–2 Observations during the Stance Phase of Gait

Gait Pattern	Heel Strike		Heel Strike to Footflat		Push-Off	
	Calcaneus	Navicular	Calcaneus	Navicular	Calcaneus	Navicular
Normal	Neutral to inverted	Up	Everts	Drops	Inverts	Rises
Late pronation (fails to resupinate)	Neutral to inverted	Up	Everts	Drops	Stays everted	Stays down
Late pronation at push-off	Neutral to inverted	Up	Stays inverted	Stays up	Inverts	Drops
Early, excessive pronation	At or near full eversion	Down	Everts	Down	Stays everted	Stays down
Abnormal supination	Neutral to inverted	Up	Stays inverted	Stays up	Stays inverted	Up

EVALUATION WORKSHEET

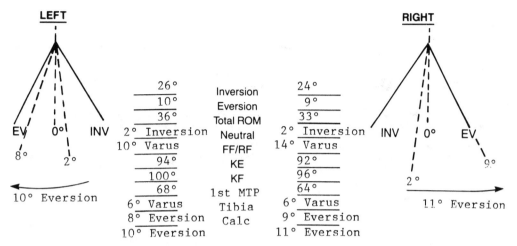

FIGURE 6-16. Case study: Summary of static evaluation findings.

temporary orthotics would be constructed that would enhance shock absorption and help to provide a rigid lever for push-off by reducing the amount of subtalar joint compensation for the various limitations.

REFERENCES

1. Root, ML, Orien, WP, and Weed, JH: Clinical Biomechanics, Vol II: Normal and Abnormal Function of the Foot. Clinical Biomechanics, Los Angeles, 1977.
2. Donatelli, RA: Abnormal biomechanics of the foot and ankle. J Orthop Sports Phys Ther 9(1):11, 1987.
3. Root, ML, et al: Biomechanical Examination of the Foot. Clinical Biomechanics, Los Angeles, 1971.
4. James, SL: Chondromalacia patellae. In Kennedy, J (ed): The Injured Adolescent Knee. Williams & Wilkins, Baltimore, 1976.
5. Elveru, RA, Rothstein, JM, and Lamb, RL: Goniometric reliability in a clinical setting subtalar and ankle joint measurements. Phys Ther 68(5):672, 1988.
6. Cantu, R, Catlin, PA, and Wooden, MJ: A comparison of two measurement tools and two techniques for measuring the forefoot/rearfoot relationship. Emory University Physical Therapy Department unpublished material, 1987.
7. Garbalosa, J, McClure, M, Catlin, PA, and Wooden, MJ: The forefoot/rearfoot relationship in the normal population. Emory University Physical Therapy Department: unpublished material, 1988.
8. Digiovanni, J, and Smith, S: Normal biomechanics of the adult rearfoot. J Am Podiatr Assoc 66:812, 1976.
9. Subotnick, S: Podiatric Sports Medicine. Futura Publishing, Los Angeles, 1975.
10. Donatelli, RA: Normal biomechanics of the foot and ankle. J Orthop Sports Phys Ther 7(3):91, 1985.
11. Tachdjian, MO: The Child's Foot. WB Saunders, Philadelphia, 1985.

APPENDIX:

Dynamic Assessment of Foot Mechanics as an Adjunct to Orthotic Prescription

I. J. Alexander, MD
K. R. Campbell, PhD

Detailed analysis of frontal plane mechanics of the foot through its examination at rest contributes significantly to the effective treatment of patients with foot and ankle complaints. A number of stress phenomena related to frontal plane deformities can be alleviated by the appropriate correction of the foot mechanics through the utilization of orthotics, and in some cases, shoe modification. Currently the assumption is made that static frontal plane deformities produce predictable alterations in the dynamic stance phase mechanics of the foot. On the basis of the static evaluation, orthotics, which are thought to correct faulty stance phase mechanics, are fabricated and modified. The effectiveness of these orthotics in relieving a variety of stress phenomena in the foot and ankle, or more proximally in the lower limb, supports the belief that the desired alterations in dynamic stance phase mechanics do occur.

Evolving advances in technology will soon provide a means to objectively document foot mechanics with a high degree of accuracy. With the two techniques described here, the usefulness of the static examination as a predictor of stance phase kinematics can be assessed, and the effectiveness of orthotic correction in altering dynamic foot mechanics can be evaluated.

The first of the two techniques measures dynamic foot pressure distribution using force platforms and has evolved over the past 30 years. The second, newer technique of three-dimensional kinematic analysis of limb motion applies to the moving foot. These two techniques make it possible to accurately document the motion characteristics of the normal, the deformed, and the neurologically impaired foot and to assess the effects of both orthotic and surgical intervention.

TECHNIQUE 1: DYNAMIC PLANTAR PRESSURE DISTRIBUTION

The assessment of dynamic plantar pressure distribution has been approached from two perspectives. The devices available record data either from a single step or to a floor-mounted device, or from multiple steps sensing pressure from transducers taped to the foot or incorporated in the shoe sole.

Two types of floor-mounted devices exist. One is based on optical recording of pressure-dependent light intensity or wavelength patterns, which, by scaling, can be converted into pressure values. The other technique is dependent on recording from an array of individual electronic transducers that are mounted on the floor. An example of this approach can be seen in Figure 6–17, which illustrates foot pressure distribution from a patient with right rigid forefoot varus and flexible compensatory hindfoot valgus and a normal left foot pressure pattern.

Shoe-mounted transducers present numerous technical problems, and the extensive modification necessary to the shoes makes the approach a relatively impractical

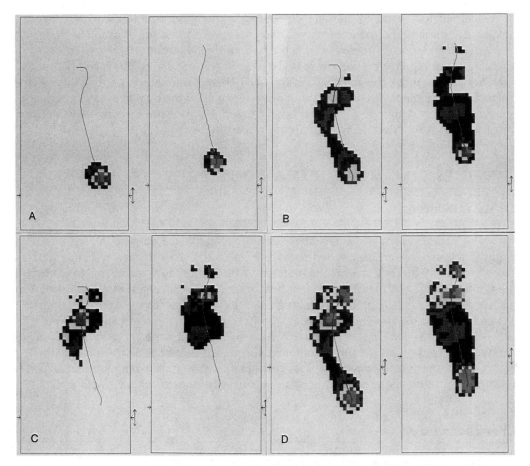

FIGURE 6–17. Sequence of foot pressure distribution in a patient with a rigid forefoot varus and compensatory hindfoot valgus (*right*) matched with stance phase pressure distribution of a "normal" subject (*left*) (*A*) Heel strike; (*B*) footflat; (*C*) heel off; (*D*) summated pressures from entire stance phase.

method of assessing plantar pressure distribution. In-shoe transducers, which are usually taped to the sole of the foot, have been utilized extensively. The quantitative accuracy of most commercially available transducers has been poor, necessitating frequent calibration. In addition, replacing transducers in the same locations on the sole of the foot can present reliability problems in serial studies.

Assessing dynamic plantar load distribution in barefoot subjects with floor-mounted devices is likely to be most helpful in studying the mechanics of normal and abnormal feet. Normal variations in foot structure and motion are reflected in different patterns of dynamic load distribution under the foot. Correlating these patterns with static structural variations noted on mechanical assessment of the foot will improve our understanding of the importance of these structural differences. In abnormal feet, the differences are magnified and the effects of therapeutic interventions to change load-bearing patterns will be more easily recognized. The in-shoe transducers or transducer mats will be most useful in evaluating the effectiveness of orthotics and shoe modification in altering weightbearing patterns under the foot.

The capabilities of currently available commercial devices are impressive. Resolution of the fixed-floor units is as good as 2×3 mm, and sampling rates of the transducer matrices are as high as 70 Hz. Sophisticated software available with some of these units offers automated center of pressure determination, whole-foot and area-specific automated determination of contact time, contact area, peak pressure, load in Newtons per cm^2, and impulse (an integration of total load and contact time). One system is even capable of storing information on preselected areas of interest, to allow comparison of identical areas under the foot before and after therapeutic intervention. Tests of the transducer type matrix have shown that reproducibility of the obtained data is high and that accuracy is within 5%. We will briefly describe two commercially available foot pressure measuring devices with quantitative capabilities.

DEVICES FOR MEASURING FOOT PRESSURE

EMED System

The EMED system is a capacitance-transducer matrix–based system with a variety of available sensor densities, two sensors per cm^2 and 4 sensors per cm^2 being utilized most frequently for foot pressure assessment. A calibration device is available to ensure continued sensor accuracy. The system has a number of collection area sizes available and is capable of collecting data at rates greater than 100 Hz. For dynamic foot pressure assessment, the usual sampling rate is 70 Hz. The EMED system can be adapted to connect to an in-shoe transducer mat which will give in-shoe pressure distribution. Early prototypes of this system do not offer the resolution of the floor-mounted device.

On an experimental basis, the floor-mounted matrices have been mounted on force platforms to allow measurement of simultaneous shear forces under the foot.

Pedabarograph

The Pedabarograph is an optics-based system that utilizes the critical light reflection technique to assess pressure distribution under the foot. The transducer-mounted glass plate of the system is illuminated from the sides and covered with a deformable plastic mat. When pressure is applied to the overlying mat, it is apposed to the glass surface and the normally internally reflected light is allowed to scatter. Greater pressure applied to the mat increases the contact area between the mat and the glass plate, producing more intense emission of light. The image is recorded through stance by a video camera. Utilizing gray scale conversion, which assigns pressure values to different intensities of light, pressure maps are generated at a sampling rate of 30 Hz. This system has the potential for measurement of simultaneous shear forces.

Both systems provide software that allows determination of area-specific peak pressure and impulse, the pressure-time integral. This allows prospective assessment of plantar pressure effects of therapeutic intervention.

TECHNIQUE 2: THREE-DIMENSIONAL KINEMATIC ANALYSIS

Kinematic analysis of stance phase of the foot using gait analysis techniques promises to provide information of even greater value than plantar pressure studies. Although a number of methods of tracking limb motion have been devised, our experience has been with computerized tracking of video camera images of retroreflective

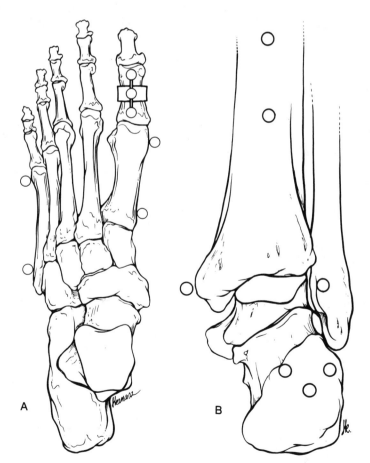

FIGURE 6–18. Posterior diagram (*left*) and a dorsal diagram (*right*) of the skeleton indicate the location of reflective markers on the foot and tibia.

markers. The subcutaneous location of many bony landmarks in the foot helps eliminate errors due to soft tissue shear so often experienced in motion studies of the more proximal limb.

For evaluation of each foot, 14 retroreflective markers are used (Fig. 6–18). Two are placed on the anterior tibia, one over each of the malleoli, three on the calcaneus, and one marker is placed over the base and the head of the first and fifth metatarsals, providing four forefoot markers. To analyze great toe motion, three markers are on wands attached to a plate wrapped over the top of the proximal phalanx of the hallux. Four cameras record the paths of each marker, and computer integration of the multiple two-dimensional pathways formulates a three-dimensional trajectory for each marker. Computerized comparison of marker positions within selected coordinate systems allows determination of the relative motion of selected marked parts. Calcaneal, mid-foot, and forefoot inversion-eversion, plantar flexion, dorsiflexion, and transverse plane rotation (calcaneal internal-external rotation), forefoot adduction-abduction can be as-sessed. Great toe flexion and extension, varus and valgus deviation, and frontal plane rotation can also be analyzed. While the accuracy of these determinations appears to be great, confirmation awaits studies made with pins placed directly into bone.

As with the quantitative study of dynamic foot pressure, three-dimensional kine-matic analysis of foot motion provides an opportunity to objectively correlate the static evaluation with actual stance phase mechanics. In addition, the mechanical effects of therapeutic interventions, both orthotic and surgical, can be evaluated using this technique.

CHAPTER 7

Evaluation of Overuse Syndromes

Bruce Greenfield, MMSc, PT

This chapter focuses on major overuse injuries of the lower extremities according to specific anatomic sites and tissues. The pathophysiology of overuse injuries is a local inflammatory response to stress. The causes of overuse injuries are either intrinsic (malalignment syndromes, muscle imbalances) or extrinsic (training error) to the patient. Intrinsic and extrinsic factors are further classified as predisposing, precipitating, or perpetuating factors. A systematic musculoskeletal assessment is therefore necessary in order to differentiate overuse injuries and to clarify the etiologic factors. Effective treatment is predicated on recognizing and correcting the underlying etiologic factors. Case studies are presented illustrating the problem-solving approach to evaluation and treatment of overuse injuries. Each case delineates and explains predisposing, precipitating, and perpetuating factors related to the overuse injury. Treatment programs that address and correct these factors are presented.

DEFINITION OF OVERUSE INJURIES

Swimming, cycling, and running continue to grow in popularity. A 1985 Gallup poll indicated that 15% of all Americans (approximately 30 million persons) jog regularly.[1] In 1984, over 100,000 persons completed marathons, and over 1 million competed in triathalons. The 1984 Ironman triathalon in Hawaii, which combines a two-mile ocean swim, 112 miles of cycling, and a marathon run, had over 10,000 applicants for 1,000 available entries.[2] Not surprisingly, injuries to the participants of these events are increasing. As far back as 1977, a *Runner's World* poll indicated that two thirds of all joggers suffer injuries to their lower extremities.[3] Marti and associates,[4] in a survey of 4,358 male joggers, found that 45.8% had sustained jogging injuries during a one-year period. Many of the injuries did not result from a single traumatic episode (i.e., a high-velocity force that produced sprain, strain, or fracture of ligaments, muscles, or bones, respectively). Instead, most of these injuries occurred insidiously, resulting from

153

overuse of various musculoskeletal tissues. Overuse injuries result from repetitive sub-traumatic forces. Breakdown of microscopic tissue occurs faster than the tissue can heal or repair itself. The results are inflammation, muscle strain, stress fractures, ligament failure, tendinitis, and tendon ruptures.[5]

Inflammatory Response

The essential component in all overuse injuries, regardless of the affected anatomic tissue, is inflammation. The repetitive force of overuse results in tissue microtrauma, which triggers inflammation.

Following injury, initial vasoconstriction and hemostasis is followed within minutes by local vasodilatation and increased intracapillary pressure, which leads to transudation of fluid. Prostaglandins, a group of vasoactive substances, cause vasodilatation and increased vascular permeability. Prolonged capillary permeability results in exudation of fluid, swelling, and pain.[6] The initial medical treatment of overuse is the administration of nonsteroidal anti-inflammatory agent, which inhibits prostaglandin synthesis.[7]

As inflammation continues, neutrophil, monocyte, and eosinophil cells migrate to the area. The neutrophil cells initiate degradation of surrounding tissue through activation of protealytic enzymes contained within their lysosomes. After a few days, neutrophil cells are replaced by monocyte cells, which in turn differentiate into macrophage cells. Macrophage cells which contain proteolytic enzymes digest cellular debris and connective tissue fragments. Lymphocyte cells are important in chronic inflammation and activate monocyte cells. Monocyte cells, which contain and release proteolytic enzymes, perpetuate the inflammatory response.

Other cells, including endothelial and fibroblast cells, migrate within a few days to the injured area and produce capillary buds and collagen, respectively, to begin the reparative process. Maturation of collagen is a relatively long-term process, and the patient must modify his or her activities for the next few weeks in order to rest the injured area. For a runner, activity modification can vary from simply decreasing training distances to actually being limited to non-weightbearing activity. An activity level is developed that allows unabated healing and scar maturation.

The clinician must recognize that inflammation is a necessary component of healing. Motion applied to the injured area during the initial inflammatory response can lead to chronic inflammation and destruction of surrounding tissues. The goal, therefore, in treating overuse injuries is to minimize chronic inflammation to allow healing.

ETIOLOGY

Factors leading to overuse injuries can be subgrouped as either predisposing, precipitating, or perpetuating (Table 7-1). These factors can be further classified as intrinsic and extrinsic.

Predisposing Factors

Predisposing factors are intrinsic to the patient and include malalignment syndromes, leg length discrepancy, and muscle dysfunction of the lower extremity. Several studies have identified malalignment syndrome in overuse injuries.[8-13] James, Bates,

TABLE 7-1 Etiologic Factors in Overuse Injuries

Predisposing (Intrinsic)	Precipitating (Extrinsic)	Perpetuating (Intrinsic and Extrinsic)
Malalignment syndromes Leg length discrepancy Muscle dysfunction	Training errors Running surfaces Shoes and equipment	Combination of intrinsic and extrinsic

and Ostering,[8] in a series of 180 patients with 232 overuse injuries, identified prolonged or excessive pronation of the ankle and foot[8] in 58% of the patients. Clement,[9] in a retrospective survey of 1,650 runners with overuse injuries, found in a majority of these runners, anatomic malalignment, including a leg length discrepancy, femoral bone anteversion, and excessive pronation of the ankle and foot.[9] Viitasale and Kvist[10] found a greater prevalence of abnormal subtalar joint pronation in runners with shin splints than in asymptomatic runners.[10] Lutter[11] reviewed 171 overuse injuries to 121 runners and found excessive pronation to be an etiologic factor in approximately 56% of the injuries.[11] Lilletvedt, Kreighbaum, and Philips[12] found a statistically greater number of malalignment problems (including tibia varum and excessive pronation) in athletes with shin splints, than in athletes without shin splints.[12] DeLacerda[13] found that a statistically significant number of subjects with excessive pronation developed shin splints after 14 weeks of controlled exercises.[13]

Overuse injuries in the lower extremities can result from excessive pronation in the foot and ankle, leg length discrepancy, and muscle dysfunction. The pathomechanical responses in the lower extremities for each of these predisposing factors are discussed below.

ABNORMAL PRONATION

The pathomechanics of excessive pronation can be understood by looking at gait and at the normal foot during heel strike. Ambulation is a series of rotations, starting at the lumbar spine, that propel the body through space. The transverse rotations of the tibia and the femur are transmitted and reduced at the subtalar joint. During the stance phase of gait, the foot does not rotate. The tibia rotates internally at heel strike and the talus of the ankle follows, resulting in pronation of the subtalar joint, or heel eversion.[14]

Normal mechanics dictate that the tibiofemoral joint extend and the lower extremity rotate externally at midstance. The calcaneus inverts and the talus is pushed by the sustentaculum tali of the calcaneus into a lateral position. The midtarsal joint locks, and the foot becomes a rigid lever for toe-off.[14]

Excessive subtalar joint pronation results in internal rotation of the tibia and delays the external rotation of the lower extremity that accompanies subtalar joint supination. Compensatory internal rotation of the femur may occur, disrupting the normal biomechanics of the lower extremity and altering patellofemoral joint tracking. Excessive pressure between the lateral facet of the patella and the lateral condyle of the femur may result.[15] Excessive pronation fatigues the anterior and posterior tibialis muscles which are attempting to support the medial border of the foot. Stress is passed upward through the foot to the medial aspect of the knee and hip. This stress may not be significant during the act of walking, but during running increased weight and rotation stresses are produced along the lower extremity. The increased stress can result in tissue fatigue and microtrauma followed by inflammation.

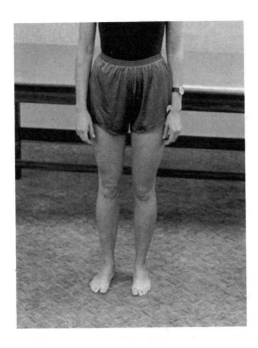

FIGURE 7–1. Miserable malalignment. Femur bone anteversion with squinting patella bone; proximal external tibia bone torsion; tibia bone varum; and subtalar joint pronation.

"Miserable malalignment" is also associated with overuse injuries.[15] Miserable malalignment, as described by James,[16] is a series of compensatory torsional and frontal plane changes in the lower extremities. Figure 7-1 shows an example of miserable malalignment, illustrating anteversion of the femur, proximal external torsion of the tibia, tibia varum, and subtalar joint pronation. Miserable malalignment with proximal external torsion of the tibia results in an increased Q angle of the extensor mechanism in the knee. An increased Q angle in the knee results in lateral tracking of the patella, and predisposes toward chondromalacia patellae.[16]

LEG LENGTH DISCREPANCY

Leg length discrepancies have been associated with various musculoskeletal problems. Giles and Taylor[17] found that over twice as many patients with low back pain have a leg length discrepancy of 10 mm or more. Bolz and Davies[18] found that in subjects with a leg length discrepancy of 0.5 cm or more, total leg strength was reduced in the short leg. Subotnick[19] examined 4,000 athletes over six years and found that 40% had either a functional or anatomic leg length discrepancy. A patient may attempt to equalize a leg length discrepancy by internally rotating the long leg. The resultant subtalar joint pronation functionally shortens the long leg. However, this posture of excessive pronation produces excessive strain along the medial structures of the ankle and knee, resulting in overuse, and pathologic changes of related soft tissues.

MUSCLE DYSFUNCTION

Muscle dysfunctions associated with overuse injuries include imbalances between the quadriceps femoris and hamstring muscles at the knee and the gastrocnemius-soleus and anterior tibialis muscles at the ankle and foot.

Muscle is the best force attenuator in the body.[20] Eccentric or lengthening action of muscle dampens the forces of weightbearing. At heel strike, the lower limb is slowly lowered to the ground. Flexion at the knee is controlled by the eccentric action of the quadriceps femoris muscle. The foot is lowered to the ground by the eccentric contractions of the anterior tibialis, extensor hallucis longus, and extensor digitorum longus muscles. The anterior movement of the tibia over the talus during midstance is controlled by the gastrocnemius-soleus muscle group.[21]

Alterations in muscle function include muscle weakness, poor flexibility, and inadequate endurance for musculoskeletal performance during specific functional activities. Alteration in muscle function results in inadequate or abnormal movement patterns during activities such as running. For example, Elliot and Achland[5] used high-speed cinematography to study the effect of fatigue on the mechanical characteristics of running in highly skilled long distance runners. They found that, toward the end of a race, the runners exhibited less efficient positioning of the foot at foot strike as well as decreased stride length and stride rate. Alteration in muscle function during running can cause bone, ligament, and tendon to be overworked, producing tissue breakdown and pathology.[5]

Hamstring muscle tightness in the presence of quadriceps femoris muscle weakness has been associated with anterior knee pain, including chondromalacia patellae.[16] In the presence of hamstring muscle tightness, patellofemoral joint compressive forces increase during the swing-through phase of gait or recovery phase of running. Quadriceps femoris muscle weakness, especially in the vastus medialis muscle, can result in lateral patellar tracking during knee flexion and extension. The result can be abnormal retropatellar stresses along the lateral facet of the patella with cartilage degeneration. Because the quadriceps femoris muscle controls knee flexion during the stance phase of walking or running, weakness can result in increased shock to the ankle and knee. Such abnormal stresses can lead to hyaline cartilage microtrauma and degeneration. Quadriceps femoris muscle weakness, therefore, places increased stress on the knee and ankle, resulting, with repetitive exercise, in overuse.[16]

Imbalance between gastrocnemius-soleus muscles and weak pretibial muscles, anterior tibialis, extensor hallucis longus, and extensor digitorum longus muscles have been associated with anterior shin splints, especially during repetitive hill running.[22] During uphill running the pretibial muscles forcefully contract in the recovery phase of running to dorsiflex the ankle, allowing the foot to clear the surface of the ground. Additionally, during downhill running, at heel strike, the pretibial muscles contract eccentrically to control ankle plantar flexion and prevent foot-slap. Overactivation of these muscles can occur in the presence of tight antagonists (the gastrocnemius-soleus muscles). The result may be microtrauma and inflammation of the pretibial muscles, tendons, and bony attachments.[22]

Precipitating Factors

In contrast to the predisposing factors, which are intrinsic, the precipitating factors in overuse injuries are extrinsic (see Table 7-1). According to Cavanaugh,[23] the average runner's pace is 3.83 meters per second, and the foot strikes the ground approximately 5,100 times each hour. The ground reaction force at midstance in running is 250 to 300% of body weight.[1] An average runner, therefore, experiences in one hour a tremendous amount of force through the lower extremities. Not surprisingly, therefore, according to James and associates,[8] training errors are associated with 60% of overuse injuries. Specifically, they found excessive mileage, the intensity of workouts, and a too rapid change in a training routine to be the major training errors. According to Clancy,[24] a series of high-intensity workouts does not allow the tissues in the lower extremity to recover from fatigue and microtrauma.

EXCESSIVE MILEAGE

Excessive mileage may culminate in fatigue of leg muscles. Muscle fatigue is characterized by impaired ability of the muscle to generate normal strength and endurance levels after vigorous exercise. Some of the biomechanical processes that are active in or responsible for the onset of fatigue are neuromuscular and chemical.[25]

Successive days of heavy training deplete glycogen stores in specific muscle fibers, such as the gastrocnemius-soleus muscles, that are used to absorb shock and propel. During midstance phase of running, the gastrocnemius-soleus muscle acts eccentrically to control movement of the tibia over the foot. The gastrocnemius-soleus muscles contract concentrically at toe-off to propel the body. The tensile loading during the contraction, combined with gravitational elongation, is extremely high. When the muscles are depleted of fluid, irritated, and repeatedly contracted, greater stress is placed on tendons, which are undergoing extraordinary stretch.[25] Microtearing of the fascicles of the tendon results in inflammation. Continued running in the presence of microtears and inflammation perpetuates the inflammatory response, thereby creating further tearing and inflammation.

RUNNING SURFACES

Hard, uneven, or sloping surfaces cause increased ground-reactive forces, altering normal biomechanics and producing injury.[24] For example, running along the transverse grade or gutter of a road causes increased pronation of the uphill foot and supination of the downhill foot. The heel of the uphill foot angles into valgus and the subtalar joint pronates. The excessive or prolonged pronation increases the stress on the foot and ankle structures and produces obligatory internal rotation of the tibia. The prolonged tibial rotation may produce strain of the medial knee structures.

As mentioned previously, uphill running requires increased dorsiflexion of the ankle during both the recovery and support phases. Increased dorsiflexion also occurs at the first metatarsophalangeal (MTP) joint, and increased tension occurs on the plantar fascia and gastrocnemius-soleus muscles. Strain along the plantar fascia results from the windlass effect,[26] which results in tightening of the plantar fascia with hyperextension of the MTP joints. This increased strain can result in microtrauma to the first MTP joint, plantar fasciitis, and Achilles tendinitis.

SHOES AND EQUIPMENT

Improper equipment selection, including inadequate running shoes, also can precipitate an overuse injury. Excessive wear along the outsole, a nonflexible outsole, and flared-in shoe last, inadequate heel cushion, and a small toe box, have all been implicated as factors in overuse injuries.[24] For example, a nonflexible outsole may reduce the ability of the foot to pronate at the midstance phase of running. A shoe with an inadequate heel cushion reduces the ability of the foot to dissipate ground reaction forces at heel strike. The result of both of these problems is an increase of forces and stress along the heel, ankle, and foot. In addition, excessive wear along the outsole of the shoe may perpetuate excessive pronation during the support phase of running. The resultant obligatory internal rotation of the leg results in increased stress along the medial structures in the ankle and knee.

Perpetuating Factors

Overuse injuries, especially in athletes, are often difficult to treat because the athlete usually resumes the same training pattern (precipitating factors) under the same pathomechanical conditions (predisposing factors) that initially caused the injury. The perpetuating factors of overuse injuries, therefore, are the combination of the precipitating and perpetuating factors discussed above (see Table 7-1). To successfully treat overuse injuries the predisposing and precipitating factors must be eliminated or modified. For each patient the clinician must evaluate lower extremity biomechanics and muscle flexibility and strength and have a thorough knowledge of the anatomic demands of the sport, the environment in which the athlete is performing, and the equipment and training techniques involved.

CLARIFYING ASSESSMENT OF THE LOWER EXTREMITIES

Evaluation for specific overuse syndromes is addressed in the following section. However, the clinician should perform a systematic clarifying evaluation of the lower extremities in all cases of overuse. This evaluation includes a comprehensive history of the injury, the patient's occupation, hobbies, exercise habits, and a thorough biomechanical evaluation of the lower extremities.

History

The initial step in evaluation is history taking. The history provides the clinician with a "road map" for the direction of the remaining clarifying evaluation. The clinician determines whether the injury was traumatic or non-traumatic. Non-traumatic injuries signal overuse and should prompt further questions concerning the patient's work and sports habits. Activities involving repetitive use of the lower extremities are determined. For runners, training methods, shoes, and training surfaces are reviewed.

Questions are asked about the area and nature of pain. The boundaries of pain are delineated, helping the clinician to isolate the involved tissues and anatomic structures. The type of pain—dull, aching, burning, throbbing—is ascertained. Generally, a superficial burning pain is a problem with muscle, tendon, or perhaps nerve; while a deep ache or dull pain could involve capsule or bone.[27] The patient is questioned about incidences of numbness or tingling, which could indicate compression neuropathy associated with conditions such as tarsal tunnel syndrome of the ankle or Morton's neuroma of the foot.[28] Questions concerning temperature change in the foot and ankle should be asked. Persistent coolness could signal compartment syndrome of the leg.[29]

The nature of the pain over a 24-hour cycle should be ascertained. Knowing what activities precipitate the pain will help the clinician determine the nature of the overuse injury. Activities and previous pain-relieving treatments such as ice, heat, rest, elevation, or aspirin provide clues for the clinician about the nature of the injury—acute, subacute, or chronic—so that appropriate and effective treatment can be planned.

Physical Evaluation

A synopsis of the physical evaluation is presented in Table 7-2. The examination includes the entire lower extremity and is not confined to the area of injury. All intrinsic factors related to overuse are evaluated.

Static postural evaluation is performed from the anterior, posterior, and lateral positions. Anteriorly, the alignment of the lower extremities is observed and the degree of torsional and/or angular malalignment is determined. "Squinting" patellas suggest femoral anteversion and are usually accompanied by an apparent genu varum, proximal external torsion of the tibia, varum of the distal tibia, and compensatory ankle and foot pronation (see Fig. 7-1).[16]

From the side, the clinician looks for genu recurvatum, which indicates a shallow femoral groove that can result in poor patellofemoral joint congruency. Poor congruency results in lateral patellar tracking, which with overuse can lead to anterior knee pain and chondromalacia patellae.

From behind, the pelvic crests, the posterior superior iliac spines (PSISs) of the pelvis, and the greater trochanters of the femurs, are palpated for any asymmetry that might indicate leg length discrepancy or a sacroiliac joint lesion. The leg-to-floor and heel-to-floor angles are measured with a goniometer (Figs. 7-2 and 7-3). These measurements give an indication of the amount of tibial varum and calcaneal eversion during

TABLE 7-2 Physical Evaluation

  I. Postural evaluation
     A. Anterior
        1. Miserable malalignment
        2. Leg length discrepancy
     B. Lateral
        1. Genu recurvatum
     C. Posterior
        1. Leg length
        2. Leg-to-floor angle (tibial varum)
        3. Heel-to-floor angle (calcaneal valgus/varum)
 II. Dynamic evaluation
     A. Walking or running on treadmill
     B. Observe movement of calcaneus and navicular bone
III. Static evaluation
     A. Q angle
     B. Patellar mobility
        1. Apprehension test
     C. Hip rotation/hip adduction-abduction
        1. Prone (femoral anteversion, femoral retroversion)
        2. Prone knee extension and flexion—adduction/abduction
        3. FABER test, hip capsule tightness/sacroiliac compression
     D. Flexibility
        1. Ankle dorsiflexion
           a) Knee straight
           b) Knee flexed 30°
        2. Hamstring muscles
        3. Ober (tensor foscia lata muscle and iliotibial band)
        4. Modified Thomas's test (iliopsoas and rectus femoris muscles)
     E. Strength
        1. Manual
        2. Isokinetic

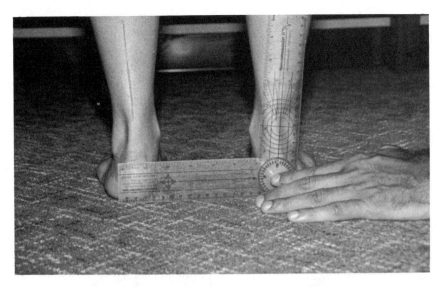

FIGURE 7–2. Leg–Floor Angle: Angle formed by a longitudinal line bisecting the distal one-third of the lower leg with a horizontal line along the ground. Represents the amount of varum in the distal tibia bone.

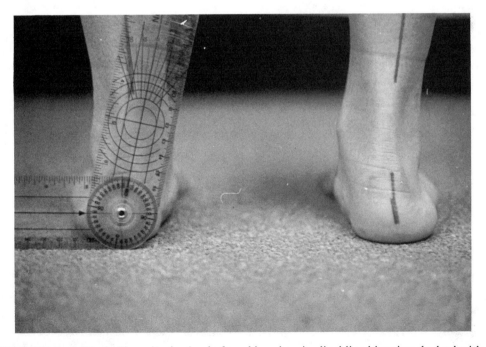

FIGURE 7–3. Heel–Floor Angle: Angle found by a longitudinal line bisecting the heel with a horizontal line along the ground. Represents the amount of eversion during standing at the subtalar joint.

weightbearing. Discussion of these measurements and their significance related to the lower quarter dysfunction is presented in Chapter 6.

The patient is observed walking, and in some instances, running. The mechanics of the subtalar joint are observed during each phase of stance. Generally, at heel strike, the joint should be in the neutral position, followed immediately by rapid pronation toward footflat. From heel-off to toe-off, resupination occurs at the subtalar joint, establishing the foot as a rigid lever for push-off.[14] Pronation beyond footflat is excessive, resulting, as described previously, in prolonged internal rotation of the tibia and femur. Stress is placed along various structures and soft tissues in the foot, ankle, knee, and hip.

The alignment of the extensor mechanism is examined by measuring the Q angle at the knee. The Q angle is measured by placing a goniometer directly over the center of the patella with one arm aimed at the anterior superior iliac spine (ASIS) of the pelvis and the other in line with the center of the tubercle of the tibia (Fig. 7-4).[16] An excessive Q angle (greater than 15° in women and 10° in men) indicates a propensity for lateral tracking of the patella during range of motion or forceful repetitive contractions of the quadricep femoris muscles.[16] The Q angle is often increased in miserable malalignment, due to external torsion of the proximal tibia, resulting in lateral displacement of the tibial tubercle.

Mobility of the patella is tested with the knee straight and at 30° of flexion. At 30° of knee flexion, the patella is secure in the femoral trochlear groove. Lateral displacement greater than one half the width of the patella indicates hypermobility with potential weakness of the vastus medialis muscle.[16] Patients with a history of a lateral dislocating patella exhibit a positive apprehension sign during forceful lateral glide of the patella (Fig. 7-5).

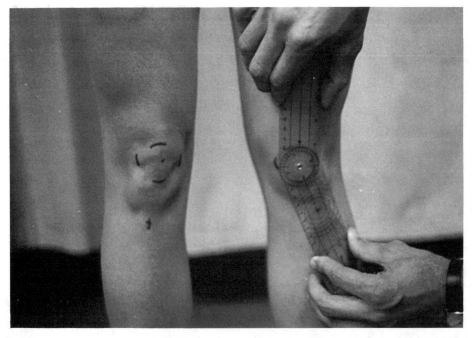

FIGURE 7–4. Q Angle: The angle formed by a line measured between the anterior superior iliac spine (ASIS) of the patella bone to the midpoint of the patella bone, and a line measured between the midpoint of the patella bone and the tibial tubercle of the tibia bone.

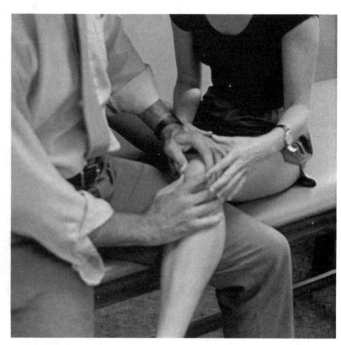

FIGURE 7–5. Apprehension sign for lateral dislocating patella.

Hip rotation is tested with the patient prone and with the knees flexed to 90° (Fig. 7-6). Excessive internal rotation suggests femoral anteversion, while excessive external rotation suggests femoral retroversion. Either condition may precipitate torsional or frontal plane compensatory changes in the lower extremities.

Flexibility tests include ankle dorsiflexion measured with the knee extended and flexed (Fig. 7-7 and 7-8). Care is taken while passively dorsiflexing the foot to maintain

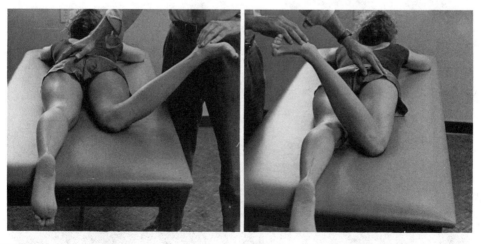

FIGURE 7–6. Hip rotation for femoral anteversion or retroversion tested prone. The hip is maintained in neutral position relative to the pelvis and the knees are flexed at 90°. Excessive outward rotation of the lower legs indicates femoral anteversion while excessive inward rotation of the lower leg indicates femoral retroversion.

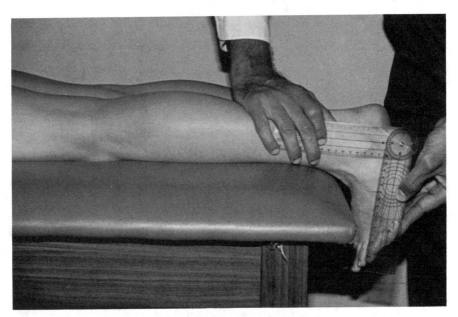

FIGURE 7–7. Ankle dorsiflexion measured with knee straight.

slight inversion. Foot eversion allows pronation to occur at the subtalar and midtarsal joints and gives a false impression of increased dorsiflexion. Other flexibility tests include the modified Thomas' test, hamstring flexibility test, and Ober test (Figs. 7-9 to 7-12). Strength tests, if necessary, are performed using one of the various isokinetic devices on the market. Important agonist-antagonist strength ratios should be ascer-

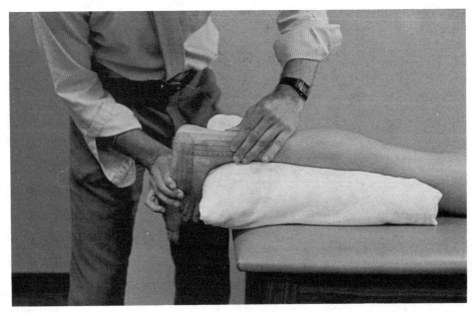

FIGURE 7–8. Ankle dorsiflexion to isolate the soleus muscle measured with knee flexed to approximately 30°.

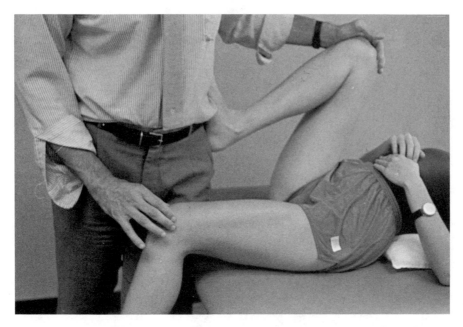

FIGURE 7–9. Modified Thomas test for tightness of the tensor fasciae latae, iliopsoas, and rectus femoris muscles.

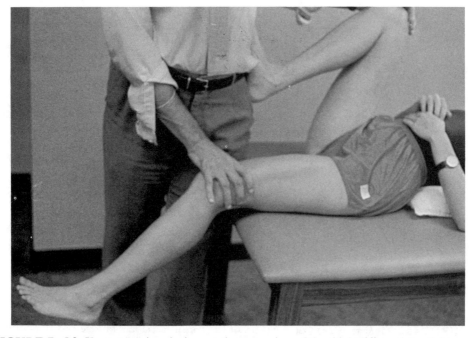

FIGURE 7–10. Knee extension during passive extension of the thigh differentiates tightness of the rectus femoris muscle from iliopsoas muscle.

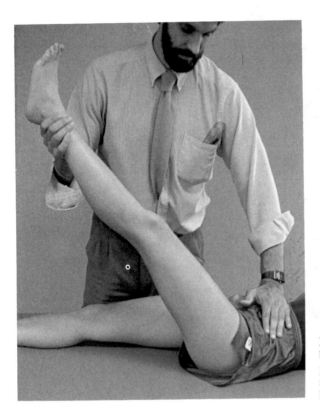

FIGURE 7–11. Hamstring flexibility: Movement of the ipsilateral pelvis and ASIS during straight leg raise indicates end range inextensibility of hamstring muscles.

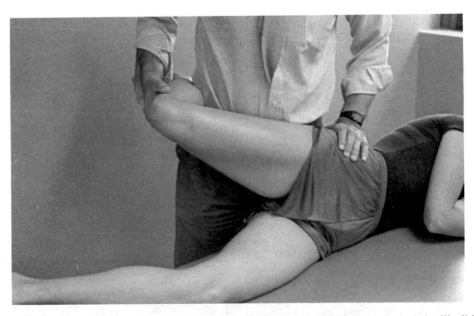

FIGURE 7–12. Ober test: Test for tightness of the tensor fascia lata muscle and the iliotibial band (ITB). The hip, with patient sidelying, is abducted and extended. Inability to passively adduct the hip indicates tightness of the tensor fascia lata and ITB.

tained for the ankle dorsiflexors and plantar flexors, the knee extensors and flexors, and the hip abductors and adductors. Normative values for some of these ratios are reported elsewhere.[30]

In summary, a thorough and systematic evaluation helps the clinician pinpoint the underlying biomechanical factors influencing the overuse injury. Correction of these factors is imperative for successful resolution of the injury and to prevent recurrence. Evaluation and differentiation of specific overuse injuries is presented below.

COMMON OVERUSE INJURIES

Overuse injuries affect different anatomic sites and tissues. A *Runner's World*[3] survey conducted in 1977 cited the most common areas of overuse in runners as the knee (25%), Achilles tendon (18%), shin (15%), ankle (11%), and heel (10%). A survey by Eggold[31] of 146 runners indicated the most common overuse injuries were knee pain (40%), plantar fasciitis (15%), Achilles tendinitis (9%), and shin splints (7%). In Clement's[8] series of 1,819 runners, the anatomic areas most affected by overuse were the knee (41.7%), lower leg (27.9%), foot (18.1%), hip (5%), lumbar spine (3.7%), and upper leg (3.6%). Specific syndromes included patellofemoral joint pain syndrome (25.8%), tibia stress syndrome (13.2%), Achilles tendinitis (6%), plantar fasciitis (4.7%), patellar tendinitis (4.5%), iliotibial friction band syndrome (ITFBS, 4.3%), metatarsal fracture (3.2%), and tibial fractures (2.6%). Finally, James' group's[7] survey of 180 runners with overuse injuries listed the following most commonly involved anatomic sites and syndromes: knee (25%), posterior tibial syndrome (13%), Achilles tendinitis (11%), plantar fasciitis (7%), and stress fractures (6%). In the knee pain group, the most common injuries included chondromalacia patella (25%), nonspecific anterior knee pain (20%), ITFBS (17%), and patellar tendinitis (7%).[7]

Based on these surveys, most overuse injuries affect the knee, lower leg, ankle, foot, upper leg, hip, and pelvis. The following case studies illustrate common overuse injuries, and their pathomechanics, clinical signs and symptoms, and conservative treatment. The case studies emphasize the problem-solving approach to treatment by identifying, defining, and addressing the predisposing, precipitating, and, hence, perpetuating factors in overuse injuries.

Plantar Fasciitis

According to Bojsen-Muller and Flagsted,[32] the plantar fascia is the most common site of heel pain in runners. The plantar fascia, or aponeurosis, is composed of central, lateral, and medial bands and originates along the medial tubercle of the calcaneus. The plantar fascia courses anteriorly along the arch of the foot, each band attaching to the sides of the proximal phalanx in each toe.[33] According to Hicks,[26] the plantar fascia is responsible for 60% of the stress applied to the foot during footflat. At toe-off, hyperextension of the MTP joints results in tightening of the plantar fascia and assists with resupination of the foot (windlass mechanism). The windlass mechanism of the plantar fascia sustains 1.7 to 3 times body weight.[26]

CASE STUDY

1: Plantar Fasciitis

Subjective. A 27-year-old male recreational basketball and tennis player complained of heel pain that was worse in the morning. The patient reported reduced pain after walking but increased pain during and after basketball or tennis. Pain was unilateral.

Objective. Palpation revealed tenderness along the medial tubercle of the calcaneus. Soft tissue edema was also palpated along the medial aspect of the calcaneus.

Trigger points were palpated along the medial arch, in the muscle of the abductor hallucis brevis. Passive dorsiflexion of the first MTP joint of the foot reproduced pain. Dorsiflexion of the ankle with the knee straight was limited to the neutral position (90°).

Forefoot varus deformities were measured at 12° in the involved foot and 10° in the uninvolved foot. Valgus of the calcaneus bones during standing was observed in both subtalar joints.

Assessment. Plantar fasciitis secondary to overstretching of the plantar fascia from its medial attachment along the calcaneus.

Predisposing Factors. Excessive pronation of the subtalar joint causes the calcaneus to move into eversion to compensate for the forefoot varus deformity, producing a stretching of the plantar fascia.

According to Lutter,[34] a majority of patients with plantar fasciitis present with either a pronated or a cavus foot. Excessive pronation of the subtalar joint results in abnormal and prolonged eversion of the calcaneus. Prolonged eversion of the calcaneus bone during footflat results in stretching of the plantar fascia. If the foot fails to resupinate at toe-off, increased strain is placed on the plantar fascia due to the windlass effect. Conversely, a cavus foot occurs in the presence of limited subtalar joint eversion. Plantar fasciitis may develop because of the intrinsic inability of the cavus foot to dissipate the weightbearing forces, particularly from heel strike to midstance. As a result, in either a pronated or cavus foot, during repetitive exercise such as running, microtears occur at the insertion of the plantar fascia on the medial tubercle of the calcaneus, resulting in localized inflammation.[34]

Achilles tendon tightness results in compensatory, increased dorsiflexion of the first MTP joint during the stance phase of gait or running. Dorsiflexion of the first MTP joint via the windlass effect stretches the plantar fascia at its insertion along the medial tubercle of the calcaneus.[35]

Precipitating Factors. Basketball and tennis: The patient averaged two hours of play daily, five days a week.

Perpetuating Factors. The above activities combined with intrinsic problems delineated as the predisposing factors to perpetuate the injury. Perpetuating factors are always a combination of predisposing and precipating factors, and therefore are not delineated in subsequent case studies.

Treatment. Ice and iontophoresis with 10% hydrocortisone were applied for 30 minutes to the inflamed area. Foot orthotics were fabricated using medial forefoot and rearfoot posts of 5–7 mm to allow the subtalar joint to function close to neutral position. Stretching exercises, by lengthening the gastrocnemius-soleus muscles of the ankle and foot, rebalance muscle flexibility in the ankle and foot during the stance phase of walking and running.

Achilles Tendinitis

Seen more often in men than women, Achilles tendinitis, with or without peritendinitis is often associated with repetitive or high-impact sports such as running, basketball, or volleyball.[36]

CASE STUDY

2: Achilles Tendinitis

Subjective: A 40-year-old male who jogs approximately 30 miles per week reported insidious onset of pain and stiffness along the posterior aspect of his ankle. Pain occurred primarily during running and subsided with rest. The patient jogged regularly along hilly terrain.

Objective. Tenderness and mild swelling were palpated along the Achilles tendon proximal to its insertion at the calcaneus. Passive dorsiflexion of the ankle with the knee straight reproduced pain. Resisted plantar flexion of the gastrocnemius-soleus muscle group was strong and slightly painful.

Structurally, the patient demonstrated bilateral forefoot varus deformities of 10°. Subtalar joint mobility was within normal limits. Static evaluation indicated bilateral eversion of 10°. During walking and running, the patient exhibited early and excessive pronation.

Flexibility tests indicated that dorsiflexion of the ankle with the knee straight was limited to 90° (neutral). With the knee flexed to 30° dorsiflexion ankle increased to 95°.

Assessment. Achilles tendinitis.

Predisposing Factors. Clement and Taunton[36] found 56% of 109 runners with Achilles tendinitis displayed *excessive pronation.* Angiographic studies indicated an area of hypovascularity approximately 2–6 cm proximal to the Achilles tendon insertion along the posterior aspect of the calcaneus.[37] Increased and excessive internal rotation of the tibia during pronation draws the Achilles tendon mediad. During running, a whipping action is created along the Achilles tendon. This action "wrings out" the hypovascular area of the tendon, resulting in microtears and inflammation.

Poor flexibility of the Achilles tendon also has been implicated in Achilles tendinitis. The gastrocnemius-soleus muscle group performs eccentrically during midstance of running to control anterior movement of the tibia over the talus. Poor flexibility of these muscles, especially during hill running, increases strain on the Achilles tendon, resulting in microtrauma. Additionally, the gastrocnemius-soleus muscles contract concentrically during push-off to propel the foot. Weakness of these muscles increases stress on the Achilles tendon and, during repetitive running, can result in microtears and local inflammation.

Precipitating Factors. Repetitive uphill running results in increased ankle dorsiflexion to allow the foot to clear the ground. Increased strain along the Achilles tendon results from poor flexibility of the gastrocnemius-soleus muscles.

These muscles contract eccentrically at midstance to control the forward momentum of the tibia. Increased speed of the tibia at midstance, during downhill running, results in increased eccentric contraction force in the gastrocnemius-soleus muscles. Forceful repetitive eccentric contractions result in breakdown of the connective tissue component of muscle, including tendon.

Treatment. The initial treatment of acute Achilles tendinitis includes ice and rest from the activity that precipitated the problem. Iontophoresis with 10% hydrocortisone is effective in reducing inflammation. An oral anti-inflammatory, such as phenylbutazone, also reduces the inflammatory reaction. After the acute symptoms subside, a gradual stretching or lengthening and strengthening program for the gastrocnemius-soleus muscles should be performed. Stretching should be gentle, using a low-load, 10-second hold. Usually 10 to 20 repetitions twice daily should be satisfactory. Strengthening can be performed using Theraband or, if indicated, isokinetic exercises. Basic tenets of isokinetics including initial submaximal contractions, progressing, as tolerated, to maximal contractions should be followed.[30]

Correction of underlying ankle and foot biomechanics includes an orthotic to control excessive pronation. Orthotics were fabricated with 5-mm forefoot and rearfoot posts. Clement and Taunton,[36] treated with orthotics the excessive pronators in 109 patients with Achilles tendinitis. In the majority of cases the results were good to excellent.

Correction of training errors involves reducing mileage and hill running and improving footwear. Footwear should include a flexible sole, such as a strip-last shoe, which provides flexibility in the midsole area and reduces stress on the Achilles tendon. The heel of the shoe should be well-padded to provide a lift for the Achilles tendon as well as shock absorption. The heel lifts, according to Clement and Taunton,[36] should be between 12 and 15 mm of thickness.

Shin Splints

According to Slocum,[38] shin splints are a common recognizable clinical entity characterized by nonsterile mechanical inflammation of the muscle and tendon and are brought about by overexertion of the muscles to the lower part of the leg during weightbearing.[39] Slocum lists the following criteria for differentiating shin splints from other disorders of the lower leg or ankle: (1) the lesion must lie at the origin, belly, or muscle-tendon junction of the ankle plantar flexors or dorsiflexors; (2) pain must be related to rhythmic, repetitive exercises; (3) classic signs of inflammation—heat, redness, swelling, tenderness—should be present at the site of the lesion; and (4) conditions resulting from direct trauma or disease must be excluded.

Therefore, shin splints may be narrowly defined as a nonsterile mechanical inflammation of the muscles and related soft tissues of the lower leg, excluding stress fractures and compartment syndromes. Depending on the affected muscles, shin splints can be anterolateral or posteromedial.[39] Anterolateral shin splits involve the pretibial muscles, including tibialis anterior, extensor hallucis longus, and extensor digitorum longus. These muscles are active during several phases of gait and running. At heel strike, the pretibial muscles act eccentrically to lower the foot and ankle, and thus can become inflamed if the running shoe has a hard heel or running takes place on a hard surface. Conversely, during the swing phase, the pretibial muscles contract concentrically to dorsiflex the ankle and clear the foot from the ground or running surface. A muscle imbalance between a weak pretibial muscle group and tight gastrocnemius-soleus muscles results in overactivation of the pretibial muscles during swing phase and at heel strike. The necessity for increased ankle dorsiflexion while running hills increases the strain along the pretibial muscles. The resultant strain on the pretibial muscles can result in microtears and local inflammation.

Posterolateral shin splints are associated with nonsterile, mechanical inflammation of the posterior tibial, flexor digitorum longus, and flexor hallucis longus muscles, and related muscle-tendon junctions. These muscles are active after heel strike, eccentrically contracting to lower the arch and assist in pronation. At push-off, in conjunction with the gastrocnemius-soleus complex, these muscles contract concentrically, propelling the foot and leg. When excessive pronation is present after heel strike, eccentric overactivation of the muscles attempts to support the medial arch and navicular bone of the foot, resulting in strain and microtears. Research has shown a strong positive correlation between excessive pronation and posteromedial shin splints.[10]

In cases where only active resisted plantar flexion is painful, one should suspect periostitis at the attachment of the medial half of the soleus muscle to the posteromedial tibia. The soleus muscle syndrome was identified as a cause of posteromedial shin splints through cadaver electromyographic (EMG) and open biopsy analysis by Michael and Holder.[40]

CASE STUDY

3: Posteromedial Shin Splints

Subjective. A 21-year-old female complained of pain along the inside of her lower legs after aerobic-type exercises. She performed high-impact aerobics two hours daily, seven days a week. She wore dancing slippers rather than an aerobic-type tennis shoe or well-padded running shoe. The pain was relieved by rest and application of ice.

Objective. Active range of motion of the involved ankle was within normal limits. Passive eversion was slightly painful; significant pain was reproduced during passive dorsiflexion of the ankle. Passive dorsiflexion of the ankle remained painful with the knee flexed to 30°. Heel raises also reproduced pain along the posteromedial aspect of the lower leg. Manual palpation of the posteromedial distal tibia reproduced the pain.

Foot evaluation using a goniometer demonstrated forefoot varus of 15° in the involved extremity and 10° in the uninvolved extremity. Range of motion of the subtalar joint was measured using a goniometer at 10° eversion and 20° of inversion, respectively, in both feet. Postural evaluation in standing indicated a valgus position from the neutral position of both calcaneus bones.

Gait assessment revealed excessive pronation of the foot during the stance phase of gait. Instability of the foot occurred during push-off. Excessive movement (pronation) during midstance occurred at the midtarsal joint.

Assessment. Posteromedial shin splints with pain during resisted plantar flexion (heel raises) of the ankle and stretch into dorsiflexion (knee flexed), probably a result of soleus muscle syndrome.

Predisposing Factors. Excessive pronation with eversion of the calcaneus in the foot during standing and jumping resulting in traction on the posteromedial fibrous attachments of the soleus muscle along the tibia.

Precipitating Factors. Repetitive jumping (two hours daily) during aerobic exercises increased stress at the attachment of the soleus muscle along the tibia, resulting in microtears and local inflammation. Inadequate rest—performing aerobic exercises daily—precluded soft tissue repair and healing of the soleus muscle.

Inadequate footwear—using dancing slippers—provided poor arch support and accentuated excessive pronation.

Treatment. Early treatment included rest from aerobic exercise, ice, and iontophoresis with 10% hydrocortisone along the posteromedial aspect of the tibia bone. Treatment time was 30 minutes. Gentle stretching, as described previously, with the knee flexed at 30° was performed daily to the soleus muscle.

Foot orthotics with 8-mm forefoot and rearfoot posts on the involved side, and 5-mm forefoot and rearfoot posts on the uninvolved side, were fabricated. The posts should correct 60% of the forefoot varus abnormality and allow the calcaneus to function close to the neutral position of the subtalar joint. The patient was instructed to purchase an aerobic shoe with a flexible, well-padded insole. A firm, wide heel counter provides good medial and lateral support to the heel.

Exercise modification included performing aerobic exercise only one hour daily, three to four times per week. This schedule precludes overstressing of tissues in the lower leg and allows for tissue recovery and repair.

Stress Fractures of the Tibia

Stress fractures are frequently seen as a cause of pain in the distal third of the posteromedial tibia.[41-42] Persistent overuse of bone that is unaccustomed to stress causes rapid focal, circumferential periosteal resorption of bone with a small cortical cavity. Not all stress fractures progress to the point of actual disruption of bone cortex. Simple cortical hypertrophy along the posteromedial cortex of the tibia may be the only sign seen on radiographic examination.[42]

CAUSES

Stress fractures result from overuse and/or overtraining. Sullivan and coworkers[43] correlated various training factors in 51 runners with stress fractures. The most common sites were the tibia, fibula, metatarsals, and pelvic bones, in that order. The majority of the runners ran more than 20 miles per week and ran on hard surfaces. Thirty-one changed training methods prior to injury; the majority increased their weekly mileage dramatically. Nineteen of the 51 runners exhibited excessive pronation. In most cases, radiographic changes showed an area of localized cortical bone thickening with periosteal and endosteal reactions. The results suggest that for many runners there is a maximum, and that to exceed it places the runner at risk for soft tissue breakdown. Additionally, malalignment of the lower extremity associated with excessive pronation is a predisposing factor.

TREATMENT

Treatment is rest from the activity that is causing the pain. Oral anti-inflammatory medicines help to reduce the inflammation. As symptoms subside, an alternative exercise program, such as cycle-ergometer or swimming, can help maintain cardiovascular fitness. Orthotics are used to correct excessive pronation of the foot. Training begins gradually, usually on a level track that has a softer surface than pavement. Running should not be resumed until symptoms resolve and radiographic evidence indicates no cortical bone defect. Serial radiographs, every two weeks after the onset of pain, are useful for diagnosis and to monitor progression of fractures. Absence of radiographic presentation (at least during initial examination), even in the presence of stress fractures, is not uncommon. Diagnostic accuracy is therefore initially enhanced by the use of a bone scan.

Compartment Syndromes

Compartment syndromes in the lower leg result when increased tissue fluid pressure in a closed fascial compartment encroaches on the circulation to nerves and muscles within that compartment. The anterior, posterior, deep posterior, and lateral compartments of the lower leg may be affected.[44,45]

SIGNS AND SYMPTOMS

Pain over the involved compartment, paresthesia over the distribution of the involved nerve, muscle weakness, and positive stretch signs of the involved muscles develop as compartment pressures become abnormally elevated.[45]

TREATMENT

Treatment includes discontinuation or modification of the activity that precipitated the problem. Acute compartment syndrome is a medical emergency necessitating immediate decompression of the involved fascial compartment. Subacute or chronic compartment syndromes may be helped with soft tissue work, including massage to promote circulation and stretch to the investing fascia. A chronic problem, however, may require a permanent modification of activity, such as reducing the weekly mileage of a runner.

Chondromalacia Patellae

Softening or fissuring of the hyaline cartilage covering the posterior surface of the patella is known as chondromalacia patellae. The cartilage breakdown results from abnormal pressure or load between the retropatellar surface and the corresponding trochlear groove of the femur. Abnormal pressure results in either too much load or too little load between the opposing articular forces. In either case, diffusion of synovial fluid through the layers of hyaline cartilage is compromised, resulting in inadequate nutrition of chondrocytes and subsequent cell death and loss of ground substance. Softening and fibrillation of hyaline cartilage increases stress along the underlying subchondral bone, which is richly innervated with pain fibers.

CASE STUDY

4: Chondromalacia Patellae

Subjective. A 16-year-old high school cheerleader presented with anterior knee pain made worse by exercise, especially running. She reportedly jogged 20 miles weekly along a flat, well-contoured macadam street in her neighborhood. The patient reported insidious onset of pain and no history of microtrauma.

Squatting activities and stair climbing were very painful. The patient reported reduced pain along her anterior knee after rest and application of ice.

Objective. There was tenderness to palpation along the lateral facet of the patella and the lateral condyle of the femur. Active range of motion of the involved knee was within normal limits when compared to that in the uninvolved knee. Patellofemoral joint crepitus was audible during knee extension and flexion. Excessive lateral glide of the patella with the knee flexed 30° elicited a positive apprehension sign. Conversely, the lateral retinaculum of the vastus lateralis muscle was tight to passive stretch. Significant atrophy was palpated in the vastus medialis obliquis (VMO) muscle. Straight leg raising was limited bilaterally by tightness of the hamstrings.

Structurally, the patient demonstrated miserable malalignment, with femoral anteversion, proximal external tibial torsion, tibia varum, and subtalar joint pronation. The result was an increased Q angle of 25° in the involved knee. The femoral anteversion was confirmed with excessive internal rotations in the hip joints. The patient also demonstrated significant recurvatum in both knees.

Evaluation of the foot indicated forefoot varus of 10° on the involved side, as compared to 8° on the uninvolved side.

Assessment. Chondromalacia of the lateral patella and lateral condyle of the femur.

Predisposing Factors. Miserable malalignment with proximal external tibial torsion resulted in an increased Q angle and lateral patellar tracking.

Excessive pronation in the stance or support phase of running and walking with obligatory internal rotation of the tibia and femur resulted in increased compression between the lateral patellar facet and the lateral trochlear groove of the femur.

Atrophy of the VMO resulted in poor medial dynamic stabilization of the patella.

Tight lateral retinaculum of the vastus lateralis muscle exacerbated lateral tracking of the patella.

The quadriceps femoris muscle contracts during forward swing in the recovery phase of running to extend the knee at heel strike. Increased quadriceps femoris muscle force may produce tight or inextensible hamstring muscles when the leg swings forward. The result is increased compressive force between the patella and the trochlear groove of the femur during running.

Precipitating Factors. Jogging 20 miles weekly along a macadam road, a relatively soft, yielding surface, is not, in this author's opinion, a training error. However, the patient did perform squatting manuevers during cheerleading that increased the patellofemoral joint compression forces.

Treatment. Treatment is designed to reduce patellofemoral joint compression forces and improve patellar tracking and control during knee flexion. Patellofemoral joint compression forces increase during increasing amounts of knee flexion. The patient is advised, therefore, to avoid activities such as stair climbing, cycling, or getting in or out of a low chair which require repetitive knee flexion or squatting. Quadriceps muscle strengthening is the most essential component of nonoperative management of patellofemoral pain. Quadriceps femoris wasting and weakness are almost constant accompaniments of chondromalacia patellae. Improved quadriceps femoris muscle strength, particularly the VMO, helps maintain the central position of the patella during knee movement in the trochlear groove of the femur. Straight leg raising or short-arc exercises performed in the final 30° of extension minimize patellofemoral joint compression forces. Straight leg raising exercises should be performed 100 times daily. Initially no weight is applied to the quadriceps femoris muscle. The patient should gradually increase weight resistance to the quadriceps femoris in one-pound increments, to a maximum of 10 to 15 pounds.

Hamstring stretching was performed daily. In addition, the patient was instructed to glide the patella medially with the knee extended. Gliding the patella medially lengthens the soft tissue structures, including the lateral retinaculum of the vastus lateralis along the lateral border of the patella.

The patient was fitted with a patellofemoral joint brace made of neoprene with a doughnut-shaped cut-out for the patella. A lateral wedge was used to buttress the lateral aspect of the patella and prevent lateral tracking or subluxation.

Orthotics were used to correct excessive pronation and correct associated rotational changes in the lower extremities. The orthotics were fabricated, posting the forefoot varus abnormalities in both feet, with medial forefoot and rearfoot posts. The girth of both posts was 5 mm.

The patient was instructed to avoid activities involving repetitive squatting and knee flexion. Her cheerleading routines were modified accordingly to avoid such harmful positions. Conservative treatment is generally very effective in relieving signs and symptoms associated with chondromalacia patellae. In a prospective study of chondromalacia patellae in athletes, DeHaven, Dolan, and Mayer[46] showed nonoperative measures were successful in 82% of 100 cases. In the same study, 66% of conservatively treated patients were able to return to unrestricted athletic activities. Gruber suggested that conservative treatment should be abandoned if no improvement is shown after three months.[47]

Iliotibial Band Friction Syndrome

The iliotibial band is a thick band of fascia that forms part of the insertion of the tensor fasciae latae and gluteus maximus muscles. It continues distally along the lateral aspect of the thigh in continuity with the lateral intermuscular septum and inserting into Gerdy's tubercle along the anterolateral aspect of the tibia bone.[33] During knee flexion greater than 30° the iliotibial band lies on or behind the lateral condyle of the femur, whereas with the knee extended, the iliotibial band lies anterior to the lateral femoral condyle.[48] Therefore, flexion and extension movements of the knee under stress produce irritation and subsequent inflammatory reaction in the iliotibial band.[48-50]

Iliotibial band friction syndrome (ITBFS) is associated with overuse syndrome resulting from friction during flexion and extension of the knee between the iliotibial band and the lateral epicondyle of the femur. The condition is usually found in runners.[51]

CASE STUDY

5: Iliotibial Band Friction Syndrome

Subjective. A 30-year-old male long-distance runner (50 miles weekly) complained of a few months' history of lateral knee pain that was worse during running. Walking with the knee extended afforded relief. The patient frequently ran along the crown of the road with his involved leg on the low side.

Objective. Evaluation of the hip indicated inextensibility of the iliotibial band to passive stretch, secondary to a positive Ober's sign. Palpation of the femoral epicondyle reproduced the patient's pain. Active range of motion of the knee reproduced the patient's pain within a given painful arc, at approximately 30° of flexion. This point in the range brings the iliotibial band into contact with the prominence of the lateral condyle of the femur.[50] Lower extremity malalignment and leg-heel and heel-forefoot relationships were normal.

Assessment. ITFBS.

Predisposing Factors. Tight tensor fasciae latae muscle and associated ITB increased friction stress of the iliotibial band along the bony prominence of the lateral epicondyle of the femur.[49,50]

Precipitating Factors. Lindenberg, Pinshaw, and Noakes[51] found that runners with ITBFS tended to run with the involved leg along the low part of the road crown.[51] Running in that position restricts pronation, thereby prolonging external tibial rotation and promoting genu varum. The result was increased stretch of the iliotibial band along the lateral epidondyle. Lindenberg's group also found that 67% of 36 long distance runners with ITBFS had recently switched to inflexible running shoes, that restrict subtalar joint pronation.[51] The authors treated many of these runners with flexible running shoes and a lateral heel wedge to promote pronation.

Treatment. Ice and ultrasound (10/watts cm^2) plus 10% hydrocortisone were applied to the inflamed area for ten minutes. Stretching of the iliotibial band, as demonstrated in Figure 7-12, was performed by the clinician with the patient's leg passively adducted. The patient was instructed to run along a level surface instead of the crown of the road.

SUMMARY

Major overuse syndromes can involve the foot, ankle, knee, and hip. They present a diagnostic challenge for the clinician. Effective treatment of the overuse injuries includes evaluation of predisposing (intrinsic) factors and precipitating (extrinsic) factors relative to the individual patient. Predisposing factors such as malalignment syndromes and muscle dysfunction result in pathomechanics that alter normal forces and stresses along various musculoskeletal tissues. Incorrect training methods and conditions precipitate tissue breakdown and injury.

The case studies presented illustrate the problem-solving approach to treatment of common overuse syndromes. Correction of the predisposing and precipitating factors is emphasized. Without correction of these factors therapeutic modalities are ineffective and superfluous.

REFERENCES

1. Mann, RA: Biomechanics of running. In Mack RP (ed): American Academy of Orthopedic Surgeons Symposium on the Foot and Leg in Running Sports. CV Mosby, St. Louis, 1982.
2. Murphy, P: Ultrasports are in, in spite of injuries. Physician Sports Med 14:180, 1986.
3. Henderson, J: First aid for the injured runner. Runners World 12:32, 1977.
4. Marti, B, Vader, JP, Minder, CE, and Abelin, T: On the epidemiology of running injuries: The 1984 Bern grand-prix study. Am J Sports Med 16:285, 1988.
5. Elliot, B and Achland, T: Biomechanical effects of fatigue on 10,000 meter running techniques. Res Quart Ex Sports 52:160, 1981.
6. Arthritis Foundation: Primer on the rheumatic diseases. JAMA 224:19, 1973.
7. Herring, SA and Nilson, KL: Introduction to overuse injuries. Clin Sports Med 6:225, 1987.
8. James, SL, Bates, BT, and Ostering, LR: Injuries to runners. Am J Sports Med 6:40, 1978.

9. Clement, DB: A survey of overuse running injuries. Physician Sports Med 9:47, 1981.
10. Viitasale, JT and Kvist, M: Some biomechanical aspects of the foot and ankle in athletes with and without shin splints. Am J Sports Med 11:125, 1983.
11. Lutter, L: Injuries in the runner and jogger. Minnesota Med 63:45, 1980.
12. Litletvedt, J, Kreighbaum, E, and Philips, LR: Analysis of selected alignment of the lower extremity related to the shin splint syndrome. J Am Podiatr Assoc 69:211, 1979.
13. DeLacerda, FG: A study of anatomical factors involved in shin splints. J Orthp Sports Phys Ther 2:55, 1980.
14. Inman, VT, Rolston, HJ, and Todd, F: Human Walking. Williams & Wilkins, Baltimore, 1981, pp 1–21.
15. Tiberio, D: The effect of excessive subtalar joint pronation on patellofemoral mechanics: A theoretical model. J Orthop Sports Phys Ther 9:160, 1987.
16. James, SL: Chondromalacia of the patella in the adolescent. In Kennedy JC (ed): The Injured Adolescent Knee. Williams & Wilkins, Baltimore, 1979, pp 214–218.
17. Giles, LGF and Taylor, JR: Low back pain associates with leg length inequality. Spine 6:510, 1981.
18. Bolz, S and Davies, G: Leg length differences and correlations with total leg strength. J Orthop Sports Phys Ther 6:123, 1984.
19. Subotnick, SI: Limb length discrepancy of the lower extremity (the short leg syndrome). J Orthop Sports Phys Ther 3:11, 1981.
20. Basmajian, JV: Muscles Alive: Their Function Revealed by Electromyography, ed 4. Baltimore, Williams and Wilkins, 1979.
21. James, SL and Brubaker, CE: Biomechanics of running. Orthop Clin North Am 4:605, 1973.
22. Subotnick, SI: The shin splints syndrome of the lower extremity. Podiatr Sports Med 66:43, 1976.
23. Cavanaugh, PR: The biomechanics of lower extremity action in distance running. Foot Ankle 7:197, 1987.
24. Clancy, WG: Runner's injuries. Am J Sports Med 8:137, 1980.
25. Solomonow, M and D'Ambrosia, R: Biomechanics of muscle overuse injuries: A theoretical approach. Clin Sports Med 6:253, 1987.
26. Hicks, JH: The mechanics of the foot. II. The plantar aponeurosis. J Anat 80:25, 1954.
27. Cyriax, J: Textbook of Orthopaedic Medicine, vol 1, Diagnosis of Soft Tissue Lesions, ed 6. Cassell, London, 1979, pp 64–103.
28. Kopell, HP and Thompson, WAL: Peripheral Entrapment Neuropathies, ed 2. Robert E. Krieger, 1976.
29. Leach, RE, Hammond, G, and Stryker, WS: Anterior tibial compartment syndrome, acute and chronic. J Bone Joint Surg 49A:451, 1967.
30. Davies, GJ: A Compendium of Isokinetics in Clinical Usage, ed 3. S and S, Wisconsin, 1987.
31. Eggold, JF: Orthotics in the prevention of runner's overuse injuries. Phys Sports Med 9:125, 1981.
32. Bujsen-Muller, F and Flagsted, KE: Plantar aponeurosis and integral architecture of the ball of the foot. Anat 121:599, 1976.
33. Warwick, R and Williams PL (eds): Gray's Anatomy, British ed 35. WB Saunders, Philadelphia, 1973.
34. Lutter, LD: Running athletes in office practice. Foot Ankle 3:153, 1982.
35. Marshall, RN: Foot mechanics and joggers injuries. N Z Med J 88:288, 1978.
36. Clement, DB, Taunton, JE, and Smart, GW: Achilles tendinitis and peritendinitis: Etiology and treatment. Am J Sports Med 12:179, 1984.
37. Lagergren, C and Lindholm, A: Vascular distribution in the achilles tendon—an angiographic and microangiographic study. Acta Chir Scand 116:491, 1958.
38. Slocum, DB: The shin splint syndrome: Medical aspects and differential diagnosis. Am J Surg 114:875, 1967.
39. Andrews, JR: Overuse syndromes of the lower extremity. Clin Sports Med 2:139, 1983.
40. Michael, RH and Holder, LE: The soleus syndrome: A cause of medial tibial stress (shin splints). Am J Sports Med 13:87, 1985.
41. Jackson, DW and Bailey, D: Shin splints in the young athlete: A nonspecific diagnosis. Phys Sports Med 3:45, 1975.
42. Devas, MB: Stress fractures of the tibia in athletes or "shin soreness." J Bone Joint Surg 40B:227, 1958.
43. Sullivan, D, Warren, RF, Pavlou, H, and Kelman, G: Stress fractures in 51 runners. Clin Orthop 187:188, 1984.
44. Reneman, RS: The anterior and lateral compartment syndrome of the leg due to intensive use of muscles. Clin Orthop 113:69, 1975.
45. Wiley, JP, Clement, DB, Doyle DL, and Taunton, JE: A primary care perspective of chronic compartment syndrome of the leg. Physician Sports Med 15:111, 1987.
46. DeHaven, DE, Dolan, WA, and Mayer, PJ: Chondromalacia patellae in athletes: Clinical presentation and conservative management. Am J Sports Med 7:5, 1979.
47. Gruber, MA: The conservative treatment of chondromalacia patellae. Orthop Clin North Am 10:105, 1979.
48. Renne, JW: The iliotibial band friction syndrome. J Bone Joint Surg 57A:110, 1975.
49. Noble, CA: Iliotibial band friction syndrome in runners. Am J Sports Med 8:232, 1980.
50. Noble, HB, Hajek, MR, and Porter, M: Diagnosis and treatment of iliotibial band tightness in runners. Physician Sports Med 10:67, 1982.
51. Lindenberg, G, Pinshaw, R, and Noakes, TD: Iliotibial band friction syndrome in runners. Physician Sports Med 12:118, 1984.

CHAPTER 8

The Diabetic Foot

Nathan Schwartz, DPM

The diabetic foot has presented, and will always present, a treatment dilemma. The foot is one of the most susceptible structures in the diabetes patient. In diabetes, vascular compromise and the lack of sensation due to nerve damage cause this amazing structure to fail. The single most destructive process to life and limb is the effect of diabetes on the circulatory system. It seems to produce the greatest pathology in the small vessels, the arterioles, venules, and capillaries. This necessitates constant monitoring and prophylactic care. This chapter discusses the pertinent anatomy, pathomechanics, and treatment of the diabetic foot, with special attention to prophylactic measures for the traumatized and infected diabetic foot.

PERIPHERAL NERVOUS SYSTEM

Four types of nerves supply the foot: cutaneus, proprioceptive, motor, and autonomic. Malfunction of one or all types, can cause or initiate pathology.

The only way the musculoskeletal system of the foot can function successfully is with an intact nervous system supplying all structures. The peripheral nervous system is constantly sending subliminal impulses to the central nervous system. The body responds, in many instances, with reflexive actions that are not brought to consciousness. The foot responds so that the stress is distributed and one area is not overloaded, thus avoiding potential trauma. In a diabetic patient, this invaluable safeguard may not function properly. Jauw-Tuen and Brown[1] found that three times as many patients were hospitalized for diabetic foot lesions initiated by neuropathy as by ischemia.

Proprioceptors of the Foot

The plantar aspect of the foot has an incredibly intricate and effective padding made up of fat held in a tubular fibrous stroma. When a bone in the foot bears weight, this fibrofatty structure dissipates the stress in all directions, protecting and acting as a shock absorber. If the toes are contracted at the metatarsophalangeal (MTP) joint, a distal positioning of the fat padding occurs, leaving the plantar surfaces of the metatarsal bones unprotected. The hyperextended position of the MTP joints and the help of the extensor muscles produce a retrograde force to plantar flex the metatarsal bones. This force further increases the plantar pressure to the head of the metatarsals (Fig. 8-1). The integument under metatarsal heads is unique. The plantar surface of the foot has the thickest skin on the body to protect the metatarsal heads and neurovascular structures. The skin on the plantar aspect of the foot can withstand extremely high pressures, up to 500 pounds per square inch (psi)[2]; however, if the nervous system is not telling the brain about the pain, pressure, and position, the structures in the foot may be subjected to irreversible damage. Even light pressure (5 psi) can cause necrosis over a long period of time. For example, a tight pair of shoes could maintain a low pressure to the foot, causing damage.

The diabetic foot may develop arthritic alterations, called Charcot changes, that result from poor sensation and lack of proprioception. During normal walking the foot is constantly protected from abnormal subluxatory motion by the proprioceptors. The pathomechanical changes that occur in diabetes represent a joint subluxing without the proper nerves signaling this altered joint position. The inability of the diabetic patient to perceive pain and trauma (which is induced by altered proprioception) causes damage in the form of microfractures at the joint surfaces. Over a period of time, repeated trauma may cause complete dislocation and destruction. Diabetes patients give a history of gross morphologic changes in their feet that occur within a very short time. A foot can collapse and become completely flat in a period of two months (Fig. 8-2).[3]

The lack of sensation has other ramifications. The person with diabetes can sustain direct physical damage without realizing it. For example, a diabetes patient who stepped on a nail while wearing a shoe did not notice that the nail had penetrated the shoe and the skin. It was not until he tried to remove the shoe that he found his foot had a nail in

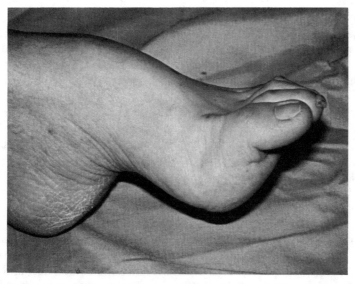

FIGURE 8–1. Pes cavus deformity. Demonstrates the retrograde force of the proximal phalanx on the metatarsal and the anterior positioning of the plantar fat pad to the metatarsal head.

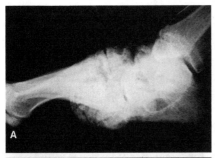

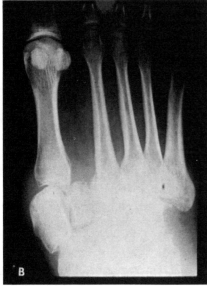

FIGURE 8-2. Examples of Charcot changes: (*A*) Severe disorganization of the tarsus and lesser tarsus. (*B*) Dislocation of the tarsometatarsal and the first and second cuneiforms.

it. The delay in removing this foreign body from the foot caused more damage than the original injury. Such insensitivity is extreme but not uncommon. Because of their inability to perceive pain, diabetics also seem to develop a cavalier attitude toward relatively serious problems and put off having ulcers treated. This behavior may be a form of denial or, simply, a manifestation of the perceived insignificance due to insensibility.

Treating infections in the diabetic foot is difficult because of the inability of parenteral antibiotics to diffuse into the infected site due to the diseased state of the small vessels.[4] In addition, the control of the diabetic state is extremely important, but the presence of infection can make this control very difficult.

Paresthesia is a form of insensitivity that can be perceived as tingling.[5,6] Diabetics often describe their numbness as painful. The degree to which this problem is disabling cannot be appreciated without experiencing this state of altered sensation. Currently, paresthesias are treated with medications that have many side effects, and the results are variable. In podiatry, the use of posterior tibial blocks has been popular. A nerve block appears to be beneficial in treating paresthesia: by paralyzing the sympathetic and sensory fibers to the posterior tibial artery, it causes increased blood flow and breaks the pain cycle. The results are still variable but have been shown to be beneficial, with few side effects.

Motor Nerves

Motor nerve loss occurs from a disorder of the motor nerve fibers or a primary myopathy. Differentiating motor nerve damage on physical examination is difficult and requires electromyographic (EMG) and nerve conduction studies. The medical course of motor nerve damage in the diabetes patient suggests a slowly progressive motor weakness that is often overlooked and mistaken for general malaise.

Autonomic Nervous System

Disturbances in the autonomic nervous system produce various problems in the foot.[7] These disorders fall into two categories: cutaneous and vascular. Disorders of the autonomic nervous system result in either anhidrosis or hyperhidrosis. Anhidrosis causes dry skin, cracks, and fissures. Fissures are very difficult to treat, often occurring about the heel, an area of poor circulation; however, elimination of fissures is necessary to avoid an infection. Debridement of hyperkeratotic tissue and the use of flexible collodion is extremely helpful in treating noninfected lesions. Hyperhidrosis is characterized by excessive perspiration; therefore, the patient is more prone to fungal and yeast infections. Such infections can be extremely serious, especially if they occur between the toes, where the potential for a break in the skin for bacterial infection is great. In the interdigital area, thrombosis of the digital vessels and platelet aggregation can occur and can result in the subsequent loss of the digit.[8] To avoid this, all diabetics must keep their feet as dry as possible, especially between the toes.

Vasodilation and vasoconstriction can result from autonomic vascular dysfunction in diabetes. Vasoconstriction is the more common of the two involvements and, to some extent, is treatable. Vasoconstriction can cause serious problems by further compromising blood flow in the small vessels of the foot (Fig. 8-3).

VASCULAR INVOLVEMENT IN DIABETES

The circulatory status of the involved limb must be assessed. If the circulation is not adequate to heal the lesion, local care is doomed to fail. Amputation or revascularization is necessary. If heat or any other modality that increases the metabolic activity is applied to an ischemic limb, premature loss may result. Many tests and instruments are used in the evaluation of the arterial circulation to the lower extremity, which means that there is no one good test or instrument. Many procedures are used in combination to give a more detailed understanding of the circulatory status.

Vascular Testing

Palpating for the pedal pulses can yield a qualitative measure of the dorsalis pedis or posterior tibial circulation, but the examiner must realize that there can be a substantial decrease in flow to the extremity even though arterial ankle pulses are good. Arterial pressures taken at the ankle level and compared with systolic pressures at the antecubital fossa can also be deceptive. False normal pressure can be recorded if there is calcification of the arterial wall. Either the Doppler ultrasonic flow detector or the pneumoplethysmograph can show a pulse wave form that can illustrate the arteries'

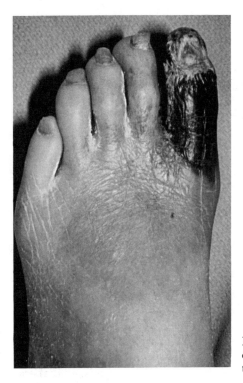

FIGURE 8–3. Dry gangrene of the first toe, caused by complete stoppage of the arterial flow to the digit.

relative elasticity. The ultrasonic flow detector is an inexpensive instrument that detects the flow of blood through the arteries by producing an audible signal.[9] By virtue of the sound produced, the relative condition of the vessel can then be determined. Similarly, the pneumoplethysmograph measures the arterial elasticity but by a different method; this instrument measures subtle changes in the volume or size of the part measured. A graph of the arterial pulsations is then produced. This instrument is more accurate than ultrasound but is expensive and difficult to use. Capillary filling time is measured with the foot elevated as a toe is pressed to squeeze out the blood temporarily. The return of color should not take more than three to six seconds. This test may produce some false negative results. Skin temperature measurements are useful if the results are asymmetric. This test can have variable results because ambient temperature can be an influence.

One must also differentiate an organic disorder, such as blockage of the lumen of the vessel, from a vasospastic condition. This can be done by temporarily dilating the vessels in question. This approach is accomplished by using an arterial tourniquet for three minutes and then releasing it. The perfusion distal to the tourniquet should increase if the condition is due to vasospasm. A detailed analysis of the peripheral vascular system is beyond the scope of this chapter. Observing your patients relative to the changes that occur in vascular disease will give you the greatest education.

PATHOMECHANICS OF INFECTION IN DIABETES

As stated earlier, the diabetic patients offer a distinct challenge. There are many reasons why these patients can develop infection that causes morbidity. To successfully eliminate the infection and prevent its recurrence the clinician must be aware of all

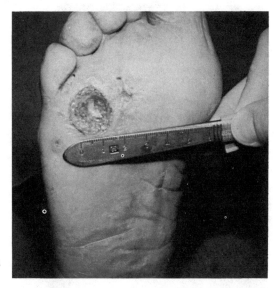

FIGURE 8–4. Mal perforans ulceration under the fourth metatarsal.

aspects of the disease. The predisposing conditions, the physiology, and the mechanics of the infection must be examined.

To effectively recognize the mechanics of infection, it is first necessary to understand the physiology of inflammation secondary to trauma. In the diabetes patient, trauma usually predisposes the patient to infection. Brand[10] has done numerous experiments with the foot pads of rats. He applied 20 psi, 10,000 times a day, simulating ordinary walking. The foot pads showed only a small rise in temperature and some swelling after the first day. When this test was repeated daily, however, ulcers and necrosis had developed by the end of a week. The repeated stress caused a gradual buildup of inflammatory cells and with diapedesis, these cells leaked into the interstitial spaces. The final necrosis began in the deeper tissues and gave the appearance of autolysis. When the repetitions were decreased to 8,000 a day and the rats were given "weekends off," there was only mild inflammation. At the end of six weeks the foot pads actually looked better than at the beginning of the test.

In diabetes patients with foot neuropathy, Boulton and coworkers[11] demonstrated abnormally high pressures beneath the metatarsal heads that were not found in diabetes patients who did not have peripheral neuropathy. The increased pressure per square inch and the inability to perceive the trauma cause the neuropathic ulcer called mal perforans (Figs. 8-4 and 8-5).

TREATMENT OF THE DIABETIC FOOT

We now specifically discuss treatment of the insensitive foot; and prophylactic measures for the traumatized and infected foot.

Treatment of Infection

The treatment of infection is an interesting topic. Infection may be regarded as a war. There is a battle between the host and the invading parasitic microorganisms, and other factors are involved as well. Without help, the diabetic patient may lose the battle

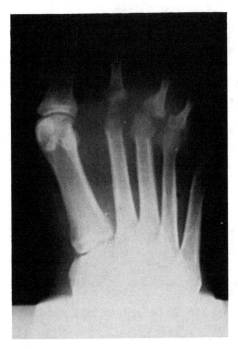

FIGURE 8–5. Osteomyelitis of the second, third, and fourth metatarsal-phalangeal joints secondary to a mal perforans.

against infection. With help and adequate circulation, that battle can definitely be won. In many instances, it may take a long time to win and the effort of a team of dedicated and trained clinicians and therapists. The patient must be able to emotionally tolerate protracted and sometimes painful therapeutic regimens. There is no doubt that this aspect may be the most difficult part of the battle; but it is necessary in order to win.

An abscess, the most common type of active infection in the diabetic foot, insulates itself from treatment by producing a protective fortress or barrier. This walling off of the infected site coupled with small vessel disease renders parenteral antibiotics ineffective. Local care—violating the barrier and gaining entry to the abscess, cleaning out the infected tissue, and establishing drainage—is necessary to eradicate the abscess. In some instances, opening the abscess is performed inadequately. There are several spaces in the foot that can become infected independently of each other. Even if a huge incision is made on the plantar aspect of the foot, an abscess can flourish on the dorsal aspect. Therefore, these feet must be assessed constantly, and if there is a cessation or regression of healing, a careful evaluation of the current therapy must be undertaken and it must be changed.

In addition, the control of the diabetic state is very important to enhance the host's ability to provide some defense against the invading bacteria and perform all of the repair. When the blood sugar level is out of control, these functions are greatly impaired. To make things worse, in the presence of infection, control of the diabetic state is extremely difficult and it is usually not until the infection is under control that the blood sugar level is within satisfactory limits.

Another aspect of this battle against infection has to be considered: the cost is very high. The expense for a three- to six-week hospital stay may reach from $15,000 to over $20,000. This reality produces an additional challenge, especially today, when there are so many pressures for cost containment. Consequently, this war may have to be fought for the most part at home or in an extended care facility, with professional treatment and supervision. The goals are to eliminate infected and necrotic tissue, establish drainage, and promote growth of granulation tissue.

Methods of eliminating necrotic, infected tissue are numerous and varied. They range from mechanical débridement to chemical débriding agents, from a scalpel to a whirlpool bath, but what happens *between* treatments is also very important. Are the bandages changed frequently, to eliminate toxic, infected exudate from the compromised area? When the foot drains via gravity, is this drainage allowed to escape or does it run back into the foot? The patient must be placed in a position that allows exudate to escape from the foot.

Dr. Brand[12] advocates the use of a total-contact short-leg cast for chronic ulcers. This method is useful and allows the patient to ambulate with protection from external stress and trauma. In addition, because the cast is well-molded and minimal padding is applied, pressure is distributed evenly and is maintained as long as the cast is worn. This total-contact cast also counteracts lymphatic congestion, which compromises the healing process.

Once the foot has healed, preventing recurrence is paramount. The foot has been compromised by the trauma of infection, and scar tissue has formed, limiting circulation and mobility of the tissues. The foot will never be as good as it was before the infection (Fig. 8-6); henceforth it will be more prone to trauma and injury. Patients must constantly monitor the condition of their feet and if a problem occurs, immediate action must be taken. Rest and proper therapy should be instituted at the first sign of a problem.

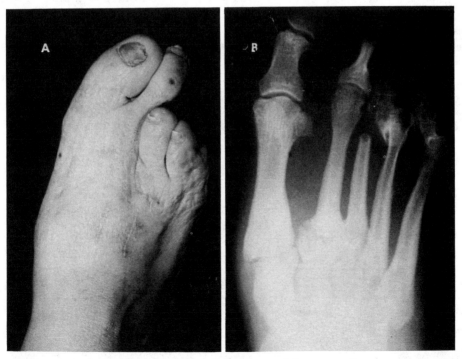

FIGURE 8-6. The clinical (A) and x-ray (B) changes of the repeated surgery to this diabetic foot in an effort to eliminate infection.

Accommodative Devices and Shoes

Accommodative devices are insoles that are placed in shoes to balance the feet, allowing pressures to be evenly distributed and permitting support of the foot. An orthotic, in contrast, supports and also controls the foot by neutralizing pronatory forces. Orthotics are discussed in detail in Chapter 9.

Accommodating shoe gear should be used by diabetic patients, and walking barefooted is prohibited. The shoe's upper should be soft, so as not to irritate any prominence or developing deformity. The accommodative insole that is used should be able to adapt to changes as well. A combination of an expanded polyethylene such as Plastazote, one-quarter inch, which permanently molds to the pressures placed on it (especially if it is heated), covered with a neoprene like Spenco that is soft and retains its shape, makes an excellent accommodative insole. This type of accommodative orthotic has saved many insensitive feet, as it not only protects the foot but also changes with additional stress. Because it adapts and conforms, the insole is accurate at any given time. In some instances, when there is an existing imbalance of the weightbearing surface, additional Plastazote must be placed in different areas so the weight can be evenly distributed during ambulation. The concept here is to put additional material in areas that are not bearing excessive weight (Figs. 8-7 to 8-10). Thinner, one-eighth inch Plastazote is excellent for this modification. The additions may be secured with contact cement and should be repeated as needed. This insole functions in vivo and is extremely forgiving (an important factor with diabetic patients).

Because of the thickness of this insole, the shoe must be able to accommodate it. Extra deep shoes are expensive and sometimes heavy. Walking shoes that come with a removable insole work well. Removing the stock innersole makes room for the device.

Shoes alone are also used in the treatment of the insensitive foot. Many advocate the use of a ridged-sole rocker-bottom shoe, as it lessens pressure at predetermined areas on the plantar surface of the foot. This change is accomplished by fashioning the apex of the rocker just proximal to the area where pressure must be relieved. These shoes are usually quite heavy, and it takes the patient a while to get used to them.

The hyperkeratotic tissue that forms as a response to increased pressure and friction should be débrided periodically, because this tissue increases the pressure, alters the mechanical properties, and causes the deeper layers of skin to retain water and become macerated. The viability of the tissue is decreased, thus predisposing the area to breakdown.

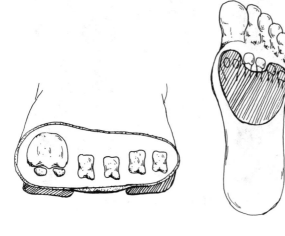

FIGURE 8-7. Accommodative padding to protect the second and third metatarsal heads.

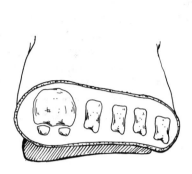
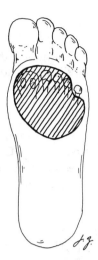

FIGURE 8–8. Accommodative padding to protect the fifth metatarsal head.

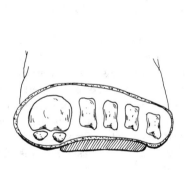
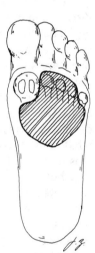

FIGURE 8–9. Accommodative padding to protect the first and fifth metatarsal heads.

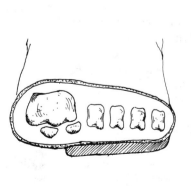
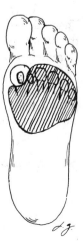

FIGURE 8–10. Accommodative padding to protect the first metatarsal head.

Surgery

Surgical intervention to eliminate osseous deformity and modify pressure is an excellent way to prevent ulceration and potential infection. Operating on patients with diabetes should lead to good healing provided that circulation is adequate. Certainly, it is easier to heal a sterile surgical wound that is closed primarily than an open, infected ulcer over a pressure point; however, the surgical sites of these patients must be watched carefully. If the nervous system is not normal, the patient is prone to injury after surgery. One of the diabetes patients upon whom I had operated had displaced the osteotomy site and fractured two other bones without noticing that anything was amiss. In spite of this, all the fractures healed, even though there was considerable displacement.

SUMMARY

Understanding as much as possible about diabetes allows an appreciation of the disease and of how it produces such dramatic changes in human anatomy and physiology. The study of diabetes patients and their foot problems is fascinating but extremely disturbing and frustrating. Although our understanding of the disease has increased, there are still many areas for investigation and the treatments are in serious need of improvement.

The best time to gather as much information as possible is when a patient is first seen. The patient's medical, family, and social history, habits, present illness, and a detailed analysis of the diabetic state are important data to gather. One must ascertain what kind of treatment has been rendered and what results were obtained. One of the most important parts of the initial evaluation is to *listen to the patient*, not only what is said but how it is said, because these patients may suffer from emotional problems associated with their disease. This observation may be one of the most important parts of the initial evaluation. As time passes and the clinician becomes more involved with the patient's treatment, there is a tendency for the clinician to lose objectivity and feel responsible for treatment failure when, in reality, patient compliance is the problem.

When patients describe their pain and discuss their problems this may be the best time to learn about the disease. There is no doubt that seasoned clinicians have gained most of their knowledge from patients by having open minds and being good listeners.

To be effective, clinicians must be extremely thorough in their physical assessment. The patient should take off both shoes and the examiner should assess the involved and the uninvolved sides to make a proper comparison. Subtleties in diabetics can be extremely revealing, when recognized. Unlike healthy patients who respond to injury and infection with inflammation, swelling, and redness, diabetics do not necessarily respond because of attenuated humoral and vascular responses. Accordingly, a diabetes patient with a foot that shows minimal changes and a break in the skin can be in a dangerous situation.

REFERENCES

1. Jauw-Tjen, L and Broen, AL, Jr: Normal structure of the vascular system and general reactive changes of the arteries. In Fairbairn, JF, Juergens, JL, Spittel, JA (eds): Peripheral Vascular Disease. WB Saunders, Philadelphia, 1972, pp 45–62.

2. Brand, PW: Patient monitoring. In Trautman, JR (ed): The Effects of Pressure in Human Tissues. North-western University Publishers, Carville, LA, 1977, pp 50–51.
3. Goldman, F: Identification, treatment and prognosis of Charcot joint in diabetes mellitus. J Am Podiatr Med Assoc 72:485, 1982.
4. Banson, BB and Lacy, PE: Diabetic microangiopathy in human toes. Am J Pathol 45:41, 1964.
5. Brown, M and Asbury, A: Diabetic neuropathy. Ann Neurol 15:2, 1984.
6. Walker, K: Peripheral neuropathy. In Davidson, J (ed): Clinical Diabetes Mellitus, A Problem-Oriented Approach. Georg Thieme Verlag, New York, 1986, pp 416–425.
7. Jurado, R and Walker, HK: Diabetic autonomic neuropathy. In Davidson, J (ed): Clinical Diabetes Mellitus, A Problem-Oriented Approach, Georg Thieme Verlag, New York, 1986, pp 426–449.
8. Lewin, ME and O'Neal, LW: The Diabetic Foot, ed 3. The CV Mosby Co, St Louis, 1983.
9. Baker, JD: Postrest Doppler ankle pressures. Arch Surg 113:1171, 1978.
10. Brand, PW: The diabetic foot. In Davidson, J (ed): Clinical Diabetes Mellitus, A Problem-Oriented Approach. Georg Thieme Verlag, New York, 1986, pp 376–382.
11. Boulton, AJM, Hardisty, CA, Betts, RP, et al: Dynamic foot pressures and other studies as diagnostic and management aids in the diabetic neuropathy. Diabetes Care 6:25, 1983.
12. Brand, PW: The insensitive foot (including leprosy). In Jahss, MH (ed): Disorders of the Foot, vol 2. WB Saunders Co, Philadelphia, 1982, pp 1266–1286.

SECTION III

Treatment Approaches to Restore Normal Movement

CHAPTER 9

Biomechanical Orthotics

Robert Donatelli, MA, PT
Michael Wooden, MS, PT

The foot functions as an important part of the lower kinetic chain and is designed to distribute and dissipate kinetic forces during the stance phase of gait. Foot orthotics are recognized as an important adjunct to the treatment of lower extremity dysfunction related to poor mechanics and alignment. The term *foot orthotics* includes many different types of orthotics—flexible, semirigid, rigid, biomechanical, sand splint, sorbothotics, functional, power soles, University of California Biomechanical Laboratory (UCBL) device, Helfet orthotics, Whitman, Roberts, Roberts-Whitman, Thomas heel, Schaffer plate, and accommodative orthotics.[1-18] For the clinician, deciding what kind of foot orthotic to prescribe can be confusing and frustrating.

For the purposes of this chapter, foot orthotics are divided into three categories: biomechanical or functional, accommodative, and pediatric. A biomechanical foot orthotic assists the lower kinetic chain in force attenuation by controlling excessive movement in the foot and ankle. Accommodative orthotics were discussed in Chapter 8. This chapter focuses on the indications, prescription, and techniques for both temporary and permanent biomechanical orthotics. A brief discussion of pediatric orthotics is also provided.

BIOMECHANICAL ORTHOTICS

The role of the biomechanical orthotic is to control excessive and potentially harmful subtalar and midtarsal joint movement. There are few objective studies demonstrating how biomechanical orthotics control excessive movement. Furthermore, very few studies discuss objective findings with successful orthotic treatment. Most studies discuss the subjective findings reported by patients using foot orthotics.[19-22] Relief from pain and the ability to return to previous levels of activity are the major criteria for determining success with orthotic therapy.

There is no evidence to indicate that the use of foot orthotics can structurally change a flatfoot deformity in adults; however, Bordelon,[23] Mereday and associates,[24] and Bleck and coworkers[25] demonstrated roentgenographic changes in children treated with foot orthotics. In all the pediatric studies, orthotics were used to correct hypermobile flatfoot.

A biomechanical foot orthotic has two important components, a forefoot and a rearfoot post. The post is a wedge on the medial or lateral side of the orthotic designed to support or control movement

Rearfoot Post

The effect of the rearfoot post on the biomechanics of the subtalar joint is not fully understood. A varus post or medial wedge is thought to limit or control eversion of the calcaneus and internal rotation of the tibia directly after heel strike.[9]

Smith and coworkers[6] reported that semirigid biomechanical orthotics reduce the amount and rate of calcaneal eversion during running. Calcaneal eversion is controlled by a rearfoot varus post. In general the semirigid and soft orthotics have a greater effect on eversion velocity than on the degree of eversion.

The results of studies relating rearfoot movement to orthotic use are conflicting. Nigg and coworkers,[26] Cavanagh,[27] and Clarke, Frederick, and Hamill[28] have shown that the rearfoot varus post significantly reduces maximum eversion. Bates, James, and Osternig[29] found no significant change in maximum eversion with the use of foot orthotics. Taunton and coworkers[30] reported a significant decrease in the total amount of eversion during the support phase of running with the use of corrective running orthotic devices. However, no significant change was noted in the amount of tibial internal rotation. In Taunton's study forefoot and rearfoot varus posts were prescribed in all the foot orthotics.

Root, Orien, and Weed[31] believe rearfoot posting should position the subtalar joint in "neutral." They also report that a minimum of 4° of pronation is necessary directly after heel strike to allow proper shock absorption and transverse plane rotation. Therefore, prescription of a rearfoot post that will allow the subtalar joint to hit near neutral and then control (but not eliminate) pronation immediately after heel strike is important.

The authors have observed that it is neither necessary nor possible for the patient to function during the stance phase from the subtalar joint's neutral position to relieve symptoms. Our preliminary studies have shown measurement techniques to be reliable in determining the neutral position, but the validity of the results remains in question.[32,33] The neutral position was determined by calculating the ratio of subtalar inversion to eversion. Neutral was defined as one third of the total subtalar joint range of motion, from the fully everted position. We have found that a thorough biomechanical evaluation, along with a trial period of temporary orthotics, will best determine the individual's need for long-term orthotic therapy.

Forefoot Posting

There is even less understanding of how forefoot posts affect the biomechanics of the midfoot and rearfoot. Shaw[34] believes the purpose of a forefoot post is to act as a crutch. The crutch holds the abnormal forefoot in a normal or nearly normal relationship to the rearfoot and the supporting surface (Fig. 9–1). The forefoot posts are

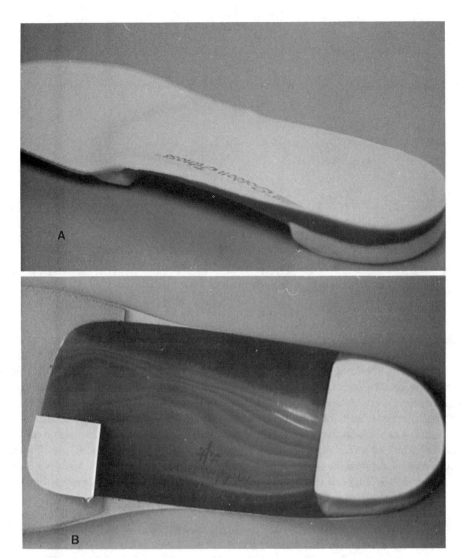

FIGURE 9–1. (A) Semi-rigid sport orthotics. (B) Extrinsic forefoot post and extrinsic rearfoot post.

prescribed for one of two deformities: forefoot varus is supported with a medial wedge; forefoot varus post, with a forefoot valgus using a lateral post.

Supporting the forefoot abnormalities reduces the need for rearfoot compensation. For example, as previously described in Chapter 2, forefoot varus is compensated for by rearfoot subtalar joint pronation. Forefoot varus, by itself, is not destructive to the foot. However, at the subtalar joint compensatory pronation results in an "unlocking" of the foot, creating hypermobility and loss of a rigid lever from midstance through push-off. This abnormal pronation of the subtalar joint allows the inverted (varus) forefoot to contact the ground for weightbearing, but the amount of pronation is excessive, and the resultant hypermobility can be destructive to the foot and to the rest of the lower kinetic chain during propulsion.

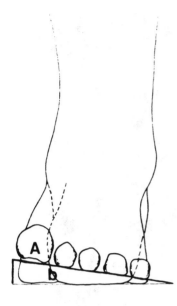

FIGURE 9–2. Forefoot post. (A) First metatarsal head; (B) Forefoot varus post or medial wedge.

Forefoot posting reduces the need for compensatory subtalar joint pronation by bringing the ground surface up to the weightbearing aspects of the metatarsal heads (Fig. 9–2). The subtalar joint does not have to pronate as much to allow the medial aspect of the foot to contact the ground. Full correction of the forefoot abnormality is not always necessary. A review of 80 patient charts indicated that the average forefoot varus post corrected 62% of the abnormality. For example, the average forefoot varus abnormality was 8.5°, so the average forefoot varus post corrected 62% of the 8.5°, or a five-degree forefoot varus post was prescribed. If forefoot varus was 10°, a 6° forefoot post was used. Conversely, with forefoot varus abnormalities of 6° or less, the forefoot post corrected 90–100% of the abnormality. The size of the forefoot post is limited by the tolerance of the patient and the constraints of the shoe.

Summary of Posting Principals

The rearfoot post is designed to alter the position of the subtalar joint from heel strike to footflat. If the calcaneus is excessively everted at heel strike, the subtalar joint is in excessive pronation. A rearfoot (medial) post will invert the calcaneus closer to its neutral position to allow the subtalar joint to pronate normally from heel strike to footflat. Conversely, if the calcaneus and the subtalar joint are excessively inverted and supinated at heel strike, a rearfoot valgus (lateral) post will evert the subtalar joint closer to its neutral position. The rearfoot post must be dynamic, that is, it must control but not eliminate subtalar joint movement. The maximum amount of rearfoot posting is usually 5–6°. Any more posting may cause the heel to ride up and out of the shoe.

The forefoot post supports the forefoot deformity by bringing the ground closer to the metatarsals, thereby reducing the need for rearfoot compensation. The forefoot post is indicated when the forefoot deformity is creating problems during the propulsive phase of stance. Generally, the maximum forefoot post that fits comfortably in a shoe is 6–8°.

In painful foot lesions, particularly those involving the metatarsal heads, posting is often not tolerated; softer materials, metatarsal pads, or relief cut-outs may have to be substituted. Posting is contraindicated in the insensitive foot, where excessive forces on plantar structures are not perceived by the patient. These forces can create lesions with resultant serious complications.

Heel Lifts

Forefoot and rearfoot posts are frontal plane corrections, whereas a heel lift (or heel platform) is a sagittal plane correction for ankle joint equinus. Whether the limitation in ankle joint dorsiflexion is caused by bony, soft tissue, or postural factors, the subtalar joint will often compensate for this limitation by pronating excessively, especially from heel rise through push-off. Adding a heel lift to the orthotic will reduce the need for compensatory pronation. Again, the maximum amount tolerated comfortably is 5–6 mm.

Temporary Orthotics

A trial of temporary orthotics (constructed from a wide variety of materials) is essential in determining the needs of the patient. Static evaluation and gait analysis determine the ideal subtalar joint neutral position, how far the patient deviates from this position, and where abnormal supination or pronation is occurring during the gait cycle. The clinician then predicts what combination of forefoot and rearfoot correction is necessary. Prior to the prescription of an expensive definitive orthotic, a temporary orthotic acts as a guide to determine accuracy and efficacy. Figures 9–3 through 9–9 outline the steps necessary for fabrication of temporary orthotics.

Permanent Orthotics

CASTING AND PRESCRIPTION

If a trial of temporary orthotics has been successful in reducing symptoms or correcting gait abnormalities and if the condition is likely to be long-term or recurrent, a permanent orthotic is indicated. The most popular type of permanent orthotic is fabri-

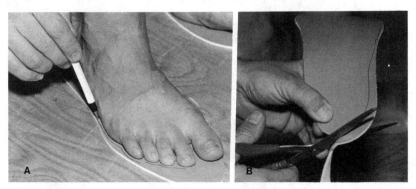

FIGURE 9–3. The foot is traced on the orthotic insert (A). The insert is cut to fit the shoe (B).

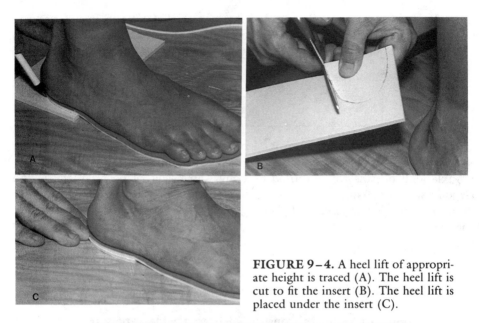

FIGURE 9–4. A heel lift of appropriate height is traced (A). The heel lift is cut to fit the insert (B). The heel lift is placed under the insert (C).

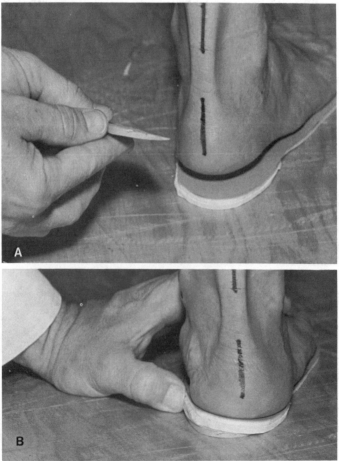

FIGURE 9–5. The degree of rearfoot post (wedge) is chosen (A). The rearfoot post is placed under the heel lift, in this case, a varus post (B).

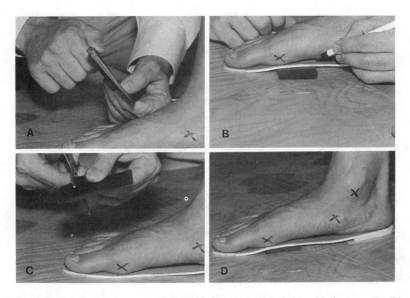

FIGURE 9–6. (A) A forefoot post of desired firmness and degree is chosen. (B) The anterior edge of the forefoot post is located under the insert and at the first MTP joint line. The post is cut to about the length of the first metacarpal. (C) The post is trimmed to fit the insert. (D) The post is placed under the insert.

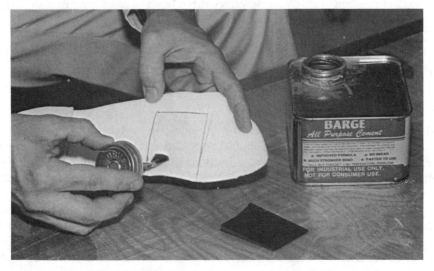

FIGURE 9–7. The lift and posts are glued to the insert.

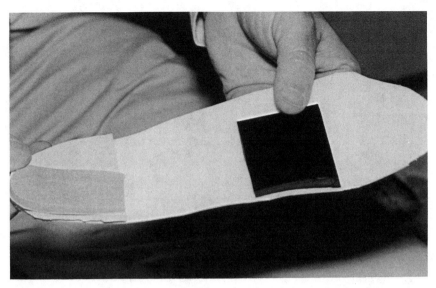

FIGURE 9–8. The finished temporary orthotic with heel lift, forefoot varus post and rearfoot varus post.

cated by an orthotics laboratory from a cast of the patient's foot. These orthotics can be made from casts or impressions taken in non-weightbearing, semi-weightbearing, or full weightbearing positions, often without benefit of measurements or posting prescriptions. Since our evaluation is concerned with determining compensations that result in deviations from the ideal neutral position, we feel the most biomechanically sound method is to cast the foot in a non-weightbearing position, with the subtalar joint held in neutral. This position captures the position of the forefoot before compensation, and allows the clinician to request from the laboratory the required amount of posting and lifting which will reduce the amount of compensation needed. Figures 9–10 through 9–13 demonstrate the neutral casting procedure with the patient in the prone non-weightbearing position. Table 9–1 describes three types of biomechanical or functional orthotics: standard, sports, and midrange.

Figure 9–14 shows a generic prescription form that lists the most important information required by orthotics laboratories. The cases presented later in the chapter give examples of how to complete the form.

IN-OFFICE FABRICATION

There are several systems that allow the clinician to fabricate a permanent foot orthotic in the office. Several factors should be considered when purchasing an in-house system. The clinician should be able to individualize the foot orthotics. The in-house orthotic should offer variable sizes, top covers, rigid, semirigid, or soft consistency, and possess the ability to post for deformities. Experiences with several in-house systems has shown the Orthofoot system to be the most adaptable. It allows the clinician to post the orthotic to correct for foot deformities. Metatarsal pads, scaphoid pads, heel cushions, heel lifts, and relief cut-outs can be incorporated into the orthotic. In addition, different top covers can be used with the orthotics, such as leather, vinyl, Plastazote, or shock-ab-

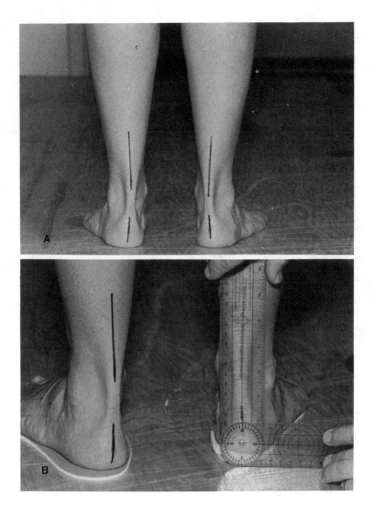

FIGURE 9–9. Patient standing, demonstrating excessive calcaneal valgus or pronation (A). With the patient standing on the temporary orthotics, the calcaneus is remeasured to determine the reduction in the calcaneal valgus (B).

sorbing material. Finally, each orthotic can vary in consistency from rigid to soft, to conform to the patient's foot.

The durability for foot orthotics fabricated in the office is questionable. However, any orthotic should be re-evaluated every one to two years, to determine durability and changes in foot abnormalities. No studies have determined the effectiveness of orthotics fabricated in the office for pain relief or correction of foot abnormalities.

PEDIATRIC FOOT ORTHOTICS

Treatment of hypermobile flatfoot in children remains controversial. A review of the literature reveals conflicting opinions, ranging from no treatment to treatment by rigid foot orthotic devices.[35-40]

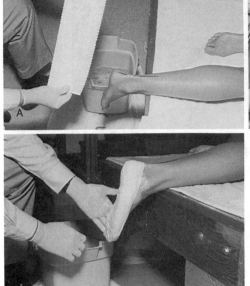
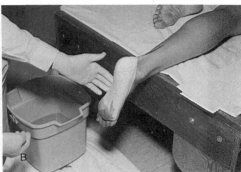

FIGURE 9–10. Two double-thickness, extra fast setting plaster splints, measuring 5 inches by 30 inches, are used (A). The first splints are placed posteriorly from the heel (B). The second splint is placed anteriorly from the toes (C).

Research

There exist few statistical data concerning the conservative care of hypermobile flatfoot in children. Penneau and associates[41] evaluated ten children radiographically. The radiographs were taken with the patient barefoot and wearing a Thomas heel, over-the-counter inserts, and two molded plastic orthotics called University of Califor-

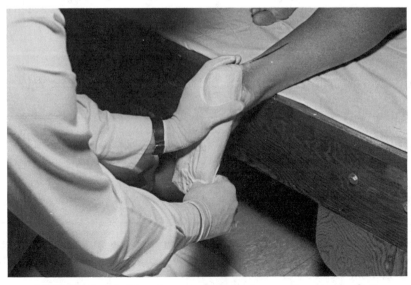

FIGURE 9–11. The plaster is smoothed to conform to the foot.

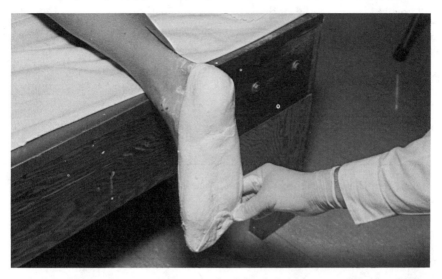

FIGURE 9–12. As the plaster sets, the subtalar joint is held in neutral by gently distracting downward on the fifth toe. <u>Note</u>: To avoid mis-shaping the cast, do not grasp the metatarsals.

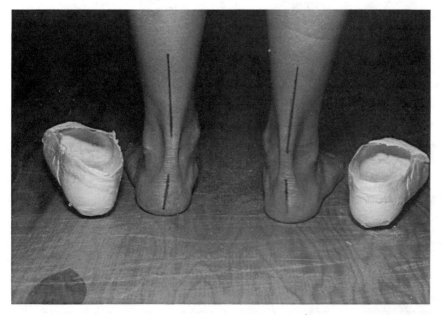

FIGURE 9–13. The casts should resemble the deformity; in this case, calcaneus valgus or pronation.

TABLE 9–1 General Characteristics of Neutral Cast Orthotics

Type	Material	Posting	Indications
Standard (functional)	Rigid plastic (Rohadur)	Extrinsic forefoot and rearfoot	Firmest control for severe pronation and hypermobility
Sports	Semirigid or plastic or fiberglass; softer rearfoot post and heel lift	Extrinsic rearfoot, intrinsic forefoot*	Very active patients, for sports activities
Midrange	Semirigid plastic soft rearfoot post and heel lift	Extrinsic rearfoot, intrinsic forefoot*	Light nonathletic activity, dress shoes

*For more control, extrinsic forefoot posts can be requested.

PERMANENT ORTHOTIC PRESCRIPTION

Therapist Info:

   Name_____

   Address_____

Patient Info:

   Name_____

   Address_____

   Occupation/Activity_____

   Age_____ Height_____ Weight_____

   Shoe Size_____ Sex_____

Orthotic Type:

_____ Rohadur

_____ Sports

_____ Semi-rigid

_____ Accommodative

_____ Children (gait plate, Roberts Whitman, etc.)

Posting Instructions

Forefoot: _____ Extrinsic   _____ Intrinsic

   Left   _____ °varus   _____ °valgus

   Right _____ °varus   _____ °valgus

Rearfoot:

   Left   _____ °varus   _____ °valgus

   Right _____ °varus   _____ °valgus

Heel Lift:

   Left   _____ inch

   Right _____ inch

Covers/extensions:

_____ Spenco

_____ Leather

_____ PPT

_____ Vinyl

Special Instructions:

FIGURE 9–14. A generic prescription form for casted orthotics. Format will vary depending on the laboratory used.

nia Biomechanical Laboratory (UCBL) devices. No significant radiographic changes in these children's feet were seen with the use of any of these foot orthotics. Bleck and Berzins[25] reported on 71 children, mean age 4.7 years, who used the Helfet heel seat and the UCBL device. They found the rate of improvement, measured by radiographs, was approximately 1° for every two months of wear. The mean duration of orthotic use was 14.5 months. Mereday, Dolan, and Lusskin[24] studied the effects of the UCBL device on ten children for two years. The children's ages ranged from 3 to 12 years. Results indicated relief from pain and improvement in gait while wearing the orthotics. However, there was no indication that structural changes resulted from the use of the inserts. Finally, Bordelon,[28] treated 50 children from 3 to 9 years of age with a custom-molded insert. The results of Bordelon's study indicated that bony deformities could be corrected by 80% with the initial fitting. The correction of bone alignment averaged 5° per year. Radiographs were taken initially and after each child had worn the orthotics for three years. Six children were evaluated after removal of the orthotics. The radiographs demonstrated that only one child showed significant loss of correction. The average time out of the orthotics was 25 months.

Orthotic Devices

The feet of children are very malleable and can be easily molded to most orthotics. The pediatric orthotic attempts to alleviate structural deformities that may lead to abnormal compensations in the foot and protects the foot during its growth period.

Several types of pediatric foot orthotics are made from rigid (fiberglass and Rohadur) or flexible (Plastizote, rubber, sponge) materials. Polypropylene, cork, and leather are intermediary materials that are neither rigid nor flexible. Orthotics commonly used for children include Whitman-Roberts orthotic, Shaffer plates, heel stabilizers, out-toe gait plates, and functional posted orthotics.[17]

The Whitman-Roberts orthotic (Fig. 9–15) is a combination of the Roberts and the Whitman orthotics. This orthotic controls or maintains a rectus heel and stimulates supination. A high medial flange is used to limit medial rotation of the talus, and a high

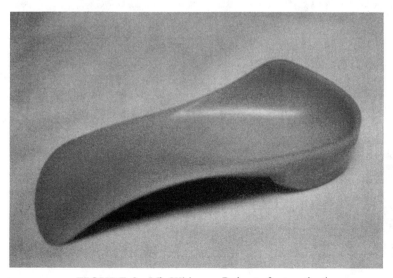

FIGURE 9–15. Whitman-Roberts foot orthotic.

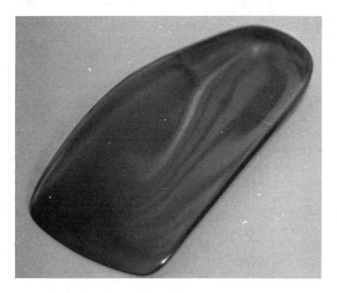

FIGURE 9–16. Shaffer plate.

lateral flange controls calcaneal eversion. The Whitman-Roberts device is useful in children over nine years of age.[17]

The Shaffer plate orthotic (Fig. 9–16) has a medial flange to support the foot and is used in older children or adolescents. The Shaffer plate does not control excessive calcaneal eversion and should not be used in severe structural collapse of the pediatric foot.

Heel stabilizers can be tolerated until 8–10 years of age. The heel stabilizers control the foot better than any other form of orthotic device. A type A heel stabilizer (Fig. 9–17) limits inversion and eversion of the calcaneus by confining the heel. There is no control of the forefoot and minimal arch support. Types A and C are designed to maximally control the heel and midfoot. Type A is used for a mild to moderately pronated foot. The medial and lateral flanges are used to support and control the rearfoot, midfoot, and forefoot. Type C differs from type B in that the medial and lateral flange extend to the first and fifth metatarsophalangeal (MTP) joints, respectively.

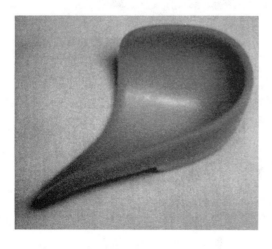

FIGURE 9–17. Type A heel stabilizer (top view).

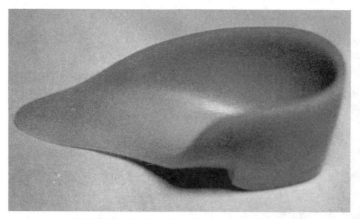

FIGURE 9–18. Type D heel stabilizer.

The type D heel stabilizer (Fig. 9–18) promotes abduction of the forefoot. The lateral plantar flange extends beyond the fourth and fifth metatarsophalangeal (MTP) joints to limit dorsiflexion of these joints. Therefore, the foot must roll inward, allowing dorsiflexion at the three medial MTP joints. The result is abduction of the forefoot, reducing a toe-in gait.

The out-toe gait plate (Fig. 9–19) functions like the type D heel stabilizer. The out-toe plate is most frequently used in children who demonstrate an in-out toe deformity and who are older than eight to ten years.

Functional type orthotics (Fig. 9–20) should be used for older children or adolescents. This orthotic does not confine the young foot sufficiently to reduce medial and lateral instabilities. Furthermore, it may be detrimental, forcing the child's foot into a posted varus or valgus position. A rectus position of the forefoot occurs when the metatarsal heads are parallel to the horizontal plane. The rectus position of the forefoot

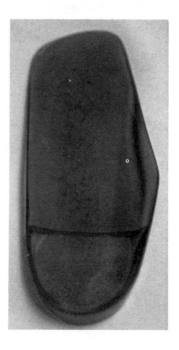

FIGURE 9–19. Out-toe gait plate (top view).

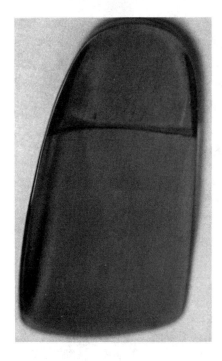

FIGURE 9–20. Functional orthotic, with a intrinsic forefoot post and an extrinsic rearfoot post. Rohadur translucent plastic material (top view).

is more desirable in attempting to correct varus and valgus deformities. Rearfoot posting is more common in pediatric orthotics to position the subtalar joint in neutral.

Summary of Pediatric Orthotic Principals

The pediatric orthotic is prescribed to control excessive rearfoot movement in the stance phase of gait. Rigid materials are more commonly used to control movement. A medial flange and a lateral flange may be prescribed in severe hypermobile flatfoot deformities. Posting of the forefoot and rearfoot is discouraged in pediatric foot orthotics. A rectus position of the child's foot is encouraged to correct varus and valgus deformities.

CASE STUDIES

This section reviews cases requiring orthotic prescription in the adult and pediatric patient.

1: Congenital Flatfoot with a Diagnosis of Talipes Calcaneovalgus

A five year old patient reported medial arch pain upon impact of jumping. Radiographic evaluation demonstrated a vertical talus and a decreased inclination angle of the calcaneus.

Upon physical evaluation ligament laxity of several joints in the lower extremities was observed. The range of motion of the subtalar joint was 35° inversion and

15° eversion. Dorsiflexion of the ankle bilaterally was measured in the non-weightbearing position at 20°. In the standing position the calcaneus was noted to be in excessive eversion. During ambulation, when excessive weightbearing occurred along the medial aspect of the foot, excessive rearfoot mobility and abnormality in the weightbearing position were noted. Figure 9–21 lists the findings of the static evaluation.

Maximum control of the rearfoot is necessary to allow the subtalar joint to function from its neutral position. If the rearfoot is stabilized, forefoot and midfoot breakdown can be avoided. The orthotic affording the most control and support to the rearfoot, midfoot, and forefoot is the type C heel stabilizer.

This patient should be re-evaluated every six months, to determine growth and structural changes. A possible progression of foot orthotics may occur over the next eight to ten years, ranging from the heel stabilizer (maximum control), to the Whitman-Roberts (moderate control), and finally, the Shaffer plate (minimal calcaneal eversion control).

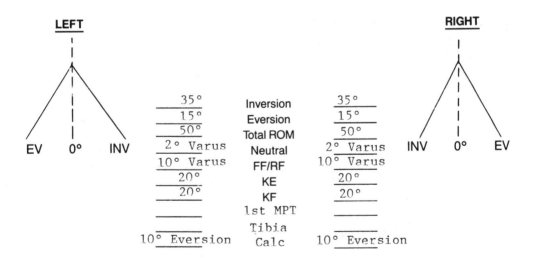

FIGURE 9–21. Evaluation form for Case 1: Congenital flatfoot talipes calcaneal valgus.

2: Plantar Fasciitis of the Right Heel and a Neuroma of the Left Forefoot, Secondary to Late Pronation During Push-off

A 42 year old male patient complained of right medial heel pain that was worst in the morning during the step taken after arising. The patient is an intense runner, averaging 60–70 miles per week. When running at the end of the day, the first two to three miles were always very painful. There was no history of knee or foot pain.

Evaluation revealed a normal medial arch in the weightbearing position, with the right foot abducted secondary to external rotation of the lower limb. No toe deformities were noted. Figure 9–22 lists the findings of the initial static evaluation. In the non-weightbearing position, with the rearfoot in neutral position, a forefoot varus of 5° was noted with a hypermobile first ray. Range of motion of the calcaneus was 10° of eversion and 20° of inversion. The left foot showed a rectus forefoot (perpendicular to the rearfoot): no varus or valgus was noted. The calcaneus range of motion was the same as on the right. Radiographic evaluation revealed a heel spur on the right calcaneal area at the insertion of the plantar fasciae. Palpation of the medial aspect of the calcaneus was tender.

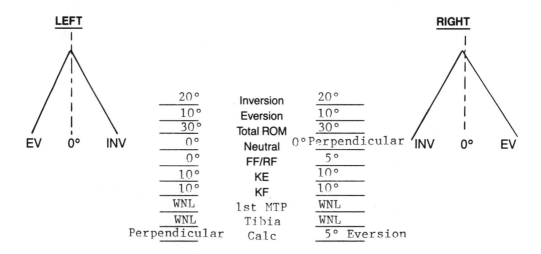

EVALUATION WORKSHEET

	LEFT				RIGHT	
		20°	Inversion	20°		
		10°	Eversion	10°		
		30°	Total ROM	30°		
EV 0° INV		0°	Neutral	0° Perpendicular	INV 0° EV	
		0°	FF/RF	5°		
		10°	KE	10°		
		10°	KF	10°		
		WNL	1st MTP	WNL		
		WNL	Tibia	WNL		
		Perpendicular	Calc	5° Eversion		

ORTHOTIC WORKSHEET

FF None°	**Varus** **Valgus**		FF 5°	**(Varus)** **Valgus**	
RF None°	**Varus** **Valgus**		RF 5°	**(Varus)** **Valgus**	
Heel Lift___mm.			Heel Lift___mm.		
Other_____			Other_____		

FIGURE 9–22. Evaluation form for Case 2: Plantar fasciitis, neuroma, late pronator.

Gait Assessment

An instability of the right foot was observed during push-off. The instability was seen at push-off, because the patient showed a heel whip at that time. The unstable first ray caused over-stretching of the plantar fascia. The right foot abducted during push-off to avoid dorsiflexion of the first MTP joint and over-stretching of the plantar fascia.

An orthotic with a forefoot post of 5° on the right, and a 5° rearfoot post was prescribed. The left orthotic was not posted because deformities were not present. The patient ran for 1.5 years without pain, during which time he set a new personal record that was five minutes faster than his previous marathon races.

After 1.5 years the patient returned, complaining of left heel pain and numbness in the lateral border of the right foot. In addition, a neuroma was present between the second and third metatarsals, and it reproduced paresthesia between the second and third toe web spaces when palpated. A forefoot varus on the left and 9° of forefoot varus on the right were measured when the patient was evaluated. Hypermobility of the first ray was noted on the right. The medial border of the left heel was also tender and painful when palpated.

The patient had obviously overextended himself during the previous 18 months. The increased running velocity produced excessive forces on the forefoot, causing further breakdown. The semirigid orthotics were unable to assist the foot in attenuation of the increased forces for longer than 18 months. The neuroma developed because of the increased shear forces between the metatarsals.

A new pair of orthotics was fabricated with a forefoot varus post of 7° on the right and 5° on the left. A rearfoot varus post of 6° was prescribed bilaterally, with 4° of motion. After running for two weeks with the new pair of orthotics, numbness and paresthesia were completely relieved on the right and 50% of the left foot heel pain was relieved.

3: Plantar Fasciitis and Heel Pain

A 38 year old laboratory technician and part-time graduate student had experienced several months of right Achilles tendon pain as well as pain on the plantar aspect of the right heel. Pain had developed insidiously as the patient became more active at work and school. The patient was diagnosed as having Achilles tendinitis and plantar fasciitis. A series of ultra-sound treatments, injections, and oral anti-inflammatory medication had been given, without success.

Assessment revealed moderate tenderness of the Achilles tendon just above its insertion into the calcaneus. Tenderness of the plantar fascia at its origin on the calcaneus was noted. Figure 9–23 shows the static evaluation measurements of the foot and ankle.

Upon gait analysis, abnormal supination throughout the stance phase of gait was observed. There was no evidence of subtalar or midtarsal joint pronation from heel strike to footflat; the foot remained supinated through push-off.

These findings indicated probable loss of shock absorption because of the abnormal supination. Temporary orthotics with 4° forefoot valgus posts were constructed. Additionally, heel lifts of about 5 mm were added, to take some tension off the Achilles tendon. A 2° rearfoot valgus post was added to help promote normal pronation from heel strike to footflat.

The patient's response to the temporary orthotics was excellent: she reported

EVALUATION WORKSHEET

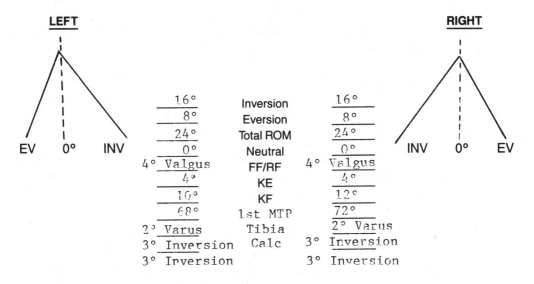

16°	Inversion	16°
8°	Eversion	8°
24°	Total ROM	24°
0°	Neutral	0°
4° Valgus	FF/RF	4° Valgus
4°	KE	4°
10°	KF	12°
68°	1st MTP	72°
2° Varus	Tibia	2° Varus
3° Inversion	Calc	3° Inversion
3° Inversion		3° Inversion

ORTHOTIC WORKSHEET

FF __4°__ ~~Varus~~ (Valgus)   FF __4°__ ~~Varus~~ (Valgus)

RF __2°__ ~~Varus~~ (Valgus)   RF __2°__ ~~Varus~~ (Valgus)

Heel Lift __5°__ mm.   Heel Lift __5°__ mm.

Other _____   Other _____

FIGURE 9–23. Evaluation form for Case 3: Achilles tendinitis and plantar fasciitis; abnormal supination.

better than 75% reduction of pain while using the orthotics. Therefore, the patient was casted for semirigid orthotics posted similarly to the temporary orthotics. In addition to promoting normal pronation, the orthotics also provided cushioning at heel strike. At the one month follow-up visit the patient reported continued relief of symptoms and was instructed to continue using the orthotics indefinitely.

4: Medial Knee Pain Associated with Jogging and Leg Length Discrepancy

A 30 year old recreation therapist presented with a three month history of right medial knee pain associated with jogging. The patient denied any direct injury, stating that pain developed after she increased her jogging mileage from 15 miles to about 25 miles per week. The pain did not respond to several weeks of rest and anti-inflammatory medications. Examination by an orthopedic surgeon revealed no evidence of ligament or cartilage injury. An isokinetic evaluation done previously indicated normal quadriceps and hamstring muscle strength. Figure 9–24 lists the findings of the biomechanical foot evaluation.

EVALUATION WORKSHEET

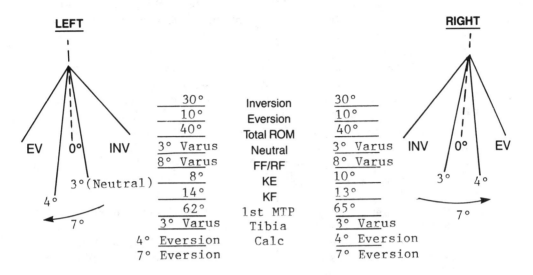

	LEFT				RIGHT	
	30°	Inversion	30°			
	10°	Eversion	10°			
	40°	Total ROM	40°			
EV 0° INV	3° Varus	Neutral	3° Varus	INV 0° EV		
	8° Varus	FF/RF	8° Varus			
3°(Neutral)	8°	KE	10°			
4°	14°	KF	13°	3° 4°		
	62°	1st MTP	65°			
7°	3° Varus	Tibia	3° Varus	7°		
	4° Eversion	Calc	4° Eversion			
	7° Eversion		7° Eversion			

ORTHOTIC WORKSHEET

FF **4°**   (Varus)
       Valgus

RF **X**   Varus
        Valgus

Heel Lift____inch

Other_____

FF **4°**   (Varus)
       Valgus

RF **X**   Varus
        Valgus

Heel Lift **3/8** inch

Other_____

FIGURE 9-24. Evaluation form for Case 4: Right medial knee pain, leg length discrepancy.

Gait analysis revealed no significant problems from heel strike to footflat, where pronation appeared to be normal; however, at push-off the calcaneus remained in an everted position, indicating inability to resupinate. In addition to these findings, the patient was found to have a ⅜ of an inch shortening of the right lower extremity.

Based on these findings, temporary orthotics with 4° forefoot varus posts were fabricated. Additionally, a ⅜ inch heel lift was added to the right orthotic. Over the next two weeks, the patient reported significant reduction in right-sided knee pain as she resumed her jogging activities. She was then casted for rigid sports orthotics with forefoot varus posts and a right heel lift, as in the temporary orthotics. One month later, the patient reported total absence of knee pain despite having increased her jogging mileage to 25 miles per week.

5: Bilateral Knee Pain Associated with Running and Bicycling

A 29 year old sales representative complained of bilateral knee pain that had persisted for several weeks and was associated with running. The patient was a triathlete who had recently increased his running mileage to about 35 miles per week, in addition to bicycling and swimming on a daily basis. He reported no history of knee pain. He stated that pain was greater on the left than on the right, but that both knees began to hurt after running 2–2.5 miles. The results of a thorough knee examination by an orthopedist were negative. Findings of the static evaluation are listed in Figure 9–25.

Gait analysis revealed signs of pronation throughout the entire stance phase. From heel strike to footflat, each calcaneus was at, or near, end-range pronation. Therefore, there was no normal pronation available from heel strike to footflat. Additionally, there was no resupination through push-off. The calcaneus remained everted, the naviculars were dropped downward and in towards the midline, and there was a sudden abduction of the foot at push-off. These findings indicated early, excessive pronation throughout the stance phase, probably secondary to forefoot varus and ankle joint equinus. Temporary orthotics were constructed. Forefoot varus posts of 6°, rearfoot varus posts of 4°, and heel lift of one quarter inch were added to each orthotic. The orthotics were designed to assist the subtalar joint of each foot at heel strike by reducing some of the excessive pronation, thus allowing the subtalar joint to pronate normally from heel strike to footflat. The forefoot posts were designed to assist with resupination at push-off by adding support to the first ray.

Over the next three weeks the patient was able to gradually resume his normal running mileage. He reported total relief of right knee pain and "signifi-

EVALUATION WORKSHEET

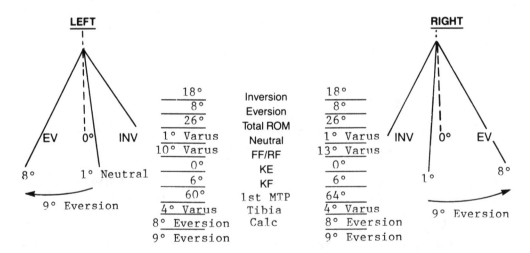

ORTHOTIC WORKSHEET

FIGURE 9–25. Evaluation form for Case 5: Bilateral knee excessive pronation.

cant relief" of the left knee pain. At that time he was casted for rigid sports orthotics with the same prescription that was built into the temporary orthotics.

SUMMARY

Biomechanical orthotics may be useful in reducing the excessive forces of weight-bearing for adults. These biomechanical orthotics are not designed to change or correct foot abnormalities but are designed to reduce pain and improve function of the foot during the stance phase of gait. The biomechanical orthotic has two components, a forefoot post and a rearfoot post. The purpose of the forefoot post is to support the forefoot deformity or bring the ground closer to the heads of the metatarsal bones. If the metatarsal heads are supported during maximum loading of the forefoot, abnormal forces can be reduced or eliminated.

The purpose of the rearfoot post is to position the rearfoot, or subtalar joint, as close as possible to a neutral position. The function of the rearfoot post is most important at heel contact. If the rearfoot post is prescribed correctly it should prevent the subtalar joint from starting the stance phase in excessive pronation or excessive supination. At the same time the rearfoot post must allow sufficient movement of the subtalar joint.

We believe that a trial period of temporary orthotics is necessary to determine a more specific orthotic prescription. A more specific prescription means less adjustment time, greater patient satisfaction, more perceptible pain relief, and better patient compliance with the use of the foot orthotics. Table 9-2 summarizes the general characteristics of neutral cast orthotics.

Orthotics are prescribed for children to control excessive rearfoot movement in the stance phase of gait. Rigid materials are most commonly used to control movement. A medial flange and a lateral flange may be prescribed for severe hypermobile flatfoot deformities. Posting of the forefoot and rearfoot is discouraged in pediatric foot orthotics.

More research is needed in the area of foot orthotics. Valid and reliable methods are needed to help determine how orthotics alter foot function during the stance phase of gait.

TABLE 9-2 Typical Progression of Orthotic Treatment

	Assessment	Treatment
Initial visit	Take history, evaluate biomechanics, perform gait analysis	Prescribe temporary orthotics (1-2 week trial)
Second visit	Re-evaluate, determine response	Adjust temporaries if necessary
Third visit	Re-evaluate, choose appropriate permanent orthotic	Cost for permanent orthotic or fabricate in-office permanent orthotic
Follow-up visits	Re-evaluate, check for fit and comfort; in children, check for growth periodically	Recast as needed

REFERENCES

1. Blake, RL and Denton, JA: Functional foot orthoses for athletic injuries. J Am Podiatr Med Assoc 75:359, 1985.
2. Eggold, JF: Orthotics in the prevention of runners' overuse injuries. Physician Sports Med 9:125, 1981.
3. Rose, GK: Correction of the pronated foot. J Bone Joint Surg 40B:674, 1958.
4. Weed, JH, Ratliff, FD, and Ross, SA: A biplanar grind for rear post on functional orthoses. J Am Podiatr Med Assoc 69:35, 1978.
5. McKenzie, DC, Clement, DB, and Taunton, JE: Running shoes, orthotics, and injuries. Sports Med 2:334, 1985.
6. Smith, LS, Clarke, TE, Hamill, CL, et al: The effects of soft and semi-rigid orthoses upon rearfoot movement in running. Podiatry Sports Med 76:227, 1986.
7. Doxey, GE: Clinical use and fabrication of molded thermoplastic foot orthotic devices. Phys Ther 65:1679, 1985.
8. D'Ambrosia, RD: Orthotic devices in running injuries. Clin Sports Med 4:611, 1985.
9. Bates, BT, Osternig, LR, Mason, B, et al: Foot orthotic devices to modify selected aspects of lower extremity mechanics. Am J Sports Med 7:338, 1979.
10. Subotnick, SI: The abuses of othotics in sports medicine. Physician Sports Med 3:73, 1975.
11. Murphy, P: Orthoses: Not the sole solution for running ailments. Physician Sports Med 14:164, 1986.
12. Odom, RD and Gastwirth, B: San splint orthoses. J Am Podiatr Med Assoc 72:98, 1982.
13. Niehaus, PL: Sorbothotics, soft tissue supplement orthoses. J Am Podiatr Med Assoc 75:46, 1985.
14. Helfand, AE: Basic considerations for shoes, shoe modifications, and orthoses in foot care. Clin Podiatry 1:431, 1984.
15. Sperryn, PN and Restan, L: Podiatry and the sports physician—an evaluation of orthosis. Br J Sports Med 17:129, 1983.
16. Nigg, BM and Morlock, M: The influence of lateral heel flare of running shoes on pronation and impact forces. Med Sci Sports Exercise 19:294, 1987.
17. MaCrea, JD: Pediatric Orthopaedics of the Lower Extremity. Futura, New York, 1985, p 317.
18. Subotnick, SI: Foot orthoses: An update. Physician Sports Med 11:103, 1983.
19. Hannaford, DR: Soft orthoses for athletes. J Am Podiatr Med Assoc 76:566, 1986.
20. Subotnick, SI: Orthotic foot control and the overuse syndrome. Arch Podiatr Med Foot Surg 2:207, 1975.
21. Carter, G: Foot orthoses: Simple prescriptions can mean dramatic pain relief. Aust Fam Physician 16:1104, 1987.
22. Scranton, PE, Pedegana, LR, and Whitesel, JP: Gait analysis: Alterations in support phase forces using supportive devices. Am J Sports Med 10:6, 1982.
23. Bordelon, LR: Hypermobile flatfoot in children. Clin Orthop 181:7, 1983.
24. Mereday, C, Dolan, CME, and Lusskin, R: Evaluation of the University of California Biomechanics Laboratory shoe insert in "flexible" pes planus. Clin Orthop 82:45, 1972.
25. Bleck, EE and Berzins, UJ: Conservative management of pes valgus with plantar flexed talus, flexible. Clin Orthop 122:85, 1977.
26. Nigg, BM, Eberle, G, Frei, D, et al: Gait analysis and sport shoe construction. Biomechanics VIA, University Park Press, Baltimore, 1978, p 303.
27. Cavanagh, PR: The Running Shoe Book. World Publications, Mountain View, CA, 1981, pp 83, 259.
28. Clarke, TE, Frederick, EC, and Hamill, CL: The effects of shoe design parameters upon rearfoot movement in running. Med Sci Sports 15:376, 1983.
29. Bates, BT, James, SL, and Osternig, LR: Foot function during the support phase of running. Am J Sports Med 7:338, 1979.
30. Taunton JE, Clement DB, et al: A triplanar electrogoniometer investigation of running mechanics in runners with compensatory overpronation. Can J Appl Sports Sci 10:104, 1985.
31. Root, ML, Orien, WP, and Weed, JN: Clinical Biomechanics, vol II: Normal and Abnormal Function of the Foot. Clinical Biomechanics Corp, Los Angeles, 1977, p 26–31.
32. Cantu, R, Catlin, P, and Wooden, MJ: A comparison of two techniques for measuring forefoot/rearfoot relationships. (submitted for publication).
33. Garbalosa, J, McClure, M, Catlin, P, et al: The relationship of the forefoot to the rearfoot in the normal population. (submitted for publication).
34. Shaw, AH: The effects of a forefoot post on gait and function. J Am Podiatr Med Assoc 65:238, 1975.
35. Cowell, HR, Drennan, JC, Hensinger, RN, et al: Childrens' foot problems and corrections. Contemp Orthop 2:526, 1980.
36. Giannestras, NJ: Foot Disorders, Medical and Surgical Management, ed 2. Lea & Febiger, Philadelphia, 1973.
37. Helfet, AJ: A new way of treating flatfeet in children. Lancet 1:262, 1956.
38. Jahss, MH: Atlas of Orthotics: Biomechanical Principles and Applications. CV Mosby, St. Louis, 1975.
39. Jahss, MH (ed): Disorders of the Foot, vol 1. WB Saunders, Philadelphia, 1982, p 1703.
40. Tachdjian, MO: Pediatric Orthopaedics. WB Saunders, Philadelphia, 1972.
41. Penneau, K, et al: Pes planus: Radiographic changes with foot orthoses and shoes. Foot Ankle 2:299, 1982.

CHAPTER 10

Physical Therapy

John C. Garbalosa, MMSc, PT

In this chapter, selected modalities and manual techniques of the physical therapy treatment for four theoretical case studies are presented to demonstrate the theory and application of the selected therapeutic techniques. The clinical decision-making model serves as the blueprint from which the selection of techniques is guided.[1]

The four case studies include a lateral ligamentous sprain, a bimalleolar fracture, calcaneal pain, and post surgical status for hallux abductovalgus (HAV) correction. Each case emphasizes a particular physical therapy technique and/or modality. The format consists of the presentation of evaluative findings, interpretation of these findings, a treatment plan, the patient response to the treatment plan, and some of the possible rationales for both the applied treatment and the observed changes.

The following material should not be taken as a definitive methodology for handling the problems presented but rather as a guideline for handling these therapeutic problems. Every effort has been made to support the clinical decisions with scientific and empirical evidence.

CASE STUDY

Case 1: Lateral Ligament Sprain

The central focus of this section is threefold: reduction of edema, restoration of movement, and prevention of reinjury of the ankle.

INITIAL EVALUATION AND FINDINGS

The initial evaluation begins with the patient's history and includes a passive range of motion (ROM) test, manual muscle test (MMT), "figure-eight" girth measurement, palpation, visual inspection, pain assessment, and other specific tests (Table 10–1).

TABLE 10–1 Case 1: Summary of Initial Evaluation and Weekly Progress

| | Passive Motion | | | | Girth Measurement (mm) | Pain Level* |
Week	Dorsi-flexion	Plantar Flexion	Inversion	Eversion		
Initial evaluation	5	10	5	5	66	9
1	5	20	5	5	61	7
2	10	25	10	10	58	0–1
3	10	25	10	10	55	0–1
4	15	47	23	10	55	0

*On a scale of 0 (no pain) to 10 (excruciating pain)

Case 1 is that of a 30-year-old recreational athlete who sustained a plantar flexion, inversion, internal rotation injury to his right ankle while playing basketball. When the injury occurred, the athlete heard a popping noise. Subsequently rapid edema about the right ankle ensued. A physician was consulted immediately after the injury by the athlete. The physician determined that there was no osseous involvement via roentgenogram. The diagnosis of the physician was moderate sprain of the lateral collateral ligaments of the right ankle.

Pain during movement of the right ankle, swelling of the right ankle, and decreased independence during ambulation were the patient's initial chief complaints. The patient described in Case 1 does not have a history of trauma to the right ankle. Using a numeric pain scale of zero to ten (with ten being excruciating pain and zero being no pain) the athlete reports a pain level of nine. Figure 10–1 is the athlete's pain drawing. The drawing includes the plantar, anterior, and lateral aspects of the right ankle and foot as the symptomatic areas.

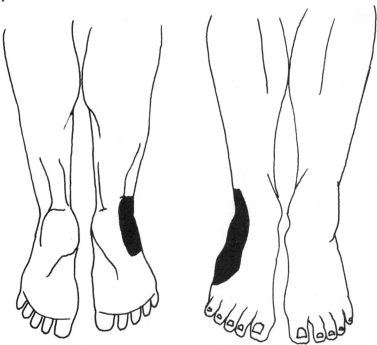

FIGURE 10–1. Pain drawing of patient in Case 1.

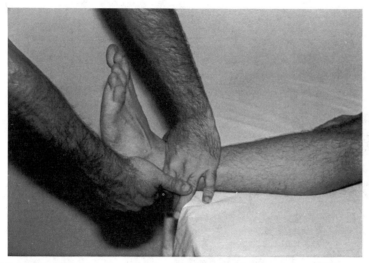

FIGURE 10-2. Anterior drawer test, Case 1: Tibia and fibula are stabilized with one hand, while other hand grasps and forces the calcaneus anteriorly.

Visual inspection by the physical therapist of the athlete's lower extremities shows them to be remarkable for severe edema about the right ankle and forefoot. Ecchymosis is also present just distal to the lateral malleolus.

A severe restriction of the active and passive ROM of the right ankle is present. Both passive and active movements reproduce the patient's pain. Passive ROM of the right ankle is 5° of dorsiflexion, 10° of plantar flexion, 5° of inversion, and 5° of eversion. The MMT of the lower leg musculature is within normal limits (WNL). Resisted eversion and plantar flexion reproduce the patient's pain symptoms, and he is unable to perform a standing toe raise with the affected limb.

Palpation of the right ankle and foot is markedly tender over the fibular attachment site of the anterior talofibular and calcaneofibular ligaments. An increase in the tissue temperature is evident over the lateral aspect of the right ankle joint.

Ligamentous stress testing of the right ankle joint does not demonstrate any increase in mobility when compared to the unaffected joint. Two ligamentous stress tests, the anterior drawer test (Fig. 10-2) and the calcaneal inversion test (Fig. 10-3) reproduce the pain complaints.[2] The figure-eight girth measurement about the malleoli, navicular tuberosity, and styloid process of the fifth metatarsal of the right ankle is 66 mm.

INTERPRETATION

The evaluative findings confirm that the lateral collateral ligaments of the right ankle—specifically the anterior talofibular and calcaneofibular ligaments—are involved. The tests of palpation, ligament stress, passive ROM, and MMT confirm the involvement of those ligaments. Theoretically, these tests isolate the anterior talofibular and calcaneofibular ligaments.[2-4] The patient's history further supports the evaluative findings, since the reported mechanism of injury is often associated with damage to the two involved ligaments.[2-5]

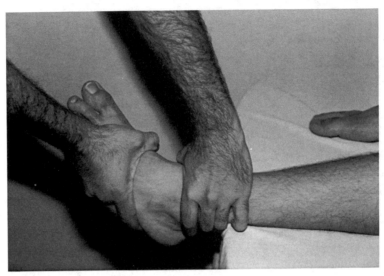

FIGURE 10–3. Inversion stress test, Case 1: Tibia and fibula are stabilized with one hand, while other hand grasps and forces the calcaneus into inversion.

TREATMENT

The primary goals of treatment are to reduce edema and improve mobility while preventing further damage to the ankle. Given these goals, treatment will initially consist of anti-inflammatory modalities. Anti-inflammatory treatments are indicated because of the presence of an active inflammatory and repair process, as evidenced by an increase in the tissue temperature and edema of the right ankle.[2–4] Mobilizing the involved ankle joint prevents the deleterious effects of immobilization.[3,4,6]

Week One

Treatment Plan. The first week of physical therapy consisted of once daily treatments of cryotherapy in combination with electrotherapy, active joint mobilization exercises, and a home exercise program. During the first week the patient was allowed to walk with axillary crutches bearing partial weight on the right ankle.

A typical treatment session during the first week began with placing the right lower extremity in an elevated position, packing the ankle and forefoot in ice, and applying high-voltage electrical stimulation (HVS) for 30 minutes. The HVS electrode pads were placed over each malleoli with the pulse rate set at 80 per second at an intensity of 150 volts and a negative polarity. After the cryotherapy treatment the patient performed 45 repetitions of active plantar flexion–dorsiflexion exercises against manual resistance, as tolerated. Next, a 10-minute light effleurage massage was applied in a caudocephalad direction, with the leg elevated. Treatment sessions ended with another 30-minute HVS and ice treatment.

At home, the athlete iced the ankle and forefoot every hour for 10 to 15 minutes and maintained the right lower extremity in an elevated position when not ambulating. The home exercise program consisted of active dorsiflexion and plantar flexion of the right ankle without resistance for 45 repetitions, six times per day. Before and after the performance of exercises, the patient iced the ankle and forefoot. This was in addition to the hourly intermittent icing throughout the day. When ambulating, a heel-to-toe partial weight bearing (PWB) gait pattern is used, and an air splint was worn. At night, the lower extremity was elevated by placing pillows beneath the foot of the mattress.

Treatment Results. At the end of the week, the passive ROM of the right ankle was 20° of plantar flexion with no changes in eversion, inversion, or dorsiflexion ROM. Ankle girth measurement is 61 mm, reduced by 5 mm. The patient's subjective pain level was 7. Palpation still revealed an increase in the tissue temperature about the lateral aspect of the right ankle.

Treatment Rationale. HVS and ice applied with the lower extremity elevated were chosen for the effects of HVS, cold, and elevation on blood flow. Cold is theorized to decrease vasodilator metabolism, encourage vasoconstriction, and increase blood viscosity.[2,7-10] Preliminary studies on the therapeutic effects of HVS are mixed.[11-14] There is some evidence in the literature that HVS alters hemodynamics.[11,12]

Reed,[12] in his animal experiment, concluded that HVS decreased the protein leakage from blood vessels via an as yet unknown mechanism. The decrease in protein leakage allows the lymphatics to remove excess fluid in the tissues and prevent further increase in fluid migration into the surrounding cells.

Michlovitz, Smith, and Watkins[11] noted a trend toward a reduction in edema and pain with the use of HVS in combination with ice; however they were unable to detect a statistically significant difference between the effects of ice used alone and ice used in combination with HVS.

Elevation of a distal extremity reduces the gravitational forces that affect the cardiovascular system.[15] Massage is also reported to enhance venous and lymphatic drainage of the lower extremity.[16]

Active and passive exercise programs are performed to reverse the effects of immobilization on the connective tissues. Several authors have noted that prolonged immobilization of a joint leads to various undesirable biochemical and biomechanical changes in the surrounding connective tissues.[6,17-23] Mobilization of a joint through its ROM may prevent them.[6,21,24] A more complete discussion of the effects of mobilization is presented in the following section.

The home program adopts the same rationale as the clinical program, with one addition: protection of the right ankle. The ankle joint is protected with an air splint and PWB with axillary crutches. The air splint provides some compression to the ankle joint (preventing further increase in edema) and prevents excessive inversion.[25,26] Partial weightbearing of the right lower extremity prevents the harmful effects of a loss of compression on hyaline cartilage. Hyaline cartilage is nutritionally dependent on alternating compression and decompression.[19,22] PWB also provides proprioceptive input to the ankle. Freeman and others[27-30] feel the loss of proprioception is one reason for the recurrence of ankle injuries.

Week Two

Treatment Plan. In the second week the physical therapy program progressed, with the addition of proprioceptive exercises (Fig. 10–4) and the use of a bicycle ergometer. During the second week, the patient was seen three times for treatment. Tiltboard exercises were performed for 10 minutes during each treatment session. HVS and icing for 30 minutes before and after exercise were applied, as in week one, as were manually resisted exercises to the dorsiflexors and plantar flexors. The patient was now allowed to fully weightbear (FWB) without using assistive devices. The air splint continued to be used whenever the athlete walked.

Gastrocsoleus stretches, toe curls, peroneal isometrics, and proprioceptive exercises were added to the patient's home exercise program. The gastrocsoleus stretching was

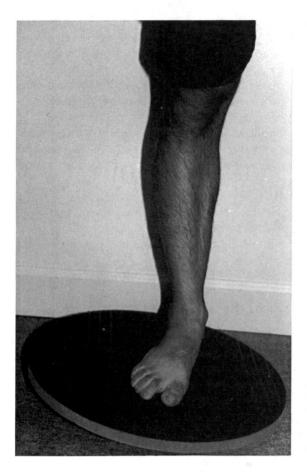

FIGURE 10–4. Proprioceptive exercises performed with Case 1 standing on a tilt board. Case 1 is instructed to bring each edge of the board (one edge at a time) in contact with the floor in a circular fashion.

performed six times per day for 10 repetitions, holding the gastrocsoleus in a stretched position for each repetition. Peroneal isometrics were performed six times per day for 45 repetitions, holding each repetition for a count of six. Toe curl exercises were performed with the patient in a sitting position with the toes resting on top of a towel lying on the floor. He curled the toes, bringing the opposite end of the towel closer to them. Toe curl exercises were performed for 10 repetitions, six times per day. The patient intermittently iced the right foot and ankle with the right lower extremity in an elevated position. Nighttime elevation of the lower extremity is also continued.

   Treatment Results. By the end of week two, the patient had minimal pain on active and passive ankle motion (pain level of 0 to 1). He continued to complain of some discomfort over the styloid process of the fifth metatarsal cuboid area. Edema was still present about the lateral aspect of the right ankle, as evidenced by the figure-eight girth measurement (58 mm). The passive ROM of the right ankle is 10 degrees of dorsiflexion, 25 degrees of plantar flexion, 10 degrees of eversion, and 10 degrees of inversion. The results of isokinetic tests of ankle dorsiflexion and plantar flexion performed at the end of the second week (as well as subsequent tests) are shown in Table 10–2. Ligament stress tests continued to show no excess of joint play. The anterior drawer test still provoked pain. No increase in tissue temperature was apparent with palpation when compared to the uninvolved extremity.

   Treatment Rationale. The absence of complications in the second week of rehabilitation allowed the physical therapy program to progress accordingly. Proprioceptive

TABLE 10-2 Case 1: Isokinetic Test Results

Tests	Plantar Flexors*		Dorsi-flexors*		Evertors†		Invertors†	
	Right (Foot-pounds)	Left	Right (Foot-pounds)	Left	Right (Foot-pounds)	Left	Right (Foot-pounds)	Left
1 (week 2)	20	56	0	20	—	—	—	—
2 (week 3)	—	—	—	—	10	21	10	22
3 (week 4)	49	54	19	21	—	—	—	—
4 (week 8)	51	54	19	21	18	20	21	22

†At 60° per second
*At 90° per second

exercises were initiated to rehabilitate the damaged mechanoreceptors in the joint capsule and accompanying ligaments.[26-28,30-32] Stimulation of the mechanoreceptor system of the injured joint may improve proprioception in the ankle. This improvement is accomplished by retraining the muscle-tendon mechanoreceptors or the undamaged joint mechanoreceptors, or both.[33] Several researchers have documented enhancement of proprioception of damaged joints through proprioceptive retraining.[28,32,33] These authors noted a decrease in position sense after inversion injury to an ankle. Following proprioceptive training using a tiltboard, position sense improves.[28,32,33]

In order to maintain the athlete's cardiovascular endurance a bicycle ergometer was used. Although cycling has not been shown to improve or maintain elite runners' conditioning, it does maintain cardiovascular endurance in moderately trained athletes.[34] It may also be effective in preventing muscle weakness in muscle groups adjacent to the injured lower extremity linkage system.[34,35] Disuse atrophy of the adjacent muscle groups as a result of immobilization of a joint has been reported.[35]

Isokinetic testing for weakness due to disuse was performed. The results of the test (see Table 10-2) showed a strength deficit of the plantar flexors of 64% and of the dorsiflexors of 100%, as compared to the uninvolved side. The patient's isokinetic test results were also below the available norms. Scranton[36] and Davies[37] have demonstrated with isokinetic testing that the right ankle plantar flexors should exhibit between 30 and 72 foot-pounds of plantar flexion and 15 and 27 foot-pounds of dorsiflexion at 90° per second.

Ligament stress testing still revealed slight involvement of the anterior talofibular ligament secondary to the reproduction of pain on stressing the ligament. The inflammatory process most probably was no longer active, as suggested by the absence of palpated elevated skin temperatures. Gastrocsoleus stretching and peroneal isometric exercises at home were implemented to improve the flexibility of the gastrocsoleus complex and retard the potential disuse atrophy of the evertors of the right ankle.[2]

Week Three

Treatment Plan. Treatment sessions during week three continued to shift from passive to active forms of treatment. The patient was still seen three times per week. Treatments began and ended with the application of ice packs to the foot and ankle, without HVS, for 20 minutes. A warm-up period, consisting of cycling on a bicycle ergometer for ten minutes, was followed by an isokinetic workout of 90 repetitions at 90° per second with the right ankle dorsiflexors and plantar flexors. The active portion of the treatment program ended with a ten-minute tiltboard workout.

An isokinetic test was done on the evertors and invertors of the right ankle at the end of the third week (see Table 10–2). Based on the results of the test, an isokinetic strengthening program was initiated with the evertors and invertors of the right foot, consisting of 90 repetitions at 90° per second.

The home program during the third week was changed to a more functional exercise regimen. A "back to run" program was implemented, which consisted of a gradual increase in running distance and agility skills. Progress in the program depends on the satisfaction of two criteria: absence of pain and of edema of the involved joint. The patient continued to ice the right foot and ankle before and after exercise and performed proprioceptive tiltboard exercises and gastrocsoleus stretching as before. Standing toe raises, for 45 repetitions six times per day, were added to the program. The use of the air splint for walking was gradually decreased.

The main focus of the treatment program is to simulate the patient's preinjury activities. His main deficits revolved around the loss of strength and reduction of cardiovascular endurance.

Treatment Results. By the end of the week, edema of the right ankle and forefoot could no longer be detected, either visually or by girth measurement. Girth of the right ankle was 55 mm. At this time he experienced minimal pain only with inversion movements. The pain was located over the styloid process of the fifth metatarsal and cuboid bones. The anterior drawer test still reproduced complaints of pain.

Treatment Rationale. Ligamentous healing allowed the initiation of isokinetic testing and strengthening of the evertors and invertors of the ankle. The tensile strength of the ligaments at this point could be assumed to be sufficient to withstand the stress of eversion and inversion exercise.[38,39] Wong et al[40] demonstrated peak torque strength of between 14–24 foot-pounds for inversion and 14–22 foot-pounds for eversion at 60° per second.[40] Because of the normative data and the contralateral isokinetic test, an isokinetic strengthening program was instituted.

The back to run program was implemented to allow the musculoskeletal system to adapt to the new stresses place on it, preventing further musculoskeletal injury. Also, the back to run program allowed the ankle to be stressed in a controlled manner, preventing premature return to full activity.[2,39,42] Further assurance of a safe return to full activity was afforded by the gradual discontinuation of the air splint.

Week Four

Treatment Plan. An isokinetic retest of the plantar flexors and dorsiflexors during week four revealed minimal deficits (49 foot-pounds and 19 foot-pounds, respectively, at 90° per second). In addition to using the bicycle ergometer for ten minutes before exercise, the patient continued to strengthen the evertors and invertors of the right ankle using an isokinetic device for 120 repetitions at 90° per second. The foot and ankle were no longer iced. A modified cuboid whip manipulation (Fig. 10–5) was performed in an effort to decrease lateral plantar pain.[43] The athlete's home program now consisted of toe raises, eversion-inversion resistive exercises using a large elastic band for 45 repetitions, tiltboard proprioceptive exercises, gastrocsoleus stretching, and agility skills. The agility skills consist of running figure-eight, back-pedaling, and zigzag patterns at varying speeds.

Treatment Results. Presently, the patient has no complaint of pain. Minimal weakness was noted. The passive ROM of the right ankle was WNL (15° of dorsiflexion, 10° of eversion, 23° of inversion, and 47° of plantar flexion). Accordingly, active treatment was discontinued. A follow-up visit was planned in four weeks for a retest of the evertors and invertors.

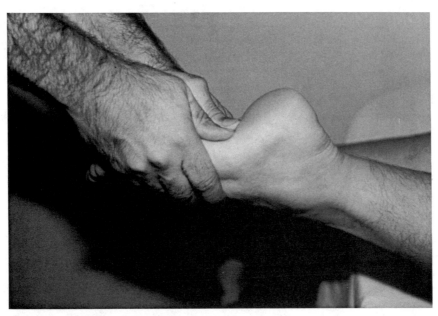

FIGURE 10–5. Modified cuboid whip manipulation. The therapist grasps the foot with both hands, placing both thumbs over the plantar aspect of the cuboid bone. From the starting position of knee flexion and ankle dorsiflexion, the therapist moves the lower leg into a position of knee extension and ankle plantar flexion and inversion while applying a superior force with the thumbs to the cuboid.

Treatment Rationale. Although the patient still had some deficit in strength, he was discharged from active treatment because of economic constraints. A follow-up visit was planned to ascertain whether the observed strength deficits were problematic. Given the inability to reproduce the athlete's lateral cuboid pain through various tests of provocation of the ankle joint and the mechanism of injury, the cuboid bone was believed to be subluxed. This subluxation was believed to be the source of the pain over the lateral cuboid area.[43]

Week 8

An isokinetic retest of the plantar flexors and dorsiflexors and evertors and invertors of the right ankle revealed clinically acceptable differences in strength (less than 10%, see Table 10–2). The patient's clinical evaluation was unremarkable, and he was discharged from active physical therapy.

Case 2: Bimalleolar Fracture

The use of mobilization techniques in the restoration of movement is the central theme of this section.

INITIAL EVALUATION AND FINDINGS

The patient in Case Two is a 26-year-old laborer who reported sustaining a bimalleolar fracture of the left ankle as a result of a fall from a ladder at home approximately 8 weeks earlier. On the date of injury the laborer was admitted to the hospital by his

TABLE 10-3 Case 2: Summary of Initial Evaluation and Weekly Progress

Week	Passive Motion*				Girth (mm)	Pain Level*
	Dorsi-flexion	Plantar Flexion	Inversion	Eversion		
Initial evaluation	0	5	0	0	60	5-9 with activity
1	5	20	5	5	59	2-7 with activity
2	9	33	10	10	57	1-8 with activity
4	12	41	18	10	57	1-8 with activity
28	5	10	5	5	58	4
29	12	25	11	10	56	0

*Measured on a scale of 0 (no pain) to 10 (excruciating pain)

physician. Open reduction with internal fixation of the fracture site was performed the same day. The postoperative hospital treatment course was uneventful. The patient reports being in a short-leg cast non-weightbearing (NWB) for 8 weeks. The cast was removed the day of his initial visit to the physical therapist.

The laborer's chief complaints were weakness, stiffness, and swelling of the left ankle. On a zero to ten numeric pain scale (with ten being excruciating pain and zero being no pain), the laborer reported a pain level of five that increased to nine with movement of the left ankle. Table 10-3 is a summary of the evaluation and subsequent weekly re-evaluation findings.

Marked atrophy of the left lower leg musculature was evident during visual inspection. The lower one third of the lower leg appeared to be slightly angulated in a varus direction. Slight edema of left ankle was also visually noted.

During the initial evaluation, the strength of the lower extremity was not tested. The passive ROM of the left ankle was 0° of dorsiflexion, 5° of plantar flexion, 0° of eversion, and 0° of inversion. Pain was present when the extremes of all motions were reached.

Edema of the left ankle was confirmed during palpation of the ankle. Minimal tenderness was reproduced over the lateral malleolus during the palpatory examination. The mobility of the incision line was not restricted in any direction. The accessory joint play motions of anterior and posterior tibiofibular glide of the talus, superior and inferior glide of the metatarsals, and anterior and posterior glide of the tibia on the fibula at the inferior tibiofibular joint were limited (Figs. 10-6 to 10-8).[43,44] Joint play is a motion necessary for normal physiologic movement. Joint play is not under the voluntary control of the patient.[43] An example of joint play is the superior glide of the proximal phalanx of the first toe on the first metatarsal at the metatarsophalangeal joint.

Figure-eight girth measurements of the left and right ankles were 60 mm and 53 mm, respectively. Figure-eight girth measurements were performed as in Case 1.

INTERPRETAION

The history provided by the laborer had important implications for future treatments and also explained some of the results seen during the initial evaluation. The use of long lever arms during mobilization techniques can be harmful. If too much force is generated by the use of long lever arms, the fracture ends could be displaced. Certain modalities, such as short-wave diathermy, are contraindicated for patients with internal fixation devices.[45]

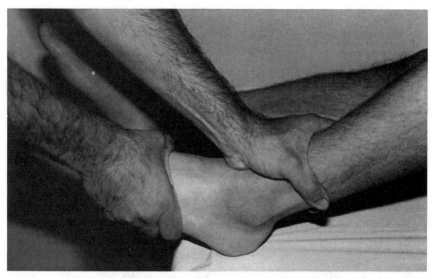

FIGURE 10–6. Tibiofibular posterior glide on talus. With one hand grasping the forefoot about the midtarsal joint, the examiner grasps and applies a posterior force on the tibia and fibula.

The extended time of immobilization can be assumed to be the cause of the observed atrophy of the lower leg musculature.[20,23,46] The deficits noted in the passive ROM of the ankle joint can be partially attributed to the period of immobilization.[6,17,18,21,23,24] Another cause of the passive motion deficits of the ankle joint may be due to the internal fixation devices.

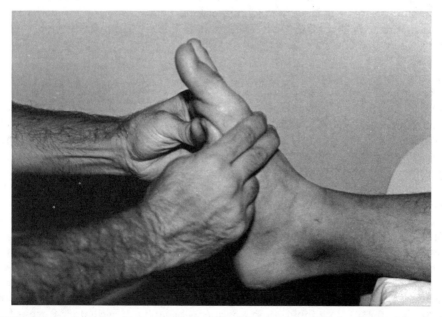

FIGURE 10–7. Superior intermetatarsal glide. The head and shaft of one metatarsal are grasped and stabilized with one hand. Other hand mobilizes the adjacent metatarsal using the same hold as the stabilizing hand.

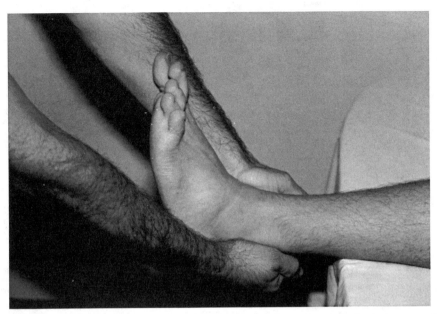

FIGURE 10–8. Posterior tibial glide on fibula. The examiner places the hypothenar eminence of the mobilizing hand over the medial malleolus and applies a posterior force. Simultaneously, the hypothenar eminence of the other hand is placed over the posterior surface of the lateral malleolus and an anterior force is applied.

TREATMENT

The primary goal of treatment is to improve the pain-free mobility of the ankle joint. Once an improvement in pain-free mobility is made, the secondary goals of increasing the strength of the lower leg musculature and increasing the patient's independence in gait can be addressed. The ultimate goal is to return the laborer to his previous functional status.

Week One
Treatment Plan. Physical therapy treatment was given on a once daily basis for the first week. The initial week of treatment consisted of warm whirlpool baths combined with active exercises in the whirlpool for 20 minutes; joint mobilization of the tibiofibular, talocrural, and intermetatarsal joints; and a home exercise program. The whirlpool exercise was drawing imaginary letters with the hallux.

Joint mobilization techniques for the inferior tibiofibular, talocrural, and intermetatarsal joints were simply a progression of the joint play test performed during the initial evaluation.[44,47] The main difference between the test and the treatment maneuvers was the addition of graded oscillations within the available joint play.[44,47] Inferior tibiofibular joint mobilization consisted of anterior and posterior glide of the tibia on the fibula (see Fig. 10–8).[44] The talocrural joint mobilizations consisted of anterior and posterior glide of the tibia and fibula on the talus (see Fig. 10–6) and long axis distraction of the talocrural joint (Fig. 10–9).[44] The intermetatarsal mobilizations consisted of superior and inferior glide of the metatarsals upon each other (see Fig. 10–7) and rolling of the forefoot (Fig. 10–10).[43,44] Mobilization treatments began with oscillatory forces of grade I and progressed immediately to grade IV forces.[47]

The home exercise program consisted of flexibility exercises, resistive exercises,

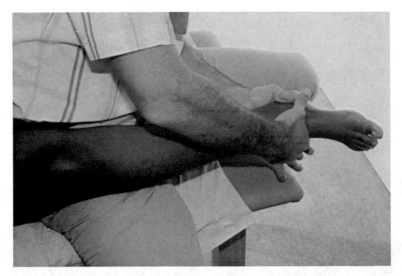

FIGURE 10–9. Long axis distraction of the talocrural joint. With the web space of one hand over the calcaneus and the web space of the other hand over the talar head, the examiner applies a force in a longitudinal direction to the lower leg.

cryotherapy, and protected gait. The flexibility exercise—gastrocsoleus stretching—is shown in Figure 10–11. To apply maximal stretch to the gastrocsoleus complex, the patient must keep the subtalar joint in a supinated position.[49,50] To ensure that this maximal stretch is attained, he was instructed to internally rotate his left lower extremity slightly and lean forward; bearing weight over the lateral aspect of the involved foot. The stretched position was held for ten seconds for ten repetitions, six times per day. Resistive exercises consist of eversion, plantar flexion, inversion, and dorsiflexion using an elastic material for resistance, performing the exercises for 45 repetitions for each motion, six times per day. The patient was encouraged to ice immediately after the

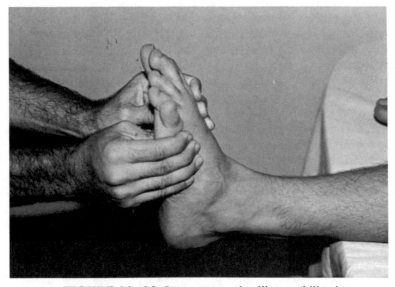

FIGURE 10–10. Intermetatarsal rolling mobilization.

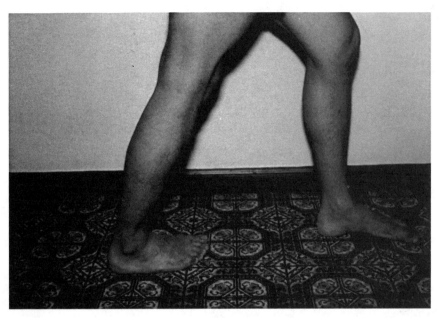

FIGURE 10-11. Gastrocsoleus stretching. Anterior leg should be flexed at the knee and hip with the posterior leg in hip and knee extension. The posterior leg should also be rotated internally slightly. The patient will then lean forward, keeping the heel of the posterior leg on the floor and the hip and knee in extension.

completion of flexibility and resistive exercises with the involved lower extremity elevated for 15-20 minutes. An air splint was applied to the ankle for walking.

Treatment Results. After the first week of treatment passive ROM of the left ankle was 20° of plantar flexion, 5° of dorsiflexion, 5° of eversion, and 5° of inversion. The patient continued to have restrictions of the joint play of his talocrural joint. Intermetatarsal joint motion was WNL. A mild edema was still noticeable over the left lateral malleolus, as evidenced by the figure-eight girth measurement of 59 mm. The patient rated a decrease in his pain level from five down to two. The pain level increased from two to seven during resistive activities with the foot (see Table 10-3).

Treatment Rationale. Warm hydrotherapy was used because the effect of heat on connective tissues is to decrease their viscosity, which helps to reduce the stiffness in the ankle joint.[8,51] Elevated tissue temperatures in conjunction with stretching are thought to cause plastic deformation in connective tissues.[8,21,50,51] A secondary response to elevated tissue temperatures is an increase in oxygen uptake and blood flow to the heated tissues. Theoretically these increases should make more nutrients available to the damaged tissues, thereby assisting in the healing process.[8,50]

During immobilization of a joint several biochemical changes occur. These changes include a decrease in glycosaminoglycans (GAG) and water content and an increase in collagen crosslink formation.[6,17,18,21,24] The decreases in GAG and water will lead to alterations in the viscous nature of connective tissue; causing an increase in the stiffness of the joint. It will also allow collagen crosslinking to occur, further diminishing the extensibility of the immobilized joint.[6,17,18,21,24]

Joint mobilization is purported to stimulate the production of GAG, thereby increasing the water content of connective tissue. The increase of both of these biochemical processes improves the mobility of the joint by decreasing the viscosity of involved tissues.[5,21] Other side effects of joint mobilization are the breaking of abnormal collagen crosslinks and the stimulation of proper collagen fiber orientation.[6,21] All of these purported effects of joint mobilization ultimately lead to an increase in ROM.

Grade I mobilizations are believed to have effects on the nociceptive system of joints. These low-amplitude oscillatory mobilizations are believed to stimulate mechanoreceptors.[3,44] Stimulation of mechanoreceptors, primarily type I and II, will have an inhibitory effect on the type IV nociceptors of the joint via certain spinal cord reflexes. Type I and IV mechanoreceptors are stimulated via grade I through IV mobilization forces.[3,44,52] Both the inhibition of pain and the reversal of the biochemical changes of immobilization improve joint mobility.

Ice after exercise was applied for two reasons: to prevent any adverse inflammatory response secondary to stretching and to maintain the plastic changes achieved during the stretch.[21,50] Maintenance of the observed clinical changes is accomplished at home by ROM exercises.

Week Two

Treatment Plan. Clinical sessions during the second week of physical therapy began with warm whirlpool treatments, as in the previous week. While in the whirlpool the patient performed gastrocsoleus stretches along with his other ROM exercises. Once out of the whirlpool, he received joint mobilization techniques of long-axis talocrural distraction, anteroposterior talocrural glide, and inferior tibiofibular joint glides to the left ankle using grade I and IV forces. He was seen three times per week for physical treatment.

After the above mobilization therapy, resistive exercises against moderate manual resistance were applied by the physical therapist. The straight plane motions of eversion, inversion, plantar flexion, and dorsiflexion were resisted for 45 repetitions in each direction. The patient complained of discomfort over the area of the left lateral malleolus with the resisted eversion and plantar flexion movements.

Upon completion of the resistive phase of the treatment the left ankle is placed in an active reflex treatment unit (ARTU)* for 20 minutes. The ARTU is a continuous passive motion, massage, and cooling device for the foot and ankle (Fig. 10–12). The extremes of all motions can be preset by the therapist to limit the degree of movement allowed by the ARTU. For the patient in Case 2, only the cooling and motion aspects of the machine were incorporated in treatment.

The home program was intensified by using a more resistive elastic material in the exercise program. The gait pattern progressed to FWB status with one axillary crutch. The laborer continued to use the air splint.

Treatment Results. At the end of week two the passive ROM was 10° of eversion, 10° of inversion, 9° of dorsiflexion, and 33° of plantar flexion. Slight edema was still noted about the lateral malleolus of the left ankle. The figure-eight girth measurement was 57 mm. Pain continued to occur with any type of resistive plantar flexion or eversion movement. Although the overall pain level was one, the plantar flexion and eversion movements raised it to seven or eight. The patient was now walking with FWB on the left lower extremity without any assistive devices except the air splint.

Treatment Rationale. The use of warm whirlpools continued secondary to the effects of heat on connective tissues, as previously mentioned. Static stretch was employed simultaneously with the whirlpool as a result of research indicating the benefits

---

*(ARTU, Universal Gym Equipment, Inc., 930 27th Avenue SW, Cedar Rapids, IA 52406)

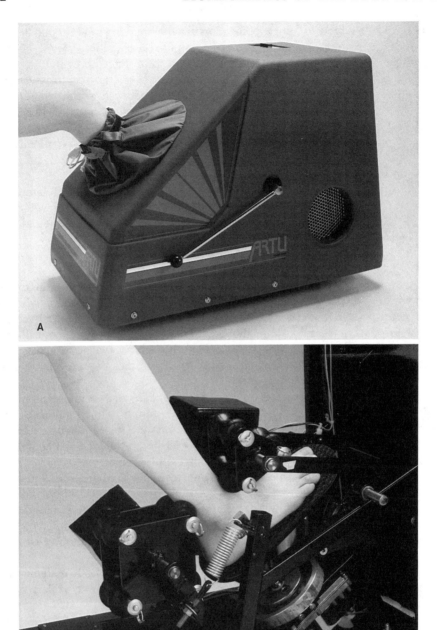

FIGURE 10–12. ARTU, active reflex treatment unit.

of prolonged low-load stretches in combination with heat.[20,21,50,51] Researchers have pointed out that low-load, long-duration stretches are more effective in attaining permanent plastic changes in connective tissues than high-load, short-duration stretches.[20,21,50,51] Joint mobilization techniques continued to be used for the same reasons previously mentioned.

Resistive exercises were now employed to regain the muscle strength of the lower extremity. Manually resisted exercises were initially employed because of weakness in the left lower leg. Given the foot-pounds needed to move the isokinetic device's extremity attachments, the therapist felt the laborer would be unable to generate enough force to use the isokinetic device. Also, the patient experienced a great deal of discomfort when performing the manually resisted eversion and plantar flexion exercises. Such discomfort is one contraindication to the use of isokinetics.[38]

Employment of the ARTU was a result of the theorized effects on mobility and control of edema by the device. As has been noted previously, applying cold will help reduce or prevent the inflammatory response.[7-10] A second reason for the use of the ARTU was its theorized effect on the maintenance and improvement of passive mobility. Theoretically, joint mobility should improve through the use of a mobilization device such as the ARTU because of the positive effects of mobilization on connective tissue.[6,8,19,20,22,39] Although sound clinical research on the efficacy of the ARTU is lacking, it does promise to be an effective adjunct in the treatment of foot and ankle hypomobility and edema.

The gait pattern had progressed to FWB because of the progress in ROM. An air splint was still used to protect the ankle joint while the joint regained its strength, mobility, and position sense. The resistive portion of the home program was increased as a result of the improvement in lower leg strength.

Week Three

Treatment Plan. Warm whirlpool treatments in conjunction with static stretching and ROM exercises continued to be administered during week three of treatment, three times per week. As a result of the restoration of joint play motions, mobilization techniques were discontinued. A submaximal isokinetic exercise program was instituted along with a low-resistance bicycle ergometer workout. The submaximal isokinetic workout consisted of plantar flexion and dorsiflexion for 45 repetitions at 90° per second (Fig. 10-13). Eversion and inversion exercises continued against moderate manual resistance for 45 repetitions (Fig. 10-14). After the strengthening exercises, proprioceptive retraining exercises using a tiltboard were implemented for 10 minutes.

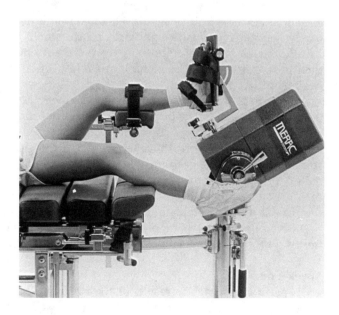

FIGURE 10-13. Inversion/eversion isokinetic workout.

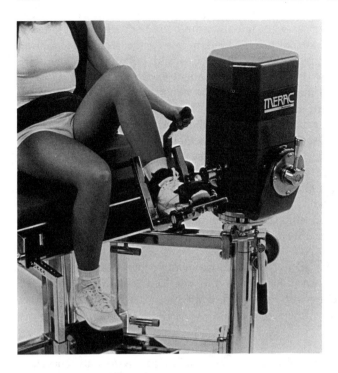

FIGURE 10-14. Plantarflexion/dorsiflexion isokinetic workout.

All treatment sessions ended with a 20 minute session of the ARTU using only the cooling and passive motion features of the instrument.

The home program progressed with the addition of proprioceptive exercises and the use of a stronger elastic material during the strengthening phase. Another change in the home program was the addition of toe raises off the edge of a step for 45 repetitions. Aside from these adjustments the home program remained unchanged.

Treatment Results. At the end of week three, the laborer continued to complain of pain (level 8) over the lateral malleolus on forceful eversion and plantar flexion movements. Passive ROM was 10° of eversion, 16° of inversion, 12° of dorsiflexion, and 40° of plantar flexion. Minimal edema remained visible over the left lateral malleolus. It was barely detectable by figure-eight girth measurement (54 mm).

Given the patient's improvement, the main objectives of physical therapy were then to reduce the level of pain, improve left lower extremity strength, and maintain cardiovascular endurance.

Treatment Rationale. Submaximal isokinetic exercises were added to the clinical program in an attempt to increase the strength of the lower extremity. Maximal resistance was not administered due to the increase in pain associated with manually resisted exercise, possibly due to the internal fixation devices. The posterolateral tendinous structures could have been pressed up against the fixation devices, causing an inflammatory response and the subsequent pain. Submaximal exercise is thought to cause less pressure against the fixation devices and therefore decreases the tendon irritation. Also, the patient did not complain of discomfort while performing this type of exercise.

Given the improvement of joint play motion, mobilization treatments were discontinued. Proprioceptive exercises were implemented with the same rationale as in Case 1.

Week Four

Treatment Plan. The results of the isokinetic plantar flexion and dorsiflexion test performed at the beginning of Week four (as well as subsequent tests) are shown in

TABLE 10-4 Case 2: Isokinetic Test Results (in foot-pounds)

Tests	Plantar Flexors*		Dorsi-flexors*		Evertors†		Invertors†	
	Right	Left	Right	Left	Right	Left	Right	Left
1 (week 4)	48	15	17	5	—	—	—	—
2 (week 28)	48	36	18	12	—	—	—	—
3 (week 30)	—	—	—	—	22	16	18	11
4 (week 31)	49	47	18	18	21	22	20	17
5 (week 33)	48	48	18	19	20	19	19	18

*At 90° per second
†At 60° per second

Table 10-4. As a result of the isokinetic test, an isokinetic exercise program was implemented, which consisted of plantar flexion and dorsiflexion for 90 repetitions at 90° per second. A bicycle ergometer was employed for 20 minutes before exercise. Whirlpool treatments were discontinued, and a static stretching program was implemented in place of the hydrotherapy. The proprioceptive and manually resisted eversion and inversion exercise regimen continued as before. A trial period of iontophoretic treatment with 1% hydrocortisone cream was initiated. The larger negative electrode pad was placed over the calf, and the smaller positive electrode pad was placed over the lateral malleolus. A 5-ma current was used for 25 minutes during the iontophoretic treatment.[53] There was no change in the home program from the previous week. The patient continued to attend physical therapy three times per week.

Treatment Results. At the end of Week four the patient had passive ROM of 12° of dorsiflexion, 41° of plantar flexion, 10° of eversion, and 18° of inversion. The isokinetic tests of his left plantar flexors and dorsiflexors revealed 15 foot-pound and 5 foot-pound of peak torque, respectively, at 90° per second (see Table 10-4). Slight edema was still visible about the lateral malleolus of the left ankle. The patient continued to complain of pain (level 8) with resistive movements of the left ankle.

Treatment Rationale. The isokinetic dorsiflexion and plantar flexion program was based on the results of the test and the patient's ability to perform maximal efforts without experiencing symptoms. The tests revealed a deficit of over 10% compared to the contralateral extremity, indicating a need to strengthen the involved muscles.

Iontophoresis with 1% hydrocortisone cream was used for the drug's anti-inflammatory and analgesic properties.[53,54] Several researchers using animal and human subjects have shown that ion transfer does occur across various membranes (e.g., skin).[55-59] Unfortunately, because of the inherent difficulties of such drug studies, the actual depth of penetration, concentration, and therapeutic levels achieved in humans have not as yet been determined.[51,54] Some attempts have been made to determine the effectiveness of iontophoretic delivery of anti-inflammatory drugs for patients afflicted with various inflammatory conditions.[60,61] Bertolucci[60] and Harris[61] have indicated in their respective studies that iontophoretic treatment with anti-inflammatory medication effectively alleviates symptoms. Further definitive research on this modality is needed to determine its clinical effectiveness.

Week Five

Treatment Plan. The clinical portion of the treatment program consisted of iontophoresis with 1% hydrocortisone cream, isokinetic exercise workouts with the plantar flexors and dorsiflexors of the left foot, bicycle ergometer workouts, and proprioceptive exercises as before. ARTU and eversion-inversion exercises were discontinued. The home exercise program remained unchanged. The frequency of treatment remained as in week four.

Treatment Results. By the end of the fifth week, ROM of the left ankle was WNL, except for inversion and plantar flexion, which lacked 6° and 5° of motion, respectively, as compared to the contralateral extremity. Pain was still being experienced on resisted eversion. Palpation over the posterolateral border of the ankle revealed point tenderness (pain level 8).

During Week five the patient saw his doctor for a follow-up visit. The physician felt that the fixation devices were irritating the posterolateral structures of the left ankle and decided that they should be removed. The patient was scheduled for surgery to remove the hardware in three months. At the physician's request, physical therapy treatments were discontinued, but the physician did instruct the laborer to continue his home exercise program.

Treatment Rationale. In the absence of any changes in the objective signs, the physical therapist felt the patient had received the maximum benefit from the ARTU and that modality was discontinued. Eversion and inversion exercises were discontinued because of the possibility that the posterolateral structures of the left ankle were being compressed against the fixation devices. This compression was believed to be the source of the patient's symptoms.

Week Twenty-Eight

Evaluative Findings. The patient returned for further treatment after the internal fixation devices were removed. After the hardware removal, the patient's leg was immobilized in an air cast for four weeks. At the end of the immobilization period physical therapy treatment was reinitiated.

Active and passive ROM of the left ankle were again restricted: 5° of dorsiflexion, 10° of plantar flexion, 5° of inversion, and 5° of eversion. The joint play motion of anterior glide of the talus was slightly restricted. Slight edema was noted about the lateral and medial maleolli. A figure-eight girth measurement of the ankle revealed a 5-mm increase in girth when compared to the unaffected ankle. Palpation of the left ankle was unremarkable. The patient's chief complaints were stiffness, edema, and minimal (level 4) pain over the lateral malleolus.

Treatment Plan. Office treatments consisted of the ARTU for 20 minutes before and after exercise, ultrasound followed by joint mobilization and static stretching, bicycle ergometer, submaximal isokinetic exercise with the plantar flexors and dorsiflexors, and manually resisted eversion and inversion. The mobilization treatment consisted of anterior and posterior tibiofibular glide on the talus using grade I and IV oscillatory forces. The home program remained unchanged from week five. The patient was seen three times per week for treatment.

Treatment Results. By the end of the week the patient had passive ROM of 25°, of plantar flexion, 12° of dorsiflexion, 10° of eversion, and 11° of inversion. No restriction was noted in any joint play motion. An isokinetic test performed at the end of the week revealed a 25% deficit of the plantar flexors and a 34% deficit of the dorsiflexors, when compared to the unaffected side (see Table 10–4). Pain was no longer noted with eversion or inversion movements of the left ankle. Figure-eight girth measurement of the left ankle was 56 mm, a 3-mm decrease from the beginning of the week.

Treatment Rationale. The ARTU was reimplemented for the device's effect on the reduction of edema. Isokinetic exercise was implemented because of the strength deficits noted.

The main goals of therapy were an increase in strength (to within 10% of the involved lower extremity's strength), the absence of edema of the involved ankle, and the restoration of pain-free ROM.

Week Thirty

Treatment Plan. An isokinetic test was performed to ascertain the strength of the evertors and invertors of the left ankle (see Table 10–4). Based on the results of that test an isokinetic exercise program was implemented (Fig. 11–18). The isokinetic program consisted of 45 repetitions at 90° per second. The ARTU continued to be used after exercise, and the bicycle ergometer, before exercise. The home program remained unchanged except for the addition of a walking program. The patient was to walk daily, increasing the distance by a quarter mile every other day until he was ambulating a maximum of two miles.

Treatment Results. The isokinetic test of the evertors and invertors of the left ankle revealed deficits of 39% and 27%, respectively. Figure-eight girth measurement of the left ankle revealed no increase in girth as compared to the uninvolved ankle (54 mm). ROM of the left ankle was 40° of plantar flexion, and all other movements were WNL. The patient had no complaints of pain in the left ankle but reported some pain over the medial aspect of the left knee.

Treatment Rationale. Because of the significant differences in strength between the involved and uninvolved extremities, an isokinetic exercise program for the evertors and invertors was initiated. Plantar flexion and dorsiflexion workouts continued because of strength deficits in these muscles.

Week Thirty-One

Treatment Plan and Results. An isokinetic retest of the lower leg musculature revealed only a 15% deficit of the evertors of the left ankle (see Table 10–4). Plantar flexion ROM continued to exhibit a loss of 6 degrees as compared to the unaffected side. The patient continued to complain of left medial knee pain that was exacerbated by increased activity (e.g., cycling, walking). The pain remained localized to the medial aspect of the left knee. A biomechanical foot evaluation (see Chapter 6) was performed (Fig. 10–15). As a result of the foot evaluation, temporary foot orthotics were fabricated, to be used for two weeks, at which time the physical therapist was to evaluate their effectiveness. During week thirty-one, the laborer was seen three times.

Based on the foot evaluation, the foot was posted medially 8 mm in the left forefoot, 4 mm in the left rearfoot, 6 mm in the right forefoot, and 4 mm in the right rearfoot (see Fig. 10–15). Active treatment for strengthening and stretching was discontinued. The patient was followed only to evaluate the effectiveness of the orthotics and to determine whether his current strength deficits were causing any difficulties.

Treatment Rationale. Given the patient's previous activity level and his home exercise program, the therapist felt that the current strength deficits were not significant enough to warrant further active treatment. The therapist felt the home program would restore the patient's strength.

Biomechanical foot orthotics were fabricated to reduce the abnormal mechanics of the lower extremity. The angulation of the lower one third of the tibia and fibula, in combination with the forefoot varus deformity, might make it difficult for the subtalar joint to compensate for the deformities.[62,63] Several studies have indicated that angular deformities of the lower leg greater than 9° can cause alterations in the mechanics of the lower kinetic chain that could produce symptoms.[62,63] To assist the subtalar joint in its compensatory role, the forefoot and rearfoot were posted medially. Theoretically medial posting decreases the amount of pronation that would otherwise occur to compensate

EVALUATION WORKSHEET

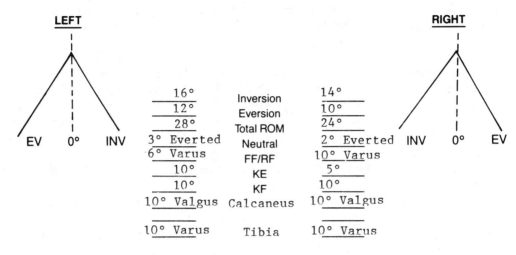

LEFT		RIGHT
	16°	14°
	Inversion	
	12°	10°
	Eversion	
	28°	24°
	Total ROM	
EV 0° INV 3° Everted	Neutral	2° Everted INV 0° EV
6° Varus	FF/RF	10° Varus
10°	KE	5°
10°	KF	10°
10° Valgus	Calcaneus	10° Valgus
10° Varus	Tibia	10° Varus

ORTHOTIC WORKSHEET

FF _6°_ Varus
       Valgus

RF _4°_ Varus
       Valgus

Heel Lift____mm.

Other_____

FF _6°_ Varus
       Valgus

RF _4°_ Varus
       Valgus

Heel Lift____mm.

Other_____

FIGURE 10–15. Biomechanical foot evaluation for Case 2. KE = Dorsiflexion with knee extended; KF = Dorsiflexion with knee flexed.

for the forefoot varus.[62-67] If no angular deformity of the lower leg is present, the subtalar joint should have enough compensatory ability to allow the lower kinetic chain to function normally.[68]

Week Thirty-Three

Permanent orthotics were fabricated using the same posting as in the temporary orthotics. At this time the patient had no complaints of pain. The excessive pronation of the subtalar joint was effectively controlled by the biomechanical orthotics. An isokinetic retest revealed a 5% deficit of the evertors only (see Table 10–4). On the basis of the results obtained from the isokinetic test and the biomechanical foot evaluation, the patient was discharged from physical therapy.

Case 3: Calcaneal Pain

The use of modalities to ameliorate pain and inflammation are the focus of this case.

INITIAL EVALUATION AND FINDINGS

The patient is a 36-year-old woman who began experiencing pain along the medial plantar aspect of her right heel approximately four weeks earlier. Figure 10–16 is the pain drawing completed by this patient. The onset of pain was insidious. The patient

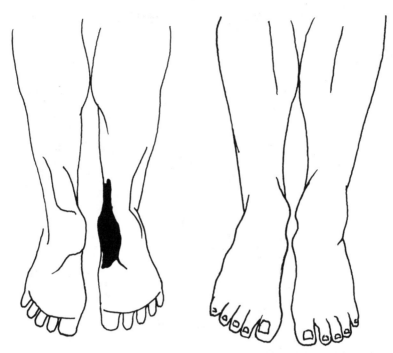

FIGURE 10–16. Pain drawing of patient in Case 3.

stated that she experienced no pain while walking but that if she sat for a prolonged period the pain would return upon standing. The pain would awaken her in the middle of the night. The pain is worse in the morning than at night. At times it radiated into the digits of the right foot. The patient rated her pain level at 8 on a numeric scale of zero to ten (ten being excrutiating pain, and zero being no pain).

On visual inspection the lower extremities were unremarkable. Decreased dorsiflexion of the right foot as compared to the left was noted during passive ROM testing. Dorsiflexion of the right foot was 5°. Results of the hyperpronation test and Tinel's sign were negative. The remainder of the evaluation was unremarkable. The hyperpronation test was performed by taking the calcaneus of the involved foot and maximally everting it. This position was maintained for 30 to 60 seconds.[69]

Palpation of the right foot revealed marked point tenderness over the plantar aspect of the anteromedial border of the right calcaneus. The patient stated that palpation over this area reproduced her symptoms. Dorsiflexing the toes and palpating the medial aspect of the calcaneus increased the severity of the symptoms.

A biomechanical foot evaluation was performed. The results are presented in Figure 10–17. Forefoot varus of 10° in the right foot and 6° in the left foot was noted. Subtalar joint motion was 24° in the right foot and 28° in the left. The left subtalar joint had 12° of eversion and 16° of inversion, whereas the right joint had 10° of eversion and 14° of inversion. Standing still, the patient demonstrated 10° of calcaneal valgus bilaterally and tibial varus of 10° bilaterally. During the gait analysis she exhibited excessive pronation at heel strike of the right foot, and the feet remained in pronation throughout the stance phase of gait.

EVALUATION WORKSHEET

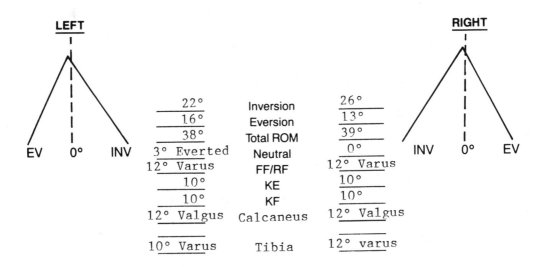

	22°	Inversion	26°
	16°	Eversion	13°
	38°	Total ROM	39°
3° Everted	Neutral	0°
12° Varus	FF/RF	12° Varus
10°	KE	10°
10°	KF	10°
12° Valgus	Calcaneus	12° Valgus
10° Varus	Tibia	12° varus

ORTHOTIC WORKSHEET

FF__7°__ Varus
         Valgus

RF__3°__ Varus
         Valgus

Heel Lift____mm.

Other_____

FF__7°__ Varus
         Valgus

RF__3°__ Varus
         Valgus

Heel Lift____mm.

Other_____

FIGURE 10–17. Biomechanical foot evaluation for Case 3. KE = Dorsiflexion with knee extended; KF = Dorsiflexion with knee flexed.

INTERPRETATION

An analysis of the evaluation findings revealed several perpetuating, predisposing, and precipitating factors. One such factor was tightness of the Achilles tendon–gastrocsoleus complex, which might cause an increase in pronation of the rearfoot.[48,49,69-71] Excessive pronation of the subtalar joint added further tensile stress, overloading the plantar fascia and possibly leading to an inflammatory condition at its insertion on the calcaneus. [69-73] The degree of forefoot varus in the right foot can be another source of strain to the plantar fascia for the same reason as a tight gastrocsoleus complex, excessive pronation.[65,66] Given the absence of signs of tarsal tunnel involvement (negative Tinel's sign and hyperpronation test) and given the results of palpation, the plantar fascia was assumed to be the source of pathology.[69,71,72]

If left untreated the inflammatory condition caused by the stress on the plantar fascia could have led to compression of the posterior tibial nerve as it divides in the tarsal tunnel into the medial and lateral plantar nerves.[69,70] Some authors feel that excessive pronation of the subtalar joint overstretches the tibial nerve and that such overstretching will itself lead to fibrotic changes within the tunnel. The increase in fibrotic changes or nerve compression ultimately causes the patient's symptoms.[69,70]

TREATMENT

The major goal of treatment was to reduce the patient's level of pain. The therapist attempts to accomplish this by controlling the abnormal mechanics of the foot, decreasing the inflammatory condition at the calcaneus and improving the flexibility of the gastrocsoleus complex.

Week One

Treatment Plan. Treatment began with iontophoresis with 1% hydrocortisone cream over the medial plantar aspect of the calcaneus followed by ice massage over the same area. Temporary orthotics were fabricated on the initial visit. The orthotics were posted medially 6 mm in the forefoot area and 4 mm medially in the rearfoot area bilaterally (see Fig. 10–17). Ultrasound treatment in combination with a static stretch is administered to the gastrocsoleus area for ten minutes.[74] The ultrasound treatment is followed by the application of cold with the patient in the same position as in the ultrasound treatment for 20 minutes. The patient was seen for three visits during the first week of treatment. She was instructed in a home exercise program of gastrocsoleus stretching and frequent ice massage to the heel during the day. At the end of week one, she reported a 50% reduction in her symptoms and a pain level of 4. The medial plantar aspect of her heel was less tender to palpation.

Treatment Rationale. The use of iontophoresis with hydrocortisone cream was implemented in an attempt to decrease the inflammatory process in the heel.[53,55,60,61,71] Ice was used following the iontophoretic treatment, to help reduce blood flow to the area, possibly reducing the amount of medication removed from the local area by the circulatory system.[7–9,71,72] Temporary orthotics were employed to decrease the excessive pronation in the subtalar joint, thereby reducing the tensile forces on the plantar aponeurosis. It was hoped that reducing the tensile forces would eradicate the precipitating factor of excessive pronation.[69,71,72,75]

Ultrasound treatments in conjunction with a static stretch were used to facilitate the increase in flexibility of the gastrocsoleus complex.[50,51,74] Wessling, Devane, and Hylton[74] noted improvement in the dorsiflexion of healthy females when this method of stretching was used. The average increase in dorsiflexion was on the order of 4.7° to 7.7° after one week of treatment. Cold was applied after stretching, to maintain the plastic deformation of the gastrocsoleus complex.[21,50,51]

In order to maintain and increase the flexibility of the gastrocsoleus complex the patient was instructed to continue with the stretching program at home. Ice was also applied at home to reduce inflammation.

Week Two

Iontophoretic treatments and gastrocsoleus stretching, as previously noted, were continued three times per week. At the end of Week two, the patient reported an 85% improvement in her symptoms. Her pain level was 2. The passive ROM of dorsiflexion was 10°. The patient reported that the temporary orthotics were very valuable in ameliorating her symptoms.

Because of the response to treatment no changes were made in the treatment program.

Week Three

Treatment Plan and Results. Semirigid permanent orthotics were fabricated using the Orthofeet* system. They were posted medially in the forefoot and rearfoot. The

---

*(Orthofeet Inc., 319 Knickerbocker Ave., Hillsdale, NJ, 07642)

forefoot and rearfoot are bilaterally posted 6 mm and 4 mm, respectively. Upon re-evaluation of the right foot, a pain level of 0 was reported. Point tenderness was no longer present. Dorsiflexion of the right foot was 10° with the knee extended and flexed. Active physical therapy treatment was discontinued as a result of the improvement.

Treatment Rationale. The choice of a permanent orthotic device was made because of the reduction in symptoms and the temporary orthotic's ability to control the abnormal mechanics in the lower kinetic chain. The patient was scheduled for a follow-up visit in three weeks.

Week Six

At the follow-up visit the patient had no complaint of symptoms. ROM measurements of the right ankle revealed 10° of dorsiflexion bilaterally. The patient was instructed to continue using the permanent orthotics and performing gastrocsoleus stretching. She was discharged from active physical therapy treatment at that time.

Case 4. Hallux Abductovalgus (HAV)

The following section emphasizes the treatment of the metatarsophalangeal (MTP) joint after surgery.

INITIAL EVALUATION AND FINDINGS

During the initial interview, the patient, a 45-year old woman, stated that she underwent surgery approximately four weeks earlier for correction of an HAV deformity in her right first MTP joint. No internal fixation device was in place in the first metatarsal, and no other significant history was reported. The chief complaints were pain (level 7-8), stiffness, and edema in the right first MTP joint.

Visual inspection of the right foot revealed a moderate degree of edema about the first MTP joint and forefoot. The incision lines over the dorsal and medial aspects of the joint were intact. The patient wore a cast shoe.

Passive and active ROM testing revealed decreased arthrokinematic and osteokinematic mobility of the intermetatarsal and first MTP joints of the right foot. Pain was felt at the extremes of flexion and extension of the first MTP joint. The ROM of the first MTP was 20° of extension and flexion to neutral (0°).

Palpation of the forefoot and MTP area of the right foot revealed marked tenderness over the joint line of the first MTP. An increase in the tissue temperature was also noted over the first MTP joint. Girth measurement at the level of the metatarsal heads of the right forefoot was 27 mm, as compared to the left forefoot, which had 23 mm.

Figure 10-18 shows the results of the biomechanical foot evaluation performed by the therapist, from which a forefoot varus deformity of 12° was noted bilaterally. In the gait evaluation, the therapist found that the patient pronated excessively late in the gait cycle, at toe-off.

INTERPRETATION

An analysis of the evaluation findings revealed the need to reduce the edema of the forefoot and improve the mobility of the first MTP joint. For normal gait to occur, at least 60° of motion is necessary in the first MTP joint.[76,77] Also, the evaluation revealed the need to control the excessive pronation in the subtalar joint, to prevent recurrence of the HAV deformity.[66]

EVALUATION WORKSHEET

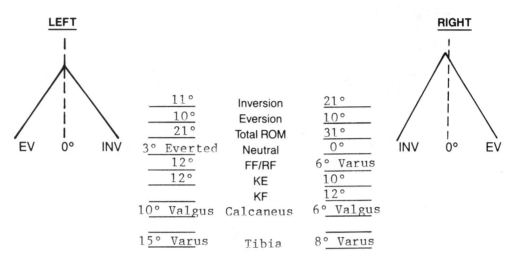

	LEFT						RIGHT	
		11°	Inversion	21°				
		10°	Eversion	10°				
		21°	Total ROM	31°				
EV	0° INV	3° Everted	Neutral	0°	INV	0°	EV	
		12°	FF/RF	6° Varus				
		12°	KE	10°				
			KF	12°				
	10° Valgus	Calcaneus		6° Valgus				
	15° Varus	Tibia		8° Varus				

ORTHOTIC WORKSHEET

FF _8°_ Varus / Valgus	FF _6°_ Varus / Valgus
RF _4°_ Varus / Valgus	RF _4°_ Varus / Valgus
Heel Lift____mm.	Heel Lift____mm.
Other_____	Other_____

FIGURE 10–18. Biomechanical foot evaluation for Case 4. KE = Dorsiflexion with knee extended; KF = Dorsiflexion with knee flexed.

Treatment

The major goals of therapy, therefore, were to increase the mobility of the first MTP to at least 60° of extension, reduce the edema of the forefoot, and prevent recurrence of the HAV deformity.

Week One

Treatment Plan. The first week of physical therapy consisted of the ARTU for 20 minutes, using the massage rollers and the cooling features of the machine. This treatment was followed by a ten-minute effleurage massage to the forefoot area with the lower extremity elevated and intermetatarsal joint play mobilization. The forefoot treatment was followed by the facilitation of passive pain-free ROM of extension and flexion of the first MTP. Figure 10–19 illustrates long-axis distraction mobilization administered to the first MTP joint using grade I oscillatory forces after the facilitation of passive pain-free ROM.[44] The treatment program ended with another 20 minute ARTU session. The patient was seen three times during the first week.

She was instructed in a home exercise program consisting of self-mobilization of MTP flexion and extension within the pain-free range. She was also instructed to keep the lower extremity elevated and to apply ice packs to the right forefoot for 10 to 15 minutes intermittently throughout the day.

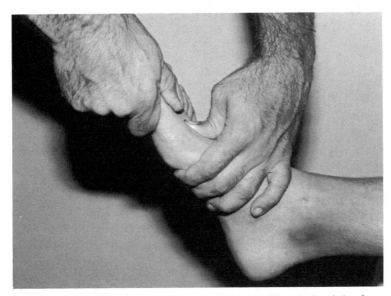

FIGURE 10–19. Long axis distraction of first MTP joint. The shaft of the first metatarsal is grasped by one hand and stabilized. The other hand will apply a longitudinal directed force to distract the MTP joint.

Temporary orthotics were prescribed. The orthotics are posted medially in the forefoot (7 mm) and rearfoot (3 mm, see Fig. 10–18).

Treatment Results. At the end of week one, the patient had 35° of first MTP extension. The girth of the forefoot was 25 mm, and the subjective pain level had decreased to 6.

Treatment Rationale. Cold and massage were applied in an effort to reduce the amount of edema in the forefoot and first MTP.[2,7,9,16,78] The mobilization program was an effort to provide nutrition to the joint, break adhesions, and realign collagen fibers along appropriate lines of stress.[19,20–22, 78]

Week Two

Treatment Plan. Clinic sessions continued to emphasize the use of cryotherapy before and after exercise using the ARTU and joint mobilization. Mobilization treatments progressed to include grade IV long-axis distraction and superior glide of the proximal phalanx of the hallux on the first metatarsal using grade I and grade IV forces (see Fig. 10–19).[43] The home exercise program progressed to walking in tennis shoes, gastrocsoleus stretching, and standing MTP stretch. Standing MTP stretch is accomplished while standing by simply raising the heel of the involved foot while keeping the hallux on the floor. The remainder of the home exercise program remained unchanged. The patient was seen three times per week.

Treatment Results. After the second week of treatment the patient had 40° of first MTP extension. The girth measurement of the right forefoot was 25 mm, a 2-mm difference from the unaffected foot.

The treatment progressed by the addition of more aggressive stretches as a result of the degree of osseous healing. At that time the therapist felt the patient could safely tolerate the standing stretch and superior glide mobilization treatment.

Weeks Three and Four

After four weeks of treatment the patient exhibited 60° of extension of the first MTP joint. No difference was detected in the girth measurement of the forefoot area, and the subjective pain rating was zero. Clinic treatments in weeks three and four remained unchanged, as did the home exercise program. The patient was seen two times per week.

During Week three, the patient was fitted with a pair of semirigid permanent orthotics that were posted identically to the temporary orthotics (see Fig. 10–18). Because the initial goals were achieved and there are no symptoms, the patient was discharged from further physical therapy treatments.

SUMMARY

Several pathological entities are identified. Some possible corresponding treatments for these pathological entities are highlighted in a clinical scenario. The scientific basis for each of the employed treatments is developed.

The reader is urged to remember that there are many ways to approach the various clinical problems discussed here. This chapter is not intended to be a definitive statement on the best (or only) way to treat the identified problems but rather as a guide with which to approach the foot using physical therapy modalities. Until such time as scientific research is available affirming the best way to treat a particular problem, clinicians must explore all feasible treatment approaches.

REFERENCES

1. Wolf, SL (ed): Clinical Decision Making in Physical Therapy. FA Davis, Philadelphia, 1985.
2. Roy, S and Irwin, R: Sports Medicine: Prevention, Evaluation, Management, and Rehabilitation. Prentice-Hall, Englewood Cliffs, NJ, 1983.
3. Kessler, RM and Hertling, D: The ankle and hindfoot. In Kessler, RM and Hertling, D: Management of Common Musculoskeletal Disorders: Physical Therapy Principles and Methods. Harper & Row, Philadelphia, 1983, p 448.
4. O'Donoghue, DH: Injuries of the ankle. In O'Donoghue, DH: Treatment of Injuries to Athletes. WB Saunders, Philadelphia, 1976, p 698.
5. Ruch, JA, Downey, MS, and Malay, DS: Ankle fractures. In McGlamry, ED (ed): Comprehensive Textbook of Foot Surgery, vol 2. Williams & Wilkins, Baltimore, 1987.
6. Donatelli, R and Owens-Burkart, H: Effects of immobilization on the extensibility of periarticular connective tissue. J Orthop Sports Phys Ther 3(2):67, 1981.
7. Kowal, MA: Review of physiological effects of cryotherapy. J Orthop Sports Phys Ther 5(2):66, 1983.
8. Lehman, JF, Warren, CG, and Scham, SM: Therapeutic heat and cold. Clin Orthop 99:207, 1974.
9. Michlovitz, SL: Cryotherapy: The use of cold as a therapeutic agent. In Michlovitz, SL (ed): Thermal Agents in Rehabilitation. FA Davis, Philadelphia, 1986, p 73.
10. Starkey, J: Treatment of ankle sprains by simultaneous use of intermittent compression and ice packs. Am J Sports Med 4(4):142, 1976.
11. Michlovitz, S, Smith, W, and Watkins, M: Ice and high-voltage pulsed stimulation in treatment of acute lateral ankle sprains. J Orthop Sports Phys Ther 9(9):301, 1988.
12. Reed, BV: Effect of high-voltage pulsed electrical stimulation on microvascular permeability to plasma proteins: A possible mechanism in minimizing edema. Phys Ther 68(4):491, 1988.
13. Mohr, TM, Akers, TK, and Landry, RG: Effect of high-voltage stimulation on edema reduction in the rat hind limb. Phys Ther 67(11):1703, 1987.
14. Walker, DC, Currier, DP, and Threlkeld, AJ: Effects of high-voltage pulsed electrical stimulation on blood flow. Phys Ther 68(4):481, 1988.
15. Sims, D: Effects of positioning on ankle edema. J Orthop Sports Phys Ther 8(1):30, 1986.
16. Beard, G and Wood, EC: Effects of massage. In Beard, G and Wood, EC: Massage: Principles and Techniques. WB Saunders, Philadelphia, 1965, p 46.
17. Akeson, WH, Amiel, D and Woo, S: Immobility effects of synovial joints: The pathomechanics of joint contracture. Biorheology 17:95, 1980.

18. Enneking, W and Horowitz, M: The intra-articular effects of immobilization on the human knee. J Bone Joint Surg 54A:973, 1972.
19. McDonough, AL: Effects of immobilization and exercise on articular cartilage: A review of literature. J Orthop Sports Phys Ther 3(1):2, 1981.
20. Perry, J: Scientific basis of rehabilitation. Instr Course Lect 34:385, 1985.
21. Sapega, AA, Quedenfeld, TC, Moyer, RA, et al: Biophysical factors in range of motion exercise. Phys Sports Med 9:57, 1981.
22. Salter, RB, Simmonds, DF, Malcolm, BW, et al: The biological effect of continuous passive motion on the healing of full-thickness defects in articular cartilage. J Bone Joint Surg 62A(8):1232, 1980.
23. Tabary, JC, Tabary, C, Tardieu, C, et al: Physiological and structural changes in the cat's soleus muscle due to immobilization at different lengths by plaster casts. J Physiol 224:231, 1972.
24. Woo, S, Matthews, JV, Akeson, WH, et al: Connective tissue response to immobility: Correlative study of biomechanical and biochemical measurements of normal and immobilized rabbit knees. Arthritis Rheum 18:257, 1975.
25. Glick, JM, Gordon, RB, and Nishimoto, D: The prevention and treatment of ankle injuries. Am J Sports Med 4(4):136, 1976.
26. Tropp, H, Askling, C, and Gillquist, J: Prevention of ankle sprains. Am J Sports Med 13(4):259, 1985.
27. Freeman, MAR: Instability of the foot after injuries to the lateral ligament of the ankle. J Bone Joint Surg 47(B)4:669, 1965.
28. Freeman, MAR: Treatment of ruptures of the lateral ligaments of the ankle. J Bone Joint Surg 47B(4):661, 1965.
29. Kay, DB: The sprained ankle: Current therapy. Foot Ankle 6(1):22, 1985.
30. Milch, LD: Rehabilitation exercises following inversion ankle sprains. J Am Podiatr Med Assoc 76(10):577, 1986.
31. Gross, MT: Effects of recurrent lateral ankle sprains on active and passive judgements of joint position. Phys Ther 67(10):1505, 1987.
32. Freeman, MAR, Dean, MRF, and Hanham, IWF: The etiology and prevention of functional instability of the foot. J Bone Joint Surg 47B:678, 1965.
33. DeCarlo, MS and Talbot, RW: Evaluation of ankle joint proprioception following injection of the anterior talofibular ligament. J Orthop Sports Phys Ther 8(2):70, 1986.
34. Moroz, DE and Houston, ME: The effects of replacing endurance running training with cycling in female runners. Can J Sports Sci 12(3):131, 1987.
35. Nicholas, JA and Hershman, EB (eds): The Lower Extremity and Spine in Sports Medicine. CV Mosby, St Louis, 1986.
36. Scranton, PE, Whitesel, JP, and Farewell, V: Cybex evaluation of the relationship between anterior and posterior compartment lower leg muscles. Foot Ankle 6(2):85, 1985.
37. Davies, GJ: Subtalar joint, ankle joint, and shin pain testing and rehabilitation. In Davies GJ (ed): A Compendium of Isokinetics in Clinical Usage and Clinical Notes. S&S Publishers, LaCrosse, WI, 1984, p 123.
38. Arem, AJ and Madden, JW: Effects of stress on healing wounds: I. Intermittent non-cyclical tension. J Surg Res 20:93, 1976.
39. Levenson, SM, Geever, EF, Crowley, IV, et al: The healing of rat skin wounds. Ann Surg 161:293, 1965.
40. Wong, DLK, Glasheen-Wray, M, and Andrew, LF: Isokinetic evaluation of the ankle invertors and evertors. J Orthop Sports Phys Ther 5(5):246, 1984.
41. Brody, DM: Part III: Rehabilitation of the injured runner. Instr Course Lect 33:268, 1984.
42. James, SL, Bates, BT, and Ostering, LR: Injuries to runners. Am J Sports Med 6(2):40, 1978.
43. Mennell, JM: Joint Pain: Diagnosis and Treatment Using Manipulative Techniques, ed 1. Little, Brown, Boston, 1964.
44. Wooden, MJ: Mobilization of the lower extremity. In Donatelli, R and Wooden, MJ (eds): Orthopoedic Physical Therapy. Churchill Livingstone, New York, 1989
45. Kloth, L: Shortwave and microwave diathermy. In Michlovitz, SL (ed): Thermal Agents in Rehabilitation. FA Davis, Philadelphia, 1986, p 177.
46. Cooper, RR: Alterations during immobilization and regeneration of skeletal muscle in cats. J Bone Joint Surg 54A(5):919, 1972.
47. Maitland, GD: Peripheral Manipulation, ed 2. Butterworths, Boston, 1977.
48. Michael, RH and Holder, LE: The soleus syndrome: A cause of medial tibial stress (shin splints). Am J Sports Med 13(2):87, 1985.
49. Tiberio, D: Evaluation of functional ankle dorsiflexion using subtalar neutral position. A clinical report. Phys Ther 67(6):955, 1987.
50. Michlovitz, SL: Biophysical principles of heating and superficial heat agents. In Michlovitz SL (ed): Thermal Agents in Rehabilitation. FA Davis, Philadelphia, 1986, p 99.
51. Warren, GC, Lehman, JF, and Koblanski, JN: Heat and stretch procedures: An evaluation using rat tail tendon. Arch Phys Med Rehab 57:122, 1976.
52. Wyke, B: The neurology of joints. Ann R Coll Surg Engl 41:25, 1967.
53. Kahn, J: Iontophoresis. In Principles and Practice of Electrotherapy. Churchill Livingstone, New York, 1987, p 153.

54. Boone, DC: Applications of iontophoresis. In Wolf S (ed): Clinics in Physical Therapy: Electrotherapy. Churchill Livingstone, New York, 1986, p 99.
55. Gangarosa, LP, Park, NH, Fong, BC, et al: Conductivity of drugs used for iontophoresis. J Pharm Sci 67(10):1439, 1978.
56. Glass, JM, Stephen, RL, and Jacobson, SC: The quantity and distribution of radiolabeled dexamethasone delivered to tissue by iontophoresis. Int J Dermatol 19(9):519, 1980.
57. Puttemans, FJM, et al: Iontophoresis: Mechanism of action studied by potentiometry and x-ray fluorescence. Arch Phys Med Rehab 63:176, 1982.
58. Tregeat, RT: The permeability of mammalian skin to ions. J Invest Dermatol 46(1):16, 1966.
59. Zankel, HT, Cress, RH, and Kamin, H: Iontophoresis studies with a radioactive tracer. Arch Phys Med Rehab 40:193, 1959.
60. Harris, PR: Iontophoresis: Clinical research in musculoskeletal inflammatory conditions. J Orthop Sports Phys Ther 4(2):109, 1982.
61. Bertolucci, LE: Introduction of antiinflammatory drugs by iontophoresis: A double blind study. J Orthop Sports Phys Ther 4(2):103, 1982.
62. Olerud, C: The pronation capacity of the foot: Its consequences for axial deformity after tibial shaft fractures. Arch Orthop Trauma Surg 104:303, 1985.
63. Ting, AJ, et al: The role of subtalar motion and ankle contact pressure changes from angular deformities of the tibia. Foot Ankle 7(5):290, 1987.
64. Donatelli, R: Normal biomechanics of the foot and ankle. J Orthop Sports Phys Ther 7(3):91, 1985.
65. McPoil, TG and Knecht, HG: Biomechanics of the foot in walking: A functional approach. J Orthop Sports Phys Ther 7(2):69, 1985.
66. Root, ML, Orien, WP, and Weed, JH: Normal and Abnormal Function of the Foot: Clinical Biomechanics, vol 2. Clinical Biomechanics Corporation, Los Angeles, 1977.
67. Subotnick, SI: Biomechanics of the subtalar and midtarsal joints. J Am Podiatr Med Assoc 65(8):756, 1975.
68. Garbalosa, JC, et al: Normal angular relationship of the forefoot to the rearfoot in the frontal plane. (submitted for publication).
69. Bordelon, RL: Subcalcaneal pain: A method of evaluation and plan for treatment. Clin Orthop 177:49, 1983.
70. Kushner, S and Reid, DC: Medial tarsal tunnel syndrome: A review. J Orthop Sports Phys Ther 6(1):39, 1984.
71. Kwong, PK, et al: Plantar fasciitis: Mechanics and pathomechanics of treatment. Clin Sports Med 7(1):119, 1988.
72. McBryde, AM: Plantar fasciitis. Instruc Course Lect: 278, 1984.
73. Sarrafian, S: Functional characteristics of the foot and plantar aponeurosis under tibiotalar loading. Foot Ankle 8(1):4, 1987.
74. Wessling, KC, DeVane, DA, and Hylton, CR: Effects of static stretch versus static stretch and ultrasound combined on triceps surae muscle extensibility in healthy women. Phys Ther 67(5):675, 1987.
75. Shikoff, MD, Figura, MA, and Postar, SE: A retrospective study of 195 patients with heel pain. J Am Podiatr Med Assoc 76(2):71, 1986.
76. Biossonault, W and Donatelli, R: The influence of hallux extension on the foot during ambulation. J Orthop Sports Phys Ther 5(5):240, 1984.
77. Bojsen-Moller, F and Lamoreux, L: Significance of free dorsiflexion of the toes in walking. Acta Orthop Scand 50:471, 1979.
78. Clanton, TO, Butler, JE, and Eggert, A: Injuries to the metatarsophalangeal joints in athletes. Foot Ankle 7(3):162, 1986.

CHAPTER 11

Biomechanics of the Foot and Ankle: Surgical Intervention

Karen S. Seale, MD

In this chapter some of the surgical options for management of several pathologic conditions of the lower extremity are discussed. These include pes cavus, pes planus, hallux valgus, hallux rigidus, deformities of the lesser toes, arthrodesis of the foot and ankle, and extrinsic abnormalities of the lower extremity. This chapter does not attempt to give specific details of every condition, or to cover all possible solutions to any given problem. Rather it is intended to help the nonsurgeon who desires a better understanding of the indications, contraindications, and mechanics of orthopedic surgery of the foot and ankle.

PES CAVUS AND HEEL VARUS

The cavus foot deformity represents a spectrum of difficulties ranging from mild elevation of the medial arch with no subjective symptoms to severe hindfoot varus, plantar flexed first ray, tight plantar fascia, and severe toe clawing. The degree and type of symptoms dictate the treatment required.

The person with mild cavus foot may have no subjective complaints and represents that segment of the population whose subtalar joint motion is decreased. Although this limited eversion and pronation is biomechanically less desirable than the more "normal" situation, not all cavus feet are symptomatic and require treatment. Surgery may be required for more severe deformities that cause symptoms that are not manageable with orthotic devices and shoe modifications. Each component of the pes cavus deformity must be carefully evaluated. A determination is then made as to the extent to which each component of the deformity contributes to the symptoms.

For example, a 24-year-old white female with Charcot-Marie-Tooth disease presented with complaints of repeated ankle sprains that had become so severe that she was unable to safely negotiate level terrain (Fig. 11-1). Treatment with appropriate

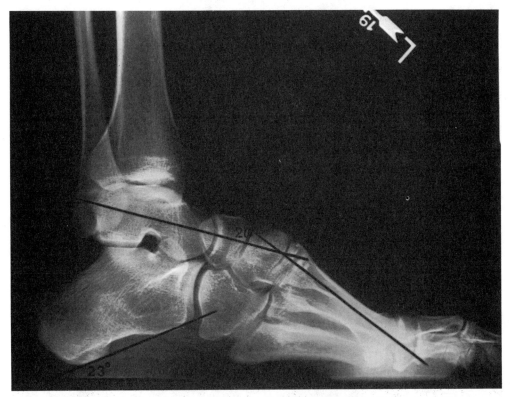

FIGURE 11-1. Pre-operative radiograph of patient with heel varus and pes cavus.

orthotic devices and shoe modifications had been unsuccessful. Biomechanical evaluation revealed three major components: heel varus, pes cavus, and mild toe clawing. Surgical options to improve the biomechanics and restore more normal function will be discussed for each component.

The patient demonstrated two factors contributing to abnormal rearfoot function, limited subtalar motion with subtalar joint neutral in varus and an increase in the angle of inclination of the calcaneus (which further accentuated the high arch).

Clinical evaluation of the midfoot revealed a tight plantar fascia, which was palpable along the longitudinal arch on passive dorsiflexion of the metatarsophalangeal (MTP) joints, and a rigidly plantar flexed first ray. The hindfoot varus locked the transverse tarsal joints. This increased the mechanical advantage of the peroneus longus as it passed around the calcaneocuboid joint to insert on the first metatarsal, accentuating plantar flexion of the first ray.

Evaluation of the forefoot revealed hyperextension deformities of all the metatarsophalangeal joints, particularly the first; mild dorsal MTP joint contractures and plantar prominence of the metatarsal heads; and flexion deformities of the interphalangeal joints.

In this particular case, attention was first directed to correction of the hindfoot varus deformity. A lateral closing wedge osteotomy of the calcaneus was performed. The tuberosity fragment into which the Achilles tendon inserts was translated laterally, thus providing a valgus shift in the biomechanical axis of the hindfoot. The tuberosity fragment was also shifted proximally to decrease the angle of inclination of the calcaneus. The osteotomy was rigidly fixed with two screws, which allowed normal function of the subtalar joint (Fig. 11-2). In addition, the plantar fascia was released from its origin on the calcaneus to prevent tethering and to allow repositioning of the calcaneal tuberosity and of the first metatarsal.

To correct the forefoot cavus deformity, a dorsal closing wedge osteotomy at the base of the first metatarsal was performed in conjunction with Jones' procedure. The metatarsal osteotomy allows elevation of the metatarsal head and improves the talometatarsal angle. Jones procedure consists of the following steps: (1) release of the extensor hallucis longus from its insertion into the distal phalanx of the great toe; (2) fusion of the interphalangeal joint; (3) release of any dorsal contracture of the MTP joint capsule; and (4) routing of the extensor tendon into the dorsal aspect of the neck of the first metatarsal. The extensor tendon now acts to help dorsiflex the metatarsal rather than to hyperextend the MTP joint, helping to eliminate the mild clawing of the great toe. The clawing of the lesser toes was not severe enough to require surgery. Surgical correction of lesser-toe deformities is discussed later in this chapter. In summary, three aspects of this patient's deformity were addressed: correction of the hindfoot varus, plantar flexion of the first metatarsal, and cock-up of the great toe.

Not all of these procedures are required by every patient with cavus foot. The person whose hindfoot is in varus but whose forefoot is plantigrade may require only a calcaneal osteotomy. In another instance, the excessive plantar flexion of the first ray may be the only problem and may require only the dorsiflexion osteotomy of the first metatarsal.

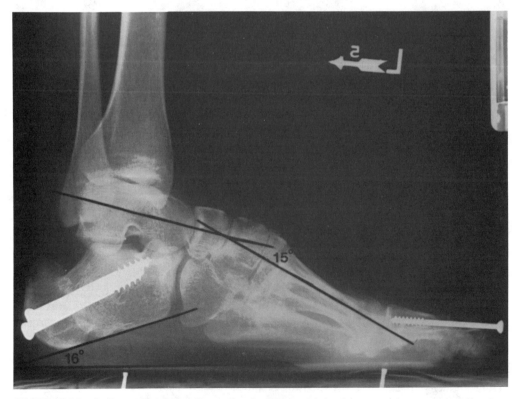

FIGURE 11–2. Post-operative radiograph of patient with heel varus and pes cavus following calcaneal and first metatarsal osteotomies and a Jones procedure.

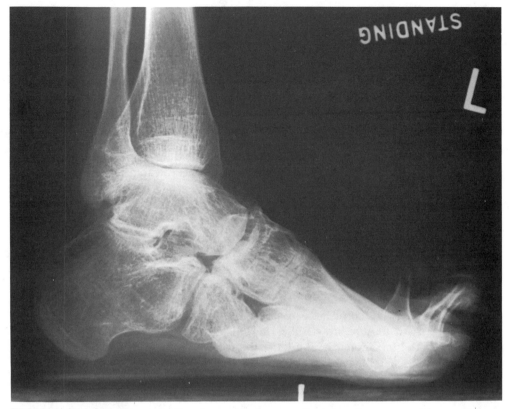

FIGURE 11–3. Radiograph of patient with degenerative joint changes requiring a triple arthrodesis to correct the deformities.

If soft tissue imbalance is contributing to the deformity, appropriate tendon transfers and soft tissue procedures can be done in place of or in conjunction with bone procedures. In considering the surgical options one should remember that the cavus foot is already more rigid than normal. Therefore, every attempt should be made to preserve or increase existing flexibility If there is evidence of degenerative joint disease in the subtalar and transverse tarsal joints (Fig. 11-3), a triple arthrodesis may be indicated. In this case, the arthrodesis is performed to correct the hindfoot varus deformity and place the foot in a plantigrade position.

A complete discussion of every surgical application to the biomechanics of the foot is beyond the scope of this chapter. An understanding of the biomechanics of the foot and a thorough examination are important in selecting the most appropriate surgical procedure for a given situation.

PES PLANUS

There are many causes of pes planus. An attempt must be made to establish the etiology so that the appropriate surgical procedure can be selected. The following causes of pes planus and the surgical considerations of each will be discussed: posterior tibial tendon rupture; tarsal coalition; Achilles tendon tightness; Charcot degeneration of the midfoot joints; hypermobile flatfoot of adulthood secondary to ligament laxity; calcaneal fracture; and rheumatoid arthritis.

Posterior Tibial Tendon Rupture

The insidious onset of unilateral, painful flatfoot in the adult is most common secondary to dysfunction of the posterior tibial tendon. The diagnosis is all too often missed. Delay in diagnosis can lead to chronic and irreversible changes in the foot. Posterior tibial tendon rupture is most frequently seen in women over the age of 40 years with no history of acute trauma.[1,2] The primary complaint is pain during the early inflammatory phase of rupture on the posteromedial aspect of the ankle, behind the medial malleolus. Once the arch has collapsed, creating excessive pronation and abnormal heel valgus, the subjective complaints may include pain over the lateral aspect of the hindfoot, which is caused by impingement of the calcaneus against the lateral malleolus, and pain in the sinus tarsi.

If the problem is diagnosed early, before chronic changes develop in the bones and soft tissues, a tendon transfer can be performed using the flexor digitorum longus. The flexor digitorum longus is incised distally and rerouted through a drill hole into the navicular bone.[2] It then supplies motor function to supinate and adduct the foot. Considerable rehabilitation is required postoperatively to store motion and strength in the transferred muscle-tendon unit, but good results have been reported.[2,3]

If treatment is delayed and the deformities of heel valgus and forefoot supination are no longer passively correctable, a soft tissue procedure is no longer an option. A triple arthrodesis is required to stabilize the calcaneus beneath the talus via a talocalcaneal fusion and to derotate and adduct the forefoot on the hindfoot by fusing the calcaneocuboid and talonavicular joints with the foot in a plantigrade position. Attempts should be made to maintain the normal function and flexibility of the foot; therefore, early diagnosis is desirable to avoid the necessity of arthrodesis.

Tarsal Coalition

Tarsal coalition is a congenital fusion of two or more tarsal bones, most commonly occuring between the talus and calcaneus or between the calcaneus and navicular. Symptoms usually occur when the patient reaches maturity, at which time the fibrous coalition ossifies, increasing the rigidity of the foot. If treatment is rendered before extensive degenerative changes occur in the surrounding joints, the coalition can be surgically excised with good results.[4] This intervention restores some motion and improves the biomechanics. Figure 11-4 is the radiograph of a 21-year-old college student who presented with symptoms of severe subtalar pain for only the last two years. He had flatfeet ever since childhood but had not had pain prior to this time. Since the radiographs demonstrated minimal degenerative joint changes, he was a candidate for surgical excision of the coalition, which united his calcaneus and navicular. Figure 11-5 is the radiograph after coalition excision.

If the condition goes untreated for many years or if the extent of coalition is such that the bones cannot be effectively separated with good results, a triple arthrodesis is required. The foot should be realigned and fused, with the heel in slight valgus and the forefoot plantigrade.

Charcot Joint Degeneration

A third cause of pes planus in adults is collapse and degeneration of joints of the hind- or midfoot secondary to neuropathy. This is most frequently secondary to diabetes. For reasons that are not yet clearly understood, the diabetic patient who has some

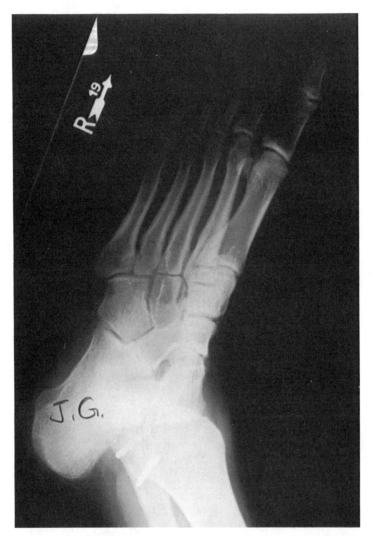

FIGURE 11–4. Pre-operative radiograph of calcaneal-navicular coalition.

degree of loss of sensation to the foot loses the structural integrity of the joints second-ary to ligament and bone destruction. Occasionally, the process can be initiated by an event as insignificant as twisting the foot or sustaining mild blunt trauma, but com-monly there is no known history of trauma. The resulting arch undergoes collapse and disintegration as seen in Figure 11-6. In the majority of cases, this condition is treated nonoperatively with compressive stockings, elevation, and non-weightbearing until the early inflammatory phase resolves and healing occurs. Surgery is required if the defor-mity causes repeated skin ulcerations over the bony prominences. Frequently, merely excising the prominences can suffice to prevent further problems, although the pes planus and abnormal biomechanics persist. Careful follow-up observation and fitting with custom-molded accommodative orthotic devices and shoe modifications are needed.

In rare instances a patient with Charcot joint degeneration may be a candidate for arthrodesis of the affected joints to correct the deformity and stabilize the foot; however, the arthrodesis poses potential risks such as infection and recurrence of the inflamma-

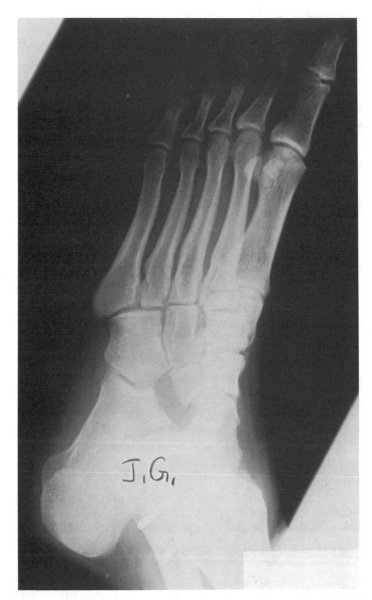

FIGURE 11–5. Post-operative radiograph after excision of C–N coalition.

tory phase of destruction. Arthrodesis requires extended periods of immobilization for healing to occur.

Hypermobile Flatfoot

As discussed in Chapter 2, flexible flatfoot is not necessarily a pathologic condition. During childhood the ligaments of the feet are normally more flexible than in adulthood. As the child matures, the tensile strength of ligaments increases to prevent abnormal pronation and excessive pes planus. However, if abnormal excessive laxity

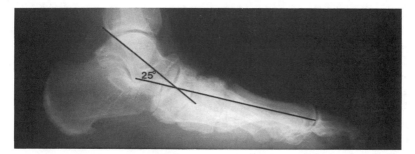

FIGURE 11–6. Radiograph of midfoot collapse secondary to Charcot joint degeneration.

persists into adulthood, abnormal stresses are placed on the hypermobile flatfoot. The presence of excessive heel valgus is frequently accompanied by contracture of the Achilles tendon, which further worsens the biomechanical situation. If regular and faithful use of custom molded-plastic orthotic devices, as described by Bordelon,[6] and a properly administered program of Achilles tendon stretching are not successful in reducing the foot deformity, then surgery can be considered.

If the problem is primarily excessive heel valgus, a calcaneal osteotomy to reduce the valgus position of the calcaneus and Achilles tendon lengthening may be all that is necessary. If the deformity is more severe and includes forefoot supination and abduction, other surgical procedures may be performed to alleviate specific deformities. Other procedures to consider include a plantar flexing osteotomy of the first metatarsal, an opening wedge osteotomy of the cuboid, and a closing wedge osteotomy of the cuneiform, to help correct the pes planus and abduction and supination deformities.[6]

Calcaneus Fractures

Fracture of the calcaneus most frequently results from a fall from a height. The calcaneus is fractured as the talus is driven, like a wedge, into the body of the calcaneus, resulting in numerous fracture patterns. Commonly, the fracture line goes through the posterior facet, leaving the medial portion of the calcaneus—the sustentaculum— relatively intact; however, the remainder of the body of the calcaneus is displaced laterally. The calcaneus loses its structural integrity and its ability to support the talus. If the foot is allowed to heal in this position, the result will be abnormal biomechanics due to excessive heel valgus and pes planus.

In recent years there has been an interest in primary operative intervention to openly reduce and internally fix calcaneal fractures. The goals of early surgery are to restore subtalar joint congruity, replace the displaced calcaneal tuberosity in its normal position, and begin early motion.

HALLUX VALGUS

Adult acquired hallux valgus is associated with imbalance of the soft tissues and abnormal bony configuration of the first cuneiform/metatarsophalangeal joint complex. Components of hallus valgus pathology can include the painful "bump," or prominent exostosis, on the medial side of the foot; lateral deviation and pronation of the great toe;

excessive metatarsus primus varus; subluxation or dislocation of the first metatarsal head from its sesamoid sling; attenuation of the medial MTP joint capsule; contracture of the adductor hallucis muscle and lateral MTP joint capsule; abnormal direction of pull of the intrinsic and extrinsic muscles of the great toe; degenerative joint disease; and associated second-toe deformities.

Adult acquired hallux valgus is found most often in women and is most likely the result of the long-term wearing of fashionable, narrow-box, pointed-toe shoes. Other associated findings, which may be implicated in the biomechanical cause of hallux valgus, include contracture of the Achilles tendon complex, pes planus, and hypermobility of the first metatarsal–medial cuneiform joint.

Over 100 different operations are described in the literature for correction of hallux valgus, and no single operation is perfect for all patients. Not every patient needs an operation, and careful patient selection is the byword. Patient personality, age, life style, expectations, degree and type of deformity, presence of arthritis, and associated findings are just some of the factors to consider before surgical intervention is undertaken. There are, however, some basic principles when approaching this complex problem.

Figure 11-7 is a schematic representation of the normal tendons acting on the first MTP joint. The action of the long and short toe extensors is normally counteracted by the long and short toe flexors, just as the abductor hallucis is counterbalanced by the adductor hallucis. This counterbalance results in normal biplanar flexion and extension of the MTP joint. Figure 11-8 represents hallux valgus in which there is lateral displacement of the long flexors and extensors, overpull of the adductor, and plantar displacement of the abductor so that it no longer efficiently resists adduction of the great toe. A rotational component pronates the toe while the metatarsal head deviates medially, thus subluxing out of the sesamoid sling. If the primary complaint is the prominent medial eminence, the deformity is mild, and relatively rapid recovery is desirable, simple surgical removal of the medial eminence can be the answer. The disadvantages are that no realignment has been accomplished and recurrence or progression of the deformity is likely.

For mild to moderate deformity in a young person, with no degenerative joint disease, consideration can be given to performing a distal metatarsal osteotomy such as a chevron osteotomy. This procedure affords limited realignment by lateral displacement of the head of the first metatarsal, removal of the medial prominence, and plication of the medial capsule. Healing is quick, and the procedure is technically less demanding than more extensive ones. Figure 11-9 is an illustration of the essential

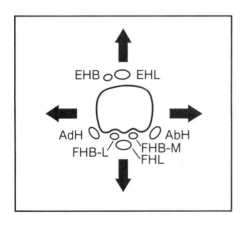

FIGURE 11–7. Schematic representation of forces acting across the normal first metatarsal phalangeal joint.

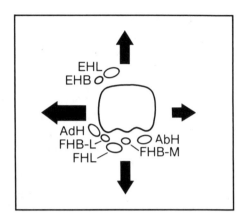

FIGURE 11–8. Forces acting across first metatarsal phalangeal (MTP) joint in hallux valgus.

features of this procedure: (1) removal of the medial prominence, (2) lateral displacement of the metatarsal head after performing the osteotomy, and (3) removal of the residual medial prominence.[1]

The procedure that has come to be known as the resection-realignment procedure is a modification of a procedure originally described by McBride.[1] It was designed to provide more extensive correction of the abnormal biomechanics of hallux valgus and is particularly useful in cases in which the deformity is more severe; that is, when MTP joint angulation is greater than 40° and metatarsus primus varus is greater than 15°. The procedure requires three incisions, through which the following steps are undertaken: (1) release of the lateral MTP joint capsule and adductor hallucis tendon; (2) removal of

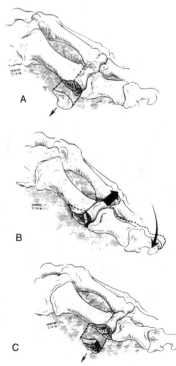

FIGURE 11–9. Schematic representation of Chevron osteotomy. (From Johnson, KA: Surgery of the Foot and Ankle, Raven Press, 1989, pg 6, with permission.)

the medial eminence and plication of the medial capsule; and (3) osteotomy at the base of the first metatarsal to correct the metatarsus primus varus. This procedure can be performed on patients of all ages, but it is better to avoid it in patients with degenerative arthritis of the first MTP joint.[2]

Presence of severe degenerative joint disease limits the surgical procedures that can be used to correct the hallux valgus deformity. Arthrodesis is an excellent procedure in the presence of degenerative joint disease, because it affords permanent correction of the deformity and elimination of pain secondary to the arthritis. The disadvantages of this procedure include the elimination of joint motion and limitation of shoe selection to heel heights of less than 1½ inches. Resection arthroplasty involves removal of the proximal one third of the proximal phalanx, which allows correction of the angulation deformity of the toe while eliminating the opposing arthritic joint surfaces. The disadvantages include shortening of the toe, decreasing the weightbearing function of the first toe, which can lead to lateral metatarsalgia, and failure to correct metatarsus primus varus. Replacement arthroplasty with a Silastic implant retains joint function and can result in good cosmesis, but it continues to be fraught with numerous problems, including excessive tissue reaction by the body to foreign materials, breakage and loosening of the implant, necessity for removal if infection occurs, and increased expense.

HALLUX RIGIDUS

Hallux rigidus, or hallux limitus, is a degenerative joint disease of the first MTP joint that causes pain and limited motion. Roentgenographic findings include osteophyte formation on the dorsal aspects of the metatarsal head and at the base of the proximal phalanx (Fig. 11-10). Hallux rigidus seems to occur more frequently in people who demonstrate a relatively flat metatarsal head than in those whose MTP joint is more rounded (Fig. 11-11). One theory to account for this difference is that when stress of narrow pointed shoes is applied to the rounded MTP joint socket, lateral deviation of the toe occurs, causing hallux valgus. When similar stresses are applied to the flat metatarsal head, pressure is applied to the articular surface in an irregular manner, leading to traumatic arthritis.[2]

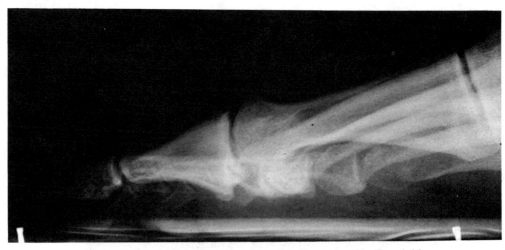

FIGURE 11-10. Pre-operative lateral radiograph of hallux rigidus.

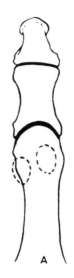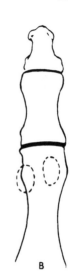

FIGURE 11–11. Schematic representation of the variations in the shape of the first metatarsal head: (A) Rounded or oval; (B) Flat. (From Mann, RA: Surgery of the Foot, CV Mosby, 1986, pg 162, with permission.)

There are three primary procedures for the treatment of adult acquired hallux rigidus, cheilectomy, arthrodesis, and replacement arthroplasty with Silastic implant. Cheilectomy involves removal of excess proliferative bone from around the metatarsal head and proximal phalanx. If this procedure fails to resolve the symptoms, or if the arthritis is too far advanced at the time of surgery, either arthrodesis or replacement arthroplasty can still be performed. Arthrodesis assures relief of pain at the sacrifice of joint motion. Replacement arthroplasty, while maintaining joint motion, can be complicated by the problems listed under the above discussion of this procedure for the treatment of hallux valgus.

MALLET TOES, HAMMER TOES, CLAW TOES

Occasionally there is confusion regarding the definitions of the lesser toe deformities. For the purpose of this discussion, the following terms are used:

1. Mallet toe is a deformity of a lesser toe in which the distal interphalangeal joint (DIP) is flexed and the proximal interphalangeal (PIP) and MTP joints are normal (Fig. 11-12).
2. Hammer toe is a deformity consisting of abnormal flexion of the PIP joint with the DIP and MTP joints in neutral position (Fig. 11-13).
3. Claw toe is hyperflexion of both the PIP and DIP joints and hyperextension of the MTP joint (Fig. 11-14).

Which procedure is best for a given deformity varies from surgeon to surgeon and patient to patient.

The following discussion includes approaches based on this author's personal experience.

Hammer toe can be classified into two categories: (1) flexible (or dynamic) and (2) fixed (or static). The categories can be distinguished by testing for contracture at the PIP joint. With the ankle in neutral position and the foot plantigrade, the PIP joint is passively manipulated into extension. If full extension can be obtained, the hammer toe

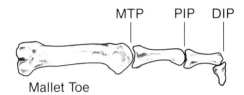

Mallet Toe

FIGURE 11–12. Schematic representation of a mallet toe.

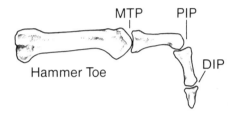

Hammer Toe

FIGURE 11–13. Hammer toe.

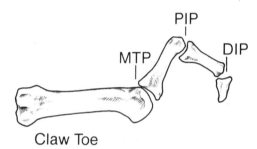

Claw Toe

FIGURE 11–14. Claw toe.

is flexible, and a soft tissue procedure such as a flexor-to-extensor tendon transfer can be performed. The procedure involves detaching the flexor digitorum longus from its insertion on the distal phalanx, splitting it along its median raphe (Fig. 11-15) and rerouting it to the dorsal aspect of the proximal phalanx (Fig. 11-16). It can now act to aid the extensor hood in flexing the MTP joint and extending the PIP joint. Some surgeons also detach the flexor digitorum brevis from its insertion at the base of the middle phalanx to remove its plantar flexing force at the PIP joint. If the PIP joint cannot be fully extended, the hammer toe deformity is considered static or fixed. This deformity can be managed by excising the distal end of the proximal phalanx. Shortening the bone is usually sufficient to allow the toe to rest in a neutral position. If a neutral position cannot be achieved, more bone must be resected or additional soft tissue releases must be performed.

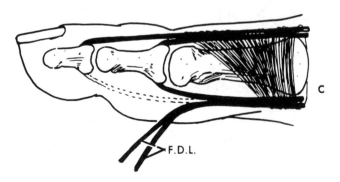

FIGURE 11–15. Schematic representation of detachment of the FDL from its insertion in this distal phalanx.

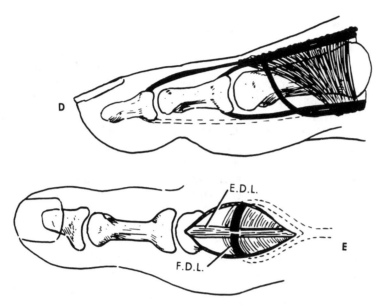

FIGURE 11–16. The FDL has been split longitudinally along its natural median raphe', each tail re-routed on either side of the proximal phalanx, and sutured to the dorsal extensor hood.

Claw toes represent the simultaneous contracture of the long flexors and extensors of the lesser toes and a muscle imbalance between the extrinsic and intrinsic muscles.[8] Claw toes usually involve multiple MTP joints, whereas mallet and hammer toes frequently occur in a single toe. Diseases with which claw toes are frequently associated are Charcot-Marie-Tooth disease, Friedreich's ataxia, diabetes, and rheumatoid arthritis. Claw toes may require release of the dorsal capsule of the MTP joints and lengthening of the extensor tendon, in addition to the procedures for treatment of hammer toes.

Mallet toe is probably caused by wearing ill-fitting shoes, which leads to contracture of the DIP joint. The problem perceived by the patient with the mallet toe is usually a painful callus on the tip of the toe. Detachment of the flexor digitorum longus from its insertion into the distal phalanx may be all that is necessary. However, if the volar plate is contracted, excision of a segment of the distal end of the proximal phalanx may be necessary to allow the toe to rest in its normal extended position.

ARTHRODESIS

Ideally, every attempt should be made to maintain motion in all the joints of the lower extremities. From Chapter 1 the reader should recall that each joint works in concert with every other joint to ensure the dissipation of rotatory, angulatory, and compressive forces generated during gait. There are certain clinical conditions, however, such as arthritis and infection, for which arthrodesis is a viable solution. If the motion of a joint is sacrificed, the surgeon must strive to place the joint in the optimal position that will minimize the ill effects of arthrodesis on the remaining functional joints.

Ankle

Although the ankle is primarily a biplanar joint for flexion and extension, it functions as a universal joint in conjunction with the subtalar joint. Elimination of ankle motion with an ankle arthrodesis places increased stress on the subtalar joint. Careful selection of the position for ankle arthrodesis becomes very important. The degree of transverse rotation should approximate that of the contralateral ankle. Thus the least amount of stress is placed on the subtalar joint. Too much internal rotation of the ankle holds the subtalar joint in a more rigid position, causing the patient to vault over a rather rigid internally rotated forefoot unless compensatory external rotation of the hip and knee joints occurs. Too much external rotation forces the patient to roll off the medial side of the foot, which applies lateral stress to the great toe, causing hallux valgus.

Neutral is the most desirable position of flexion and extension, assuming normal muscle strength and equal leg lengths exist. Some clinicians suggest that 10° of plantar flexion in females may be desirable, to allow for the wearing of a higher heeled shoe. However, more compensatory plantar flexion than dorsiflexion occurs at the midfoot joints. Thus, the patient is allowed more versatility if the ankle is fused in the neutral position. Too much dorsiflexion should be avoided because this causes concentration of forces upon ground contact over a small area of the heel, which can cause pain. The optimal varus-valgus position of ankle arthrodesis is 5° to 7° of valgus in relation to the entire tibia. Too much varus places excessive stress on the fifth metatarsal and can cause pain and calluses.

Subtalar Joint

The subtalar joint uniquely translates the transverse rotation passing from the tibia into the foot. Proper alignment of this joint in fusion is critical. Slight valgus tilt of 5° to 7° will allow the body weight to pass medially to the calcaneus, placing little stress on the lateral ankle ligament and maintaining some flexibility in the transverse tarsal joints. This allows even weight distribution across the foot. Too much valgus can result in excessive strain along the medial longitudinal arch, causing pain. Too much varus causes strain of the lateral collateral ankle ligament and excessive pressure under the lateral border of the foot, and imparts rigidity to the transverse tarsal joints.

Transverse Tarsal Joints

The calcaneocuboid and talonavicular joints work in concert with the subtalar joint and with one another. If motion is eliminated in any one of these joints, motion in all three is essentially eliminated. When either or both of the transverse tarsal joints are fused, the subtalar joint should be held at 5° and the forefoot in a plantigrade position. Too much supination results in pain under the lateral border of the foot. Too much pronation results in stress under the first metatarsal head and the sesamoids.

First Metatarsophalangeal Joint

Arthrodesis of the first metatarsophalangeal joint can result in minimal loss of function if done in the proper position of 10° to 15° valgus and 25° to 30° of dorsiflexion. The greater the degree of dorsiflexion, the higher the shoe heel that can be worn,

However, too much dorsiflexion can result in rubbing in the top of the shoe at the interphalangeal joint when flatter shoes are worn. Insufficient dorsiflexion results in the need to vault over the great toe, resulting in hyperextension of the interphalangeal joint and in callus formation.

EXTRINSIC ABNORMALITIES OF THE LOWER EXTREMITY

As has been emphasized repeatedly in this book, each bone and joint in the kinematic chain works in concert with every other component. Extrinsic abnormalities of the hip, knee, femur, and tibia can exert a deleterious effect on the ankle and foot. The effect of each of these proximal components on the distal component must be considered in the patient evaluation and treatment. The surgical implications of four clinical problems are presented: femoral anteversion, tibial torsion, leg length discrepancy, and angular deformities of the tibia.

Femoral Anteversion

Femoral anteversion is exaggerated internal torsion of the femur affecting rotational alignment of the lower extremity. This common developmental deformity of children causes toeing in. Some rotational malalignment corrects spontaneously, independent of exercise or braces, as the child matures. In rare cases, the deformity is severe enough to require surgery. Tachdjian recommends that surgery be reserved for the child eight years and older whose hip cannot be externally rotated beyond neutral, and whose functional disability and cosmetic appearance warrant correction.[6] An external rotation osteotomy may be performed at (1) the subtrochanteric region using a blade plate; (2) at the diaphysis using an intramedullary nail; or (3) at the distal metaphysis using pins or plate fixation. The bone is cut, the foot is rotated externally so that equal amounts of internal and external rotation of the foot are achieved, and the cut ends of the femur are fixed in a stable configuration until healing occurs.

Tibial Torsion

Internal tibial torsion can occur alone or in conjunction with femoral anteversion and is another spontaneously cause of in-toeing. Unlike femoral anteversion, most cases correct with growth. In the rare child whose internal tibial torsion persists past eight years of age, surgery can be performed. A derotation osteotomy of the tibia, similar to that for femoral anteversion, is performed to realign the transmalleolar axis at 25° of external torsion. Internal tibial torsion should be differentiated from Blount's tibia vara, which usually requires early bracing and surgical correction.

Leg Length Discrepancies

There are many causes of structural leg length inequality including congenital anomalies, tumors, infection, trauma, and neuromuscular disease. The options for surgical management include retarding or permanently arresting the growth of the longer limb in the skeletally immature patient, shortening the longer limb, and lengthening the shorter limb. Some of the factors considered in the surgical evaluation include decisions about the skeletal site at which the leg length discrepancy occurs, the age of patient, the amount of discrepancy present and the total amount of discrepancy anticipated, etiology, the condition of the soft tissues, the predicted eventual total body height (if patient is skeletally immature) the presence of structural or functional compensation in the spine, the abnormality of gait, the degree of coordination, and the requirement for a lift.

If leg length discrepancy occurs in a child who has sufficient remaining growth potential in the shortened limb, the ideal solution would be selective and unilateral epiphyseal stimulation of the affected limb to allow growth of the short leg to "catch up" to the normal one. Unfortunately, a safe and reliable technique of epiphyseal stimulation is not yet available.

Premature fusion of one or more of the physes of the limb that is longer allows the short extremity to equalize the disparate leg lengths as normal growth occurs. Using a complex system including serial limb measurements with orthoroentgenography, determination of skeletal maturity, relative size of the individual, and rate of growth, a growth prediction chart can be used to help determine at which anatomic site (femur or tibia) and at what age surgical growth arrest, or epiphysiodesis, can be most successfully employed. The surgical principles of epiphysiodesis include careful removal of the physis and packing of the space with bone graft to obliterate the growth plate.

Angulatory Deformities of the Tibia

Two of the most frequently seen angulatory deformities of the tibia that cause clinical symptoms are tibial shaft malunion and genu varum.

TIBIAL MALUNION

Tibial malunions following fracture can occur at any level of the tibia. The more proximal the malunion, the greater the magnitude of angulatory deformation and the greater its effect on foot and ankle biomechanics. The arthrokinematic system of the foot and ankle is more effective at compensating for a valgus deformity of the tibia than for a varus deformity. Tibia varum can result in excessive strain on the lateral aspect of the ankle and cause pain and calluses along the lateral border of the foot.

Surgical management includes corrective osteotomy, preferably at the level of greatest angular deformity, to bring the foot into correct alignment with the knee and hip.[8] The osteotomy can be performed to correct any rotational malalignment that might exist. The bone is fixed with either an intramedullary rod, internal screws and plates, or external devices until healing occurs. The surgical options for the skeletally mature patient whose leg length inequality is severe enough to require surgery are limited to lengthening the short leg or shortening the long leg. Once again, this decision is dependent upon age, site and etiology of discrepancy and the condition of the soft tissue, among other factors.

Resecting a segment of the femur or the tibia and fibula provides a way to shorten the long limb. Leveling of the knees is an important cosmetic consideration. Ideally, if the loss of length of the short side has occurred at the tibial level, shortening the longer, contralateral, tibia is preferable. However, shortening of the tibia is complicated by several factors. The muscles of the leg can become permanently weakened if more than three centimeters of bone is removed.[9] The surgery is more complex, because resection of portions of both the tibia and the fibula is required and the leg is at risk for compartment syndrome.

Shortening the femur offers fewer potential complications than the above procedure, and can be done in any number of ways. A current popular technique is the use of an intramedullary saw which allows resection of the desired amount of the shaft of the bone without requiring a separate incision on the thigh. Using the closed technique, an intramedullary rod is passed through the same incision through which the saw is inserted over the greater trochanter. Femoral bone healing is more rapid and predictable than tibia healing, and there are fewer complications of muscle weakness, infection, and malunion.

Theoretically, lengthening the short leg makes more sense from a cosmetic and biomechanical standpoint. However, bone lengthening, especially of the tibia, has been fraught with complications, such as overstretching, interference with the blood supply, insufficient fixation of the fragments, and problems of operative technique.[9] One of the most exciting current developments in limb lengthening has been the introduction of the Ilizarov technique of corticotomy and gradual bone lengthening. This technique involves subcutaneous fracture of the cortex of the bone and gradual distraction of the fragments using an external fixation device. Lengthening of up to 12 cm of the femur and 15 cm of the tibia has been reported, with fewer complications than with previous techniques.[10]

A combination of lengthening the short limb and shortening the long limb can be used to enhance symmetry of both limbs, and this approach can reduce the potential complications of either technique used alone.

GENU VARUM

Genu varum can occur gradually as a result of asymmetric wearing away of the medial compartment of the knee secondary to osteoarthritis, rheumatoid arthritis, or tibial plateau fracture. If genu varum exists in conjunction with arthritis limited to the medial compartment of the knee, consideration can be given to a proximal tibial osteotomy. This surgery corrects the angular deformity, preserves the joint, and more evenly distributes weightbearing stresses from the medial to the lateral compartment. However, if arthritis exists in the patellofemoral or lateral compartment, total knee arthroplasty should be considered. At the time of joint replacement, attention must be directed to correcting the varus malalignment with the appropriate soft tissue and bone techniques, to prevent failure of a malaligned prosthetic joint.

SUMMARY

I will prescribe regimen for the good of my patients according to my ability and my judgment and never do harm to anyone.

Hippocrates of Cos

Before intervening with surgery that alters the biomechanics of the foot and ankle, the wise surgeon may well ponder these words of Hippocrates. Surgery is undertaken only if nonoperative or conservative measures have failed or are considered inappropriate for a given condition. As with any invasive procedure, the risks associated with surgery must be weighed against the potential benefits. Only after careful and thorough evaluation of the clinical condition can the surgeon embark on surgery. Our understanding of this aspect of medicine is far from complete, and as technology and research in biomechanics of the foot increase, so will our knowledge and success.

This chapter was written to allow the clinician to gain an appreciation for the circumstances under which surgical interventions are undertaken to assure maximal biomechanical efficiency of the foot and ankle complex. Factors contributing to surgical treatment of pes cavus, pes planus, hallux valgus, hallux rigidus and toe deformities were presented. Circumstances under which arthrodeses of the ankle, subtalar joint, transverse tarsal joint and first metatarsal phalangeal joint are performed were reviewed. Last, a surgeon's perspective on specific extrinsic abnormalities in the lower limb was presented.

REFERENCES

1. Johnson, KA: Tibialis posterior tendon rupture. Clin Orthop 177:143, 1983.
2. Mann, R and Specht, L: Posterior tibial tendon ruptures: Analysis of eight cases. Foot Ankle 2:6, 350.
3. Mann, R and Thompson, F: Rupture of the posterior tibial tendon causing flat foot. J Bone Joint Surg 67A:556, 1985.
4. Scranton, P: Treatment of symptomatic talocalcaneal coalition. J Bone Joint Surg 69A:533, 1987.
5. Swiontkowski, MF et al: Tarsal coalitions: Long term results of surgical treatment. Pediatric Orthopedics 3:287, 1983.
6. Bordelon, RL: Surgical and Conservative Footcare. Slack, Thorofare, NJ, 1988, pp 72–73.
7. Johnson, KA: Surgery of the Foot and Ankle. Raven Press, New York, 1989.
8. Mann, R: Surgery of the Foot. CV Mosby, St Louis, 1986.
9. Tachdjian, MO: Pediatric Orthopaedics, vol 2. WB Saunders, Philadelphia, 1972.
10. Paley, D: Current techniques in limb lengthening. J Pediatr Orthop 8:73, 1988.

INDEX